WITHDRAWN 19/06/24.

BEHAVIOURAL AND MENTAL HEALTH RESEARCH: A HANDBOOK OF SKILLS AND METHODS

BEHAVIOURAL AND MENTAL HEALTH RESEARCH: A HANDBOOK OF SKILLS AND METHODS

edited by

Glenys Parry

*Department of Psychiatry, University of Southampton
and
Department of Psychotherapy, Royal South Hants. Hospital,
Southampton, SO9 4PE*

Fraser N. Watts

MRC Applied Psychology Unit, Cambridge, CB2 2EF

with a foreword by

Sol Garfield

LAWRENCE ERLBAUM ASSOCIATES, PUBLISHERS
Hove and London (UK)   Hillsdale (USA)

Lawrence Erlbaum Associates Ltd., Publishers
27 Palmeira Mansions
Church Road
Hove
East Sussex, BN3 2FA
U.K.

British Library Cataloguing in Publication Data

Behavioural and mental health research
  A handbook of skills and methods
  1. Medicine. Psychiatry. Research. Methodology.
  I. Parry, Glenys II. Watts, Fraser
  616.89'0072

  ISBN 0-86377-115-7
  ISBN 0-86377-121-1 pbk

Typeset by Acorn Bookwork, Salisbury, Wiltshire
Printed and bound by BPCC Wheatons, Exeter

Contents

Foreword

As indicated in their preface to the book, the editors have attempted to prepare a volume on research methodology that is geared especially for graduate students and professionals in the mental health fields. The aim was for emphasis to be on the practical aspects that are sometimes glossed over or omitted in more advanced treatises that emphasise research design and statistical analyses. In my opinion, the editors have been successful in fulfilling their objective. At the same time, with the collaboration of a number of research specialists, they have covered practically every pertinent topic in terms of research methods in the mental health field.

There are currently so many different procedures and methods of statistical analysis available to potential investigators that it is difficult for any researcher, let alone inexperienced and would-be researchers, to be acquainted with or knowledgeable about all of them. It is also true that merely reading the present handbook will not make the reader an expert researcher or even an expert on any particular type of procedure or method. However, a familiarity with the contents of the chapters in the book will enable the reader to become acquainted with the diversity of methods that are available to the investigator, and should help him or her to be able to make a more informed selection of the most appropriate procedures to be used for a particular study. Some methods are presented that may be of special interest or applicability to clinicians who want to make some initial attempts to evaluate their clinical work. The chapters on preparing a research project, selecting and developing measures, qualitative research, single case research, and patient series would appear to be of particular relevance in this regard.

In addition to these chapters there are also some others that may be of special interest to graduate students and to others who are relative beginners in conducting research and in preparing reports of research. Although most graduate training programmes have several courses on research design and statistical methods, there is usually little or no formal instruction on the preparation of research reports. The chapter by Glenys Parry on *Writing a Research Report*, therefore, should be helpful to students with regard to this aspect of research. In fact, apart from actually getting started on a workable research project, writing a decent research report appears to give students the most difficulty. Having graduate students delete unnecessary verbiage and reducing the length of their research reports to a third of their original size is always a trying experience. This chapter should help in preparing students to anticipate this problem and to lessen its impact.

The chapter by Chris Colbourn, *Using Computers*, also covers an area that is of increasing importance for researchers and I believe it is a welcome addition to a text on research methods. I also should mention the very first chapter in the book: *More Fun, Less Stress: How to Survive in Research*. This is a delightful, disarming, yet honest introduction to some of the problems encountered in doing research.

As I read through the manuscript of the Handbook, I was impressed not only with the variety of materials, methods, and procedures that exist today, as contrasted particularly to the 1940s when I began my career as a clinical psychologist, but also with the existing gaps in my own knowledge. As I have already indicated, none of us can be fully expert or fully knowledgeable about all the current research topics and areas. That, of course, is the obvious reason for publishing an edited handbook instead of a single or co-authored book. In a similar fashion, if I were to teach such a course for graduate students, I would attempt to have at least a few of the topics covered by guest lecturers who were relative experts, at least as compared to me. I might also have the students choose one method or topic for a special project or report. Each of the chapters has a number of references that can be consulted in terms of such an assignment. In this fashion, students can be introduced to the variety of issues and methods that currently characterise research in the mental health area, and also pursue more intensively a particular topic of interest.

Thus, as I have indicated, this Handbook is a very welcome addition to the very few books that are currently available as useful introductions to research methods and procedures in the area of mental health. Since the authors all appear to be British researchers and the chapter on writing a grant application is essentially oriented to British granting agencies, it would appear that the Handbook is addressed primarily to British graduate students and mental health professionals. This is understandable—indeed my own textbooks on clinical psychology generally emphasised professional developments in the United States almost exclusively. Perhaps such a phenomenon is inevitable. However, I hope that the book will also be read be clinical researchers and graduate students who are not British. Research, after all, should not be limited by national boundaries. In reading this Handbook, for example, I noted references to a number of British studies with which I was not familiar. Luckily, we share a common language and thus I was able to broaden my own knowledge.

In closing, let me state again that I believe the present book fulfills the editors' objectives and should be a useful source of information concerning the planning and conducting of mental health research. The topics covered are relevant, the content is clinically oriented, and the writing is clear.

Sol L. Garfield, Ph.D.
Professor Emeritus of Psychology,
Washington University,
St. Louis, Missouri.

Preface

We are frequently consulted by colleagues and students for advice about research, as are all the contributors to this book. Although a number of excellent texts are available on research design and analysis, we continue to find a need for something rather different. Most of the people who consult us are psychologists, psychiatrists, social workers or graduates training in these disciplines. Their need for guidance arises in two main contexts—they are either conducting research or reading about someone else's. We wanted to provide a book which would be helpful in both enterprises. As behavioural scientists working in the mental health field, we were also aware of how many social and applied psychologists would find such a book useful.

Mental health professionals who are conducting research need information about the practicalities of how to do it, at least as much as advice about an appropriate research design. Most books on research methods do not give much insight into research skills. Our coverage of skills includes the basics: how to prepare a project, how to choose or develop measures, how to use computers, how to analyse data, how to write a research report. We have also included less obvious topics which we find are just as important—how to enjoy the research and so avoid a stressful research experience, and how to apply for funding. Each of these chapters is written with an honest appreciation of the realities of the research enterprise. These 'tricks of the trade' are seldom written down. Sometimes they are handed on from supervisor to student during research training, but many of our readers may not have had the opportunity to learn them at first hand.

Many health professionals, when faced with a research problem, will consider only a narrow range of possible methods to explore it. All too often, the research question seems to be determined by knowledge of a particular method (e.g. experimental group comparisons). We would prefer the research problem to dictate the choice of method. Research should be like detective work, starting with a question and working towards an answer; the report of the research should be the story of how the question was answered. The 'rules' of research methodology are really just tips about how to arrive safely and securely at a solution to the problem. We have tried to make sure that guidance on research is presented here, not as a set of arbitrary requirements, but as practical help in doing successful research.

A recurrent problem with psychological research is that it can too easily become trapped in particular paradigms. The range of research approaches available is actually very broad. Unfortunately, most 'research methods' textbooks confine themselves to quantitative methods using group designs, and they also assume quite an advanced level of statistical knowledge. A particular research problem in the mental health field may be best explored by using a qualitative, language-based method rather than a quantitative, statistical one. Alternatively, the study of single cases or using one of a related family of intensive designs may be called for. Quite often, a method is needed which can be successfully used in a clinical situation to yield results directly applicable to clinical practice, for example, evaluating clinical services or investigating a patient series. Behavioural researchers will be able to recognise the relevance of these clinical examples to work in their own fields.

Although separate volumes about qualitative methods, epidemiology, single case research or service evaluation are available, they are often inaccessible to the beginner. We have found a need for one volume which covers a range of available research approaches to mental health problems. Each of our contributors is an established researcher in his or her field. In this way we hope to bring a breadth of experience to the reader, and a deeper knowledge of each particular skill or method than could be achieved by a single author.

For every mental health worker engaged in research, there are several who are not. This is particularly true in those fields which require extensive resources, such as outcome research and epidemiology. However, everyone in the field of mental health needs to be an intelligent consumer of research findings. Making sense of other people's research is a skill in itself, and we know it is one which many find difficult. The present book should be helpful. It is much easier to evaluate a research report when one understands the basics of research design, measurement, analysis and interpretation.

Finally, many books are written in technical language which is daunting to the would-be researcher. We believe it is possible to explain most basic research skills and methods using ordinary language, and that where technical terms are unavoidable, they can be explained. We wanted a book which was 'user friendly'—accessible to the beginner, yet valuable to the more experienced.

We were quite clear what kind of a book was needed: a handbook rather than a textbook, a book for the desktop rather than the bookshelf. Whether we have achieved it, we shall leave the reader to judge.

Glenys Parry and Fraser Watts

About the Editors

Glenys Parry is Regional Tutor in Clinical Psychology for Wessex and also works in a multidisciplinary psychotherapy department as a Top Grade clinical psychologist. She holds an honorary Senior Lectureship in the Faculty of Medicine, Southampton University.

Fraser Watts is a Senior Scientist with the Medical Research Council, at the Applied Psychology Unit in Cambridge. He is also currently Deputy President of the British Psychological Society and a past Chair of the Division of Clinical Psychology.

Part I: Skills

1 More Fun, Less Stress: How to Survive in Research

Ray Hodgson and Stephen Rollnick
Whitchurch Hospital, Cardiff.

It is often said that stress is a feature of modern life. Therefore, stress management unsurprisingly is a bandwagon which is rapidly gaining momentum. Most airports and supermarkets display numerous books and articles on how to cope and how to succeed. It is very easy to find a self-help book which provides very practical advice on how to overcome stress, marital problems, alcoholism or all of these together. There are shelves full of paperbacks on how to succeed in management and how to delegate, with a strong emphasis on how to succeed without stress and without really trying. This is all well and good; but what has been published that will help the young, lively, questioning researcher who has great expectations but a lack of practical experience? As far as we know the answer is very little. The avowed aim of this chapter is therefore to provide what has come to be known as a 'brief intervention' which might help to prevent learned helplessness.

In the style of the non-conformist minister, John Wesley, we will begin by preaching doom and gloom, hellfire and damnation. Trouble awaits those unwary souls who believe that research flows smoothly and naturally from questions to answers via a well-organised data collection system. This is certainly not the case. Even the most experienced, systematic and hard-working research worker will have to face trials and tribulations before a project is successfully concluded. Hence to prevent relapse into more comfortable lifestyles, the problems encountered in carrying out a research investigation must be clearly anticipated. The following may appear to be simply a list of aphorisms but actually they are laws of nature. Ignore them at your peril!

1.   GETTING STARTED WILL TAKE AT LEAST AS LONG AS THE DATA COLLECTION

This is not a problem provided that everybody is aware that this is the case and forward planning takes this law into account. Settling upon a key question, choosing a population or client group, devising questionnaires and a research design, guiding the proposal through the appropriate ethical committees and obtaining the co-operation of others are just a few of the time-consuming activities that seem to continue until somebody says that's enough. There may be a PhD at stake, and so one member of the team keeps adding extra conditions or novel questionnaires to make sure that his/her PhD has a strong base. The questions to be asked and the methods of answering them will repeatedly change. Complicated subsidiary projects will be grafted on until everybody is happy. We know of one study that took over 4 years to get started and about 2½ years to collect the data. Although we were not closely involved we do know that the team members began to imagine that the project would never get off the ground and yet, when finally published, the study turned out to be very influential. The job satisfaction of the research team would have been much greater had they known about rule number one.

2.   THE NUMBER OF AVAILABLE SUBJECTS WILL BE ONE-TENTH OF YOUR FIRST ESTIMATE

It is well known that if a particular disorder is being researched then people suffering from that problem seem to leave the district. The wider the net is spread the further they go. Recently, a trainee clinical psychologist in South Glamorgan decided that obese subjects would be very easy to obtain, and so obesity was chosen as the topic of his dissertation. You would imagine, as he did, that many people suffering from obesity would welcome the opportunity to discuss their problem with a psychologist and to obtain some advice on changing habits and self-management. Discussions with GPs indicated that at least forty subjects would be referred within a couple of months and the trainee was almost overcome by a sense of joyful anticipation. Six months later a desperate situation arose when the deadline for data collection had passed and still only three suitable clients had been referred.

Obtaining subjects is like betting on a horse. The most realistic assumption to make is that your expectations will turn out to be wrong.

3. COMPLETION OF A RESEARCH PROJECT WILL TAKE TWICE AS LONG AS YOUR LAST ESTIMATE AND THREE TIMES AS LONG AS YOUR FIRST ESTIMATE

A piece of research will almost never take less than the first estimate unless it is drastically cut down to size. Of course it should be recognized that the first estimate will be a function of personality and cognitive style. Pessimists will tend to over-estimate the time needed to carry out a variety of research tasks. Our deliberations have taken this into account but it is a very minor factor since only optimists get involved in research. Very often a project takes so long that it is never completed, but we have left these failures out of the calculation when formulating the above equations.

4. A RESEARCH PROJECT WILL CHANGE TWICE IN THE MIDDLE

One common misconception of the research process is responsible for a great deal of frustration. It is a popular view that a research worker progresses as smoothly as Sherlock Holmes from questions to answers via the systematic gathering of evidence. This is not the case, as the following typical example demonstrates. A few years ago, we decided to test out the effectiveness of Drinkwatchers groups for problem drinkers attempting to control their drinking. We obtained a small grant from the Medical Research Council and started to advertise. All we needed were thirty subjects from amongst the estimated 10,000 problem drinkers in South Glamorgan. One hundred and sixty problem drinkers answered the advertisement which deliberately did not provide details of the type of help that we were intending to provide. Of these only eight volunteered to join a Drinkwatchers group, three turned up to the first meeting and one of these came to the second. There was no choice but to abandon our original plans. Since one of us had been appointed for a year to carry out a small-scale study our only option was to change the project. Our first change of direction focused upon our advertising and the general messages that we were communicating (e.g. alcoholism, alcohol and health, or alcohol and fitness). Such an investigation turned out to be unrealistic and the project ended up answering the question: what sort of help do problem drinkers really want?

Unlike Conservative prime ministers, research workers have to respond flexibly when their cherished models begin to break up and well-laid plans go haywire. Funding bodies as well as apprentice researchers should be made aware that even the most experienced research workers have to do U-turns and S-bends in the middle of a project.

5. THE HELP PROVIDED BY OTHER PEOPLE HAS A HALF-LIFE OF TWO WEEKS

It is very difficult to say No when an enthusiastic and earnest research worker accosts you in the corridor. On the other hand, it is very easy to forget a promise to help. Most research projects rely upon some co-operation from others but it is wise to assume that actions won't speak as loud as words. If you are relying on ratings from nurses, spouses or GPs then you will have to set up a regular monitoring system to ensure that these tasks are carried out to your satisfaction.

6. THE TEDIUM OF RESEARCH IS DIRECTLY PROPORTIONAL TO ITS OBJECTIVITY

Some research workers manage to make use of interesting and productive research strategies such as the semi-structured interview and naturalistic observation of social interactions. Unfortunately, some questions are not amenable to this sort of methodology but have to be answered by devising experimental investigations involving very specific objective and tedious measurements. It is not easy to sustain 6 months of research activity which comprises giving a battery of reaction time tests to 100 subjects or observing speed of drinking in alcoholics. Most research involves some activities that are repetitive and boring, but then so do most jobs. Cabinet makers, space explorers and circus clowns all have to put up with a great deal of tedium if they are going to succeed in their chosen profession. This must be recognised so that ways of coping with the boredom can be devised.

7. THE EFFORT OF WRITING UP IS AN EXPONENTIAL FUNCTION OF THE TIME SINCE THE DATA WERE COLLECTED

Not everybody writes up as soon as, or even before, the data have been collected. If the raw data lie in a filing cabinet for a year then they are likely to stay there for 2 years. If they lie there for 4 years they will never escape and will certainly never be written up. One of us has a folder entitled 'The inhibitory effects of mental set' which contains data collected a quarter of a century ago and never written up. It is difficult to understand why these data were not thrown away 20 years ago.

8. EVIDENCE IS NEVER ENOUGH

Although research is beset with difficulties the rewards justify the effort. Good, strong evidence from good solid research is the best way to change conceptual frameworks as well as the behaviour of policy makers and practitioners. Or is it? Unfortunately, rigid views are not susceptible to change even when the evidence is overwhelming. One very good example of this phenomenon is provided by the debate between Priestley, Lavoisier and other eighteenth-century chemists, about the existence of phlogiston. When metals are burned or calcinated the modern view is that they are turned into oxides as they combine with oxygen in the air. According to the phlogiston theory a totally different process occurs since a metal is not an element but a compound which gives out phlogiston when heated. Now a crucial test would be to weigh the metal before and after calcination. The phlogiston theory would be falsified if the metal actually gains weight when it is burned. This experiment was carried out and the phlogiston theory was certainly not supported. Calcination of a metal leads to an increase in weight. It turned out that such apparently conclusive evidence did not convince the phlogiston supporters since they responded by suggesting that phlogiston must be a substance having a negative weight or that the departure of phlogiston increased the density, and therefore the weight, of the substance which held it.

One piece of evidence is never enough and an important research finding could well be ignored if it conflicts with the prevailing view. The debate about controlled drinking for alcoholics is a good example which should make a fascinating field of study for future philosophers of science.

There are many other laws which should be taken into account. For example, every research worker will have regrets: they will regret that they didn't include a particular measure or a particular intervention. Research workers will spend too long squeezing every last pip out of a data set. On the other hand, most of them will spend too little time plotting graphs and getting to know their data. We must now remember, however, another law of nature which we have recently uncovered: those people who teach research methods and those who write chapters about research spend too much time concentrating on problems and not enough time on solutions. Bearing this law in mind we will now change the focus of our attention.

Our views have been coloured by our own interest in relapse and particularly the work of Alcoholics Anonymous. Every year thousands of research workers start off with good intentions and high ideals. They want to push forward the frontiers of science and to help their fellow human beings. Unfortunately, most of them give up the ghost before the year is out and relapse into a more settled way of life. There are a few simple ways of preventing such a relapse process, and most of them have been adopted by AA. The first is the most important.

A. FORM A TEAM

It is almost impossible to carry out research when working alone, especially if there are strong pressures to do everything but research, as there are in the NHS for example. In the summer of 1935 Bill Wilson, a New York stockbroker, and Robert Holbrook Smith, a doctor in Akron, Ohio, worked together to overcome their drinking problems and were able, together, to achieve and maintain the sobriety that had been so elusive while each battled alone. The subsequent evolution of Alcoholics Anonymous is a remarkable success story. From its inception in 1935 AA has grown into a worldwide organisation claiming well over one-million active members. Most members of AA attend one or two groups every week and rely upon the support of like-minded people with similar problems. We believe that the best way of getting research completed is to form a team of three or four people who are interested in answering similar questions. They should meet once a week to set specific objectives and solve specific problems. Such a team can work very efficiently. They can share out a variety of tasks such as identifying appropriate measures, reading the relevant literature and speaking with key people. More importantly, such a team develops a sense of cohesion and enthusiasm. Where two or three are gathered together a sense of purpose develops which can resist the strong personal and social pressures to relapse.

The next best alternative is to form a support group: a network of people working in the same locality but researching different areas and asking different questions. Ideally, a small research team would also be members of a larger support group. This larger group would make sure that they keep up with developments in computing, statistics, measurement and methodology; and this larger support group might link up with other groups in different locations. Both of us have worked alone and also in a team. The experiences are totally different, and it is our contention that most research, and certainly most PhD research, flounders simply because of the lack of adequate social support.

B. ONE DAY AT A TIME

This famous AA catch-phrase economically captures a basic element of self-contol or self-management. It is easy to be overwhelmed by the size of the task, and focusing upon smaller goals has a number of important consequences. As Weick (1984) observes:

Deliberate cultivation of a strategy of small wins infuses situations with comprehensible and specific meaning (commitment), reinforces the perception that people can exert some influence over what happens to them (control), and produces changes of manageable size that serve as incentives to expand the repertory of skills (challenge). Continued pursuit of small wins could build increasing resistance to stress in people not originally predisposed toward hardiness.

One of the examples given by Weick is the success of the US Environmental Protection Agency in the early 1970s. The first administrator, William Ruckelshaus, decided not to draw up policies and plans to clean up all aspects of the environment but went instead for a relatively small win. Prior to the formal opening of the agency he discovered an obscure 80-year-old law relating to water pollution which permitted him to take a number of cities to court. On the first day of the Agency's formal existence he announced five law suits against major American cities. There then followed a long series of successes that resulted in the strengthening of the Agency and additional resources as well as the increased enthusiasm to take on slightly larger goals.

The fact that going for small wins increases commitment, control and hardiness is sometimes difficult to translate into the field of research but the following guidelines are suggested:

1. Avoid the massive multicentred study. If an error of judgement is made early on there will be an enormous waste of resources.
2. Always try to cut a study down to size and go for relatively quick results. It is better to have six people working on a 1-year project than one person working on a 6-year project.
3. Don't imagine that you have to follow the tradition of writing a large and comprehensive literature review before starting work on a study.
4. A small win that does not shake the world could lead to a big win. In any case, it is better than a large flop.

Of course, large-scale research has to be done but only after carrying out enough small-scale work to be almost certain that the large-scale study will be a success.

C. KEEP IN MIND THE PAYOFFS

It is very easy to sink into a routine of collecting data and coping with the day-to-day problems of research whilst forgetting the reasons for starting the project in the first place. Such a state of mindless persistence is a recipe for relapse. One basic process in self-control is to bear in mind the future consequences of today's activities (Horan, 1971). What are the positive outcomes that might reasonably be expected if the research project is completed? Of course the basic reason for carrying out a piece of research is to answer a question or solve a puzzle. The more important the question is considered to be the greater will be the motivation to complete the study, so it is important to focus upon a burning issue when planning a project. Discovering something new is certainly the biggest reward of research. Nevertheless, research is also associated with a wide range of pleasurable experiences over and above the intellectual stimulation of solving puzzles and these should be kept in mind especially when the burning question begins to look more like a dying ember.

Consider the example of Heartbeat Wales, which is a community programme designed to reduce high levels of heart disease throughout the principality. This project has been in existence for about a year and has not yet uncovered any world-shaking facts about changing human behaviour. Even so the project team has been rewarded in a large number of ways.

First, they have increased the level of awareness about healthy lifestyles throughout Wales. For example, Heartbeat Wales' health surveys have produced local information which communities are taking very seriously. Second, they have written a great deal for professional journals and the mass media. Third, they are now recognised experts in the field and are asked to lecture and to advise other programmes (e.g. the English Heart Programme). Of course Heartbeat Wales is not representative of other research projects since it is also a campaign. Nevertheless, many other projects lead on to a wide range of benefits. Often they can raise awareness and research workers do become the 'experts' who are frequently consulted. Furthermore, research involves thinking. Thinking sometimes produces ideas, and ideas can lead to publications, lectures and new research projects.

One Medical Director of the World Health Organisation insists that research workers affiliated with the WHO should be considering the 'products' that can result from their research over and above the final research publication. These products could be questionnaires, self-help manuals, guidelines for treatment, speculative articles, review articles, guidelines for community projects and proposals for further research. He recognises that a 5-year wait for a definitive article is not the best way of maintaining enthusiasm for a study. Rewards have to be built in along the way.

There are many benefits associated with research, and all research projects have a range of spin-offs. We are proposing that one way of preventing relapse is to regularly bring them to mind.

D. AVOIDING HELPLESSNESS

Many skills are needed in carrying out research and they have to be learned if a feeling of helplessness is to be avoided. It helps to know a good deal about experimental designs and methodology. Basic principles of reliability and validity will have to be considered. Data will have to be analysed possibly using a computer program. In our experience many researchers fall by the wayside because they feel that they lack knowledge and experience in these areas. Other chapters in this book are intended to provide this type of knowledge, and we suggest that the best way to ensure that some of these skills are well learned is to offer to give a course of lectures, in 6 months time, on basic statistics and methodology. Some of the advice that we have given in this chapter has been tongue in cheek but we make this suggestion in all seriousness, bearing in mind that your audience will have to be carefully chosen.

E. DOUBTING AND QUESTIONING

Our final piece of advice is very simple. Research is all about doubting, questioning and enquiring. Even the laws described earlier in this chapter can be questioned, and a good research worker is someone who is always asking questions and coming up with ideas that fly in the face of prevailing views. Sometimes the questioning leads to radically different approaches and models. For the past 50 years it has been held that alcoholics must be abstinent for life but now this view is being questioned. Early behaviour therapists questioned the prevailing view that curing a phobia by desensitisation or exposure would only cure the symptom and subsequently result in catastrophic consequences. The traditional response to mental illness has been hospitalisation, but the wisdom of institutionalisation is now being questioned.

It follows that one of the most basic methods of maintaining motivation and enthusiasm for research is to develop attitudes which take into account the possibility that research will lead to radical approaches in the future. To take one example, in 50 years time the National Health Service will be very different. Unless our own views are very wide of the mark there will be more work carried out in the community, with a wider range of professionals being responsible for services and greater emphasis on prevention. Changes in our traditional systems will occur more speedily if a large number of health workers are repeatedly questioning current practices, researching ways of making changes and developing an attitude of mind that welcomes a questioning spirit and welcomes appropriate changes. Maintaining a sense of wonder about human behaviour and human institutions as well as a vision of the continuous process of change that can and should be influenced by good evidence is perhaps the best way of maintaining enthusiasm for research.

THE RESEARCH GAME

Before concluding this chapter we would just like to provide one very simple method of surviving in the research field without really trying. Table 1.1 shows young researchers everything that is needed to make a name for themselves if they are researching psychological phenomena. In all fields of exploration and discovery those lucky individuals who are able to put a catch-phrase or title to a new phenomenon will not only survive but will be put on a pedestal by their colleagues. We will now reveal how this can be accomplished. It is often thought that research workers discover a phenomenon and then put a name to it, but actually the reverse is true. We have discovered that impressive-sounding labels are first of all generated and then a search is mounted for a phenomenon that fits the label. This is how many psychological phenomena were originally discovered including cognitive dissonance, erogenous zones, the inverted Oedipus complex, the reinforcement retroaction paradox, waxy flexibility, dementia infantalis, critical fusion frequency and the abstinence violation effect. Now, for the

TABLE 1.1
Buzz-word generator

1. Dementia	Retroaction	Complex
2. Abstinence	Self-	Therapy
3. Perceived	Restructuring	Fixation
4. Oral	Violation	Efficacy
5. Learned	Dependence	Questionnaire
6. Anal	Helplessness	Syndrome
7. Instrumental	Dissonance	Effect
8. Cognitive	Autonomous	Paradox
9. Reinforcement	Oedipus	Frequency
10. Inverted	Infantalis	Self-actualisation
11. Critical	Relativist	Construct
12. Functional(ly)	Flicker	Orientation

To form acceptable and influential psychological terminology randomly choose one number for each of the three columns. For example, 4 3 2 = Oral Restructuring Therapy; 6 1 8 = Anal Retroaction Paradox; 8 6 5 = Cognitive Helplessness Questionaire.

first time, we are publishing the buzz-word generator that was used to produce these and many other labels within the field of psychology. The words displayed in Table 1.1 can be put together in over 2000 ways and only 55 combinations have so far been used to label psychological phenomena. If you play around with this buzz-word generator your perceived self-efficacy will be enhanced and from an instrumental relativist orientation your future functionally autonomous self-actualisation will be guaranteed.

REFERENCES

Horan, J J. (1971). Coverant conditioning through a self-management application of the Premack Principle: its effects on weight reduction. *Journal of Behaviour Therapy and Experimental Psychiatry*, **2**, 243–249.

Weick, K. E. (1984). Small wins: Redefining the Scale of Social Problems. *American Psychologist*, **39**, 40–49.

2 Preparing a Research Project

Edgar Miller
*Department of Clinical Psychology, Addenbrooke's Hospital,
Cambridge CB2 2QQ.*

For those setting out on clinical research for the first time the biggest difficulty is often that of identifying a suitable problem that is both researchable in practical terms and that is likely to lead to worthwhile results. There are no rules for doing this that are guaranteed to lead to a high-quality end result. So far it has not proved possible to operationalise inspiration! What this chapter aims to do is very much more modest. This is to set out some general principles which it is hoped will help those inexperienced in clinical research to achieve better results than they might otherwise have done.

Encountering research in its final form as an impressive paper in a prestigious journal gives a certain indication as to how research develops. The published paper starts with a review of the literature which then leads logically into an elegant hypothesis derived from that review. An experiment or investigation is then designed to examine the hypothesis. The results are then analysed with confidence and lead on to conclusions concerning the question that prompted the investigation. This is a nice, neat and logical progression. Needless to say this is a very formalised account of what typically goes on. The researcher may have thought of the hypothesis first with only the vaguest knowledge of the literature. The experiment may originally have been much bigger in scope, and what is reported is only those aspects of the data that seem to be interpretable. The execution of the project may have included a great many vicissitudes that the final account fails to describe.

Although the course of research generally rivals true love in not running smoothly it is usually sensible to try to follow a certain logical progression, even though some good clinical research obviously does not follow this sequence. For example, it is generally advisable to have a reasonable background knowledge of the relevant literature before embarking on the details of any investigation. This is not always possible. Sometimes opportunities arise suddenly and the investigator has to do something quickly or miss the opportunity altogether (e.g. when a patient with a very rare and exotic condition turns up out of the blue and something has to be done immediately). This happened to the writer when a case of transient global amnesia was admitted one lunchtime still in a profoundly amnesic state. This condition is very rare, and the patient's amnesia is expected to recover within a few hours at most.

Putting aside instances like this, the sequence may run more or less along the following lines. First, the researcher identifies a particular problem to investigate in very general terms, e.g. benzodiazepine dependence or incontinence in psychogeriatric patients. Secondly, background information is acquired about the topic, most commonly from the literature, including what has been discovered (or not discovered) so far. Next a specific question or hypothesis needs to be formulated and, finally, the investigation or experiment is designed in such a way that it will offer a reasonable examination of the question chosen. These last two stages really tend to be the two sides of the same coin. The experimental design is very much determined by the hypothesis under consideration and a good hypothesis is, amongst other things, one that will lead to a suitable research design. With the reservations already alluded to, these four stages form a convenient base around which to organise subsequent discussion.

SELECTING A PROBLEM AREA

This is the crucial first step, but is also the aspect about which it is most difficult to offer advice. Researchers select problems on which to work for a variety of different reasons, and not all of these are particularly logical. That the researcher actually identifies a suitable problem area is of greater importance than the means by which this decision is achieved.

A common basis for selecting a problem area is the inherent interest that it holds for the individual. Providing it can lead to useful results, interest is certainly not a bad basis for selecting a research topic. It is very difficult to research a topic that appears tedious and dull. Nevertheless, the initial attractiveness of an area may lead to unfortunate decisions when used as the sole criterion for determining the topic. Just why some men should develop couvade (the husband having symptoms such as morning sickness and pains like labour pains whilst the wife is pregnant and giving birth) may be a fascinating question, but it has severe limitations as an area for clinical research. Instances of couvade are only rarely encountered in clinical practice and even more rarely still is it a problem of such magnitude as to warrant intervention.

It is often advisable to consider research topics other than those of initial attraction. A very useful approach is to consider problems that are frequently encountered in clinical practice. These are not only likely to be of immediate practical importance but will also provide a flow of suitable subjects on which to carry out research. Monitoring one's own clinical practice carefully can provide a fund of ideas. For example, the writer once had a period in which a series of referrals arose requiring advice as to whether a brain-damaged individual was safe to drive again. In general there is very little established knowledge on which a decision of this kind might be based and it is a problem not infrequently encountered by clinical psychologists working in neurological/physical rehabilitation settings as well as by other professionals (e.g. physicians) working in the same fields. Any further information that might help decision making would therefore be of real practical value.

Not only may relatively underinvestigated problems be encountered but clinical practice can also identify important but little understood features of otherwise well-researched topics. For example, it might be noted that one particular type of patient under treatment by cognitive or behavioural methods seems to be especially poor at carrying out 'homework' assignments. Trying to determine just why this should be the case could result in knowledge that could be used to enhance the efficacy of therapeutic interventions.

A topic identified from clinical practice, like that of assessing the suitability of patients to drive, may at first sight be of little intrinsic interest. However, some careful consideration of the problem as well as background reading can produce an interest in the most unlikely things. Something like incontinence in psychogeriatric patients may have very low initial appeal but, as this writer has recently found, external pressure to look at this problem does reveal features of interest even in this most unlikely of topics. Even if the first topic identified from routine practice is rejected further monitoring will always throw up additional problems.

Research topics can be suggested in a number of other ways. The scientific and professional literature is continually throwing up ideas. To cite another example, a review paper by Barraco and Stettner (1976) has suggested that memory/learning may be adversely affected by the administration of antibiotics in experimental animals. Similar effects in humans could be of considerable significance. Such effects are most likely to occur where antibiotics are prescribed on a long-term basis. This sometimes happens to dermatological patients with severe and unremitting acne. Such patients are often teenagers and many will be in the later stages of schooling where cognitive functioning needs to be at its best.

Yet another source of ideas for research can come from new service developments. Most services change from time to time as new ideas for service provision are developed and incorporated into practice. These changes are rarely evaluated properly. Recently the psychogeriatric service in Cambridge refurbished an old ward and decided to use some of the beds for intermittent relief rather than for long-stay cases. The idea was that providing intermittent relief (say, for 2 weeks in every 10) would help the supporters in the community to cope better and so act to cut the need for long-term admissions. It is important to know if this goal can be achieved since, if it is, there would be a good case for converting more long-stay beds to intermittent relief.

One word of caution needs to be entered here. Many researchers end up by studying problems that are essentially trival. Just because an anomalous result can be found in the literature does not mean that further investigation of that problem will necessarily lead to findings of any practical value. Similarly, the ready availability of certain clinical techniques does not mean that further exploration of their application is of value. To take but one example, the presence of neuropsychological test batteries has resulted in these being applied to almost any clinical population that comes to hand, ranging from depressed psychiatric patients to subjects with diabetes mellitus. That the resultant pattern of scores may show some superficial features in common with some neuropsychological groups often has no practical significance and, in any case, the finding may defy satisfactory interpretation (Miller, 1983).

Just where the initial ideas for research come from is not really important as long as the idea is suitable in that it leads to research that can be carried out within the confines of the clinical setting and which will lead to worthwhile results. Nevertheless, the best ideas for clinical research often follow from taking an enquiring and critical attitude towards everyday clinical practice. By its very nature clinical practice requires the practitioner to go beyond what is known and make assumptions about the nature of problems, the mechanisms that underlie them, and the means by which they can be resolved. Examining these assumptions, at least where this is practicable, leads to useful research with direct implications for practice and which can be carried out on subjects that are immediately to hand.

THE BACKGROUND

Having identified a general topic it is advisable to gather background information. This usually comes from the scientific literature, especially other reported studies of the same or similar topics, but it can also be derived from discussing the problems with others who share an interest in the same general area. In this search for background information certain things are of particular significance. Obviously, it is sensible to know what has been established, or not established, so far. Previous investigations in the same general area will also give some idea of the kinds of methodology that might be useful, the pitfalls that may need to be avoided, and the sorts of measures that might be used.

Most of this depends upon a literature search. Again there are no really hard and fast rules about this, but certain things are worth bearing in mind. Getting started may be difficult, especially if the problem is a little unusual and rather circumscribed, with relevant papers and books not coming to hand very readily. After a while the problem more commonly becomes one of coping with the vast amount of relevant, or potentially relevant information. Once a start is made and some access to the relevant literature is achieved, the question then typically becomes one of when to stop chasing further background information.

Initially the abstracting journals are often very useful. As well as *Psychological Abstracts* there are the medical abstracting journals which can often be at least as useful for clinical psychologists. The main ones are *Exerpta Medica* and *Index Medicus*. Many libraries can also obtain computer searches by 'Medlars' but this is essentially a search of *Index Medicus* based on identification of articles by keywords. Inevitably some material of interest is missed because it does not have the relevant keyword(s) assigned to it. Looking through the index of one or more of these abstracting journals over a year or two will usually turn up something or even the most obscure topic. This source will itself cite references which will in turn often be useful.

Once some idea of the basic key references has been obtained the *Science Citation Index* may be of value. This starts from specific references and then lists the current sources citing this reference. Thus someone wanting to consider the impact of the family on discharged schizophrenics may identify the paper by Vaughn and Leff (1976) on expressed emotion. Looking up this reference in the *Science Citation Index* would then show which authors had cited this paper and who, therefore, might also be dealing with the same general problem.

The real need is then to develop a picture of the state of knowledge in the relevant field including what seems to be well established, what is not so well established, what controversies exist and where the main gaps in useful knowledge lie. Eventually the search for additional background information will reach a stage where newly indentified material will be adding little of consequence to this overall picture. This is the point at which it then becomes safe to start formulating questions or hypotheses for further investigation. On the other hand, if this search has by itself alone lead the enquirer to a new and much enhanced understanding of the nature of the problem area that prompted the search, then writing a review article may be a useful preliminary outcome. Not all research includes the collection of new data (a literature search is research of a kind) and the ability to present and systematically summarise a complex and varied literature so as to be able to draw out implications for clinical practice can be a very useful achievement in itself.

In considering the literature it should be remembered that authors' conclusions about their own data are not necessarily correct and can sometimes fail to take into account other possibilities or even be totally misleading. Sometimes there is a good case for re-analysing data to check how well the conclusions can be substantiated. Furthermore, the development of meta-analysis (see Chapter 9) has created new scope for collating the results of separate investigations statistically. Again, this may be a useful preliminary before trying to gather new data.

FORMULATING A QUESTION OR HYPOTHESIS

The next stage is to select a specific question or hypothesis for investigation. Essentially the ideal question is one which, if answered properly, would lead to new information of clinical value and that would add to existing knowledge. There are no firm rules for achieving this but a useful guide is provided by the 'so what?' test. Even if the question proposed for investigation could be answered definitely, then 'so what'? Would the clinician actually be better placed to deal with a certain kind of problem or, at least, would the clincan be a step nearer to being better placed? Trying to determine whether one suggested subtest pattern on the WAIS is better at distinguishing people with dementia than another is a researchable question. If there are reasons to believe that no WAIS subtest pattern is likely to achieve a good enough level of reliability in distinguishing early dementia to be of any clinical value (Miller, 1980) then is the answer to this question worth obtaining?

To answer the question posed usually means devising an investigation, and a researchable question is also one that can be investigated given the limitations under which the investigator has to work—physical, ethical, financial or whatever. The limitations that are most important in practice typically centre around the availability of suitable subjects and the ability to carry out the necessary manipulations or procedures. Investigating commonly encountered problems can help ensure a supply of subjects, but practical or ethical considerations usually greatly reduce the things that can be done as part of the investigation. Such things as the inability to have an ideal control group or to carry out an adequate follow-up may limit what can be done and therefore what questions can be adequately answered. Other methodological constraints may be of significance. For example, it may not be possible to obtain or devise a suitable measure to meet the purpose of the investigation. Some of these problems are much less tractable than others in that practical limitations can sometimes be circumvented by using an alternative research design whilst an inability to measure the key variable in a satisfactory way may be insurmountable.

It has been suggested above that to be of value the question chosen should yield new information or break new ground. This is so eventually, but if the question that the investigator would like to answer means building directly on to a finding in the literature that is not well replicated then it can be a good thing sometimes to start by trying to replicate the finding in the investigator's own setting. This can achieve a number of things. If the original finding is important enough to lead on to other things then a replication may well be useful in itself. Secondly, the replication establishes that the investigator can obtain the effect that is being depended upon. A replication, or near-replication, also gives the experimenter experience in working in the general problem area, use of possible methodology, etc. This can itself help to suggest better questions for further investigation. This can be of particular value to new researchers starting to feel their way.

Finally, it is probably important for inexperienced researchers to remember that usually any one investigation can only produce a very small step forward. It is often tempting to try to hit the jackpot first time and try to produce a result of outstanding importance. Since experienced and distinguished research workers only very rarely do this, novices are well advised to set modest goals that might be within their grasp. Establishing the cause of schizophrenia or the ideal treatment for anorexia nervosa at the first attempt is highly unlikely!

DESIGNING THE INVESTIGATION

Having decided upon a hypothesis to test or question to answer there now comes the critical problem of designing the actual experiment or investigation. Most psychologists will have been through undergraduate and even postgraduate courses with titles like 'statistics and experimental design'. These courses generally say a lot about statistics and very little about design. They thus often give the erroneous impression that the design of investigations is little more than the problem of selecting a suitable statistical model with the best experiments using a sophisticated form of analysis of variance. This may be a caricature of what is taught but it is much less of a caricature of the beliefs many students derive from such courses. In fact the problem of designing an experiment is primarily one of logic. The statistical model employed, if such is required, is selected because it matches the logic of the investigation. To go straight for the statistical model implies that the experimental logic implicit in the statistical model is suitable for the question which it is hoped to answer. If the logic has not been thought out first then it is impossible to say whether the logic implicit in the statistical model is appropriate.

This is not in any way to decry statistics which are an essential tool in many investigations. The aim is merely to set them in their proper context as tools of analysis rather than as a factor determining how the experiment should be designed in the first place. In fact some experienced investigators suggest that it can be helpful to imagine beforehand the kind of data that might be derived from the experiment and to try to interpret them. This can help to detect deficiencies in the design before the investigation is carried out. Nevertheless there is no substitute for having a clear grasp of the logic of what is being attempted.

The key concept in design is 'control'. Essentially, control refers to the ability to relate the outcome of the investigation (i.e. changes in the dependent variable) to the factors that are of particular interest to the investigator. Thus if the aim is to show that changing the environment on a psychogeriatric ward has an effect on the behavioural competence of residents, then the investigator needs to be reasonably sure that any changes produced really are the consequence of altering the environment and not to some other extraneous and unwanted factor (e.g. a change in nursing staff on the ward that happened at about the time the general environmental change was introduced). This ability to relate one set of factors to another is referred to as 'internal validity' by Cook and Campbell (1979).

Another important aspect of any investigation is what Cook and Campbell (1979) refer to as 'external validity'. Except under very rare circumstances investigators are not just concerned with those particular subjects in the particular setting in which the study is carried out. The hope is to draw some sort of conclusion applicable to, say, other psychogeriatric patients in other residential units. For the most part this ability to generalise from the result is dependent upon using subjects that are as far as possible typical examples of their kind and studied under typical circumstances.

A problem arises because there can be advantages in having very clearly defined groups of subjects. For example: chronic schizophrenics within a certain age range, having been resident in hospital for a certain length of time, who clearly meet certain diagnostic criteria, who have never had any other psychiatric label applied to them, etc. This makes it clear to others exactly what the population studied was and makes for easy replication of the investigation by others. In addition, using a homogeneous group of subjects reduces the within-group variance, thus enhancing the statistical power of the experiment. The question then arises as to how typical of long-stay patients generally labelled as 'chronic schizophrenics' such a narrowly defined sample would be?

The extreme of this situation arises when studies (often single case or of small numbers of subjects) are carried out on very 'pure' examples of a particular problem. For example, if the interest is in what mechanisms underlie compulsive checking behaviour then many cases encountered in clinical practice will have other features, such as some degree of depression. A pure case with only checking may then be of particular interest for study since the results will not be contaminated by these other factors. However, generalisation to more typical cases must take into account the possible confounding effects of such things as depression. In general terms the study of relatively pure cases is useful for teasing out the mechanisms controlling some form of abnormal behaviour, but this is at the price of weak generalisation to more typical examples with regard to such things as the ease and extent to which the indentified mechanisms can be manipulated as part of a therapeutic intervention.

Another important consideration is the 'power' of any experimental design in the sense of its ability to detect an effect if the looked for effect really does exist. This is called 'statistical conclusion validity' by Cook and Campbell (1979) but this can be misleading because the general issue of the power of the investigation to detect the effects sought is still present even if no formal statistical procedures are being used. Thus if it is intended to increase detection of post-natal depression in the 6 months after birth from a current level of 6% to be nearer the real rate of, say, 10–15% (e.g. Cox, Connor and Kendell, 1982) then introducing an experimental screening procedure that might improve detection by about a further 2% at best, and expecting to get a definite indication of improvement after screening 40 consecutive cases, would be extremely hopeful to say the least. In general power can be achieved by improving the sensitivity of the measures and by either increasing the number of subjects or by increasing the number of observations/data recorded from each subject in single-case or small N designs (see Cohen, 1977, for a full discussion of power analysis).

A final general consideration is that of the measures used. Do these really reflect the things that they are supposed to reflect? For example, in looking at anxiety is the investigator really concerned with state or trait anxiety and is the measure of anxiety being used of the right kind? Different measures tend to be useful in different contexts. Thus the considerable stability of IQs derived from the major intelligence tests can be of value under some circumstances. This stability, however, makes them relatively insensitive to change and therefore not good as dependent variables where the aim is to detect some small change. Given the considerable problems of measurement in psychological research it is often sensible to avoid having to rely on single measures, and including an alternative measure of the same function can act as a useful insurance against problems with the first.

Besides these questions of logic, practical limitations also have to be taken carefully into account in planning clinical research. Two commonly encountered problems are a shortage of suitable subjects and the fact that it is not always possible to use what might be considered the ideal type of experimental design because of either practical or ethical reasons. Examples of the latter are where in looking at the effect of changing a ward environment it is not practically possible to get an adequately matched control ward and it is not considered either practical or ethical to return the experimental ward to its pre-intervention state to see if an obtained effect is reversed.

As has already been stated earlier in the chapter, selecting problems commonly encountered in clinical practice is one way of trying to ensure an adequate flow of subjects. Where an adequate number of subjects are not available researchers can adopt two strategies. One is to use 'analogue research' as when college students reporting a fear of spiders are used to study ways of treating phobias. Analogue research of this kind does have its limitations (Miller and Morely, 1986; see also Chapter 8) but will not be considered any further because it is not really clinical research as conceived here.

The other strategy is to rely on small N or even single-case designs. These intensive designs usually rely on obtaining a large amount of data from subjects over a prolonged period of time and demand the use of suitable measures (e.g. measures that do not have large practice effects where the subject obtains the maximum level of performance after a few administrations). The fact that single-case studies typically go on over long periods of time makes them susceptible to interference from uncontrolled changes in the environment (i.e. the longer an experiment goes on the more chance there is that something will happen that can upset the experiment, especially if it is being carried out in the natural setting). As indicated above these designs are best for examining underlying mechanisms but they are weak at indicating what the typical patient's response to some form of intervention might be. For a more detailed discussion of such designs see Chapter 12.

The other major practical problem in clinical research is that it is not always possible to carry out what would be the ideal experimental design. For example, if a ward-based intervention is being used then it may not be possible to find a similar ward containing identical patients. The logic of experimental design might suggest pooling the patients from two wards and reassigning them to wards at random. There are usually strong practical and ethical objections to such a procedure. Thus it may be necessary to work with a control that differs in a potentially relevant way from the experimental ward/subjects (e.g. in having different levels of severity of disorder or different lengths of time resident in hospital). This then necessitates working with quasi-experimental designs (Cook and Campbell, 1979; see also Chapter 10). In general quasi-experimental designs tend to have good external validity. Because they are typically carried out in the 'real life' setting and with typical subjects generalisation to other clinical samples is good. (It is indeed the restrictions imposed by working in 'real life' settings with typical subjects that force the investigator to opt for a quasi-experimental design in the first place.) The most serious limitation for quasi-experimental designs relates to internal validity. In other words it is less possible to be sure that changes observed really are the consequence of the manipulations that were applied. Quasi-experimental designs are discussed in Chapter 10.

ETHICAL ISSUES

Ethical issues should be considered at an early stage of planning research. Researchers need to ensure that the research they are planning is ethical in essence, as well as that detailed aspects of the procedure do not raise any specific ethical problems. Researchers should be familiar with an accepted set-up of ethical guidelines, such as the American Psychological Association's (1981) Ethical Principles of Psychologists (especially section 9 on research with human participants). Where any doubts arise, the comments of an independent colleague should be sought at an early stage. The role of obtaining ethical approval in preparing a grant application is referred to in Chapter 7.

Each field of psychological research raises its own characteristic ethical problems. For example, animal research raises particularly distinctive problems that have recently been much discussed; social psychology research raises issues about deception more commonly than other areas of psychology. In clinical research, there are two particular problems that recur regularly. One relates to the ability of particular groups of clinical participants to give free and informed consent. There is quite an extensive literature on specific populations, of which Kinard's (1985) discussion of the ethics of research with abused children is a good, recent example. Another recurrent ethical problem in the clinical field concerns providing or withholding treatment in the course of research; see for example Garfield's (1987) discussion of eithical issues in psychotherapy research.

FINAL COMMENTS

Fundamentally research is an intellectual exercise. No matter how elegant or sophisticated the procedures adopted or the form of the statistical analysis, what emerges will be trivial or worthless, unless the investigator has phenomenal luck, without the whole business carefully and logically thought through beforehand. The best clinical research emerges from a critical and questioning attitude to clinical practice and the problems that emerge from clinical practice. It also relies on the investigator's familiarity with the current state of knowledge in the relevant field, an ability to generate sensible and researchable questions as well as a keen appreciation of the logic used in trying to answer these questions. If this, admittedly tall order can be achieved the rest tends to fall into place. Even if some technical problems remain it leaves the investigator properly equipped to approach other experts, such as statisticians, with a reasonable hope of getting appropriate and helpful advice which will resolve the outstanding technical issues.

REFERENCES

American Psychological Association (1981). Ethical principles of psychologists. *American Psychologist*, **36**, 631–638.

Barraco, R. A. & Stettner, L. J. (1976). Antibiotics and memory. *Psychological Bulletin*, **83**, 242–302.

Cohen, J. (1977). *Statistical Power Analysis for the Behavioral Sciences*. New York: Academic Press.

Cook, T. D. & Campbell, D. T. (1979). *Quasi-Experimentation: Design and Analysis Issues for Field Settings*. Chicago: Rand McNally.

Cox, J. L., Connor, Y. & Kendell, R. E. (1982). Prospective study of the psychiatric disorders of childbirth. *British Journal of Psychiatry*, **140**, 111–117.

Garfield, S. L. (1987). Ethical issues in research on psychotherapy. *Counseling & Values*, **31**, 115–125.

Kinard, E. M. (1985). Ethical issues in research with abused children. *Child Abuse & Neglect*, **9**, 301–311.

Miller, E. (1980). Cognitive assessment of the older adult. In J. E. Birren and R. B. Sloane (eds) *Handbook of Mental Health and Aging*. Englewood Cliffs: Prentice Hall.

Miller, E. (1983). A note on the interpretation of data derived from neuropsychological tests. *Cortex*, **19**, 131–132.

Miller, E. & Morley, S. (1986). *Investigating Abnormal Behaviour*. London: Weidenfeld & Nicolson.

Vaughn, C. E. & Leff, J. P. (1976). The influence of family and social factors on the course of psychiatric illness. *British Journal of Psychiatry*, **129**, 125–137.

3 Selecting and Developing Measures

Graham E. Powell
University of Surrey, Guildford, Surrey, GU2 5XH.

WHAT IS MEASUREMENT?

Psychological measurement is most commonly encountered in the form of psychological *testing* or *assessment*.

This branch of science and psychology has a fascinating history, dating back at least to the early Chinese some 22 centuries BC (Du Bois, 1966; 1970). They formally attempted to assess the capabilities of their civil servants and developed a system that lasted for 3000 years. In more recent history, the late nineteenth century saw the emergence of an interest in individual differences and how to test them. Galton (1879) published the results of 'psychometric experiments' in one of the first volumes of *Brain*, James Cattell opened his laboratory in Pennsylvania, and Alfred Binet began work on his famous intelligence scale. Early in the twentieth century several factors combined to create an urgent interest in their work. In particular, it became crucial to assess persons for military, industrial and educational purposes for both economic and social reasons. Psychological testing, then, has its roots in the need to make decisions about people. 'Standardised' tests were developed which had a manual describing the exact way to administer the test, defined the precise materials to use, had an objective scoring system, and which could be shown through controlled studies to contribute to better decision making.

Psychological *measurement*, on the other hand, is a broader topic relating to a more general interest in how to describe and ultimately understand the way that a person functions. Psychologists as experimental

27

scientists are called upon to measure an ever-increasing diversity of behavioural, social, cognitive, biological and environmental parameters. In the social sphere, for example, even a cursory glance at the published literature is revealing; there are attempts to measure such disparate things as facial expression, speed of eye movements, embarrassability, stressfulness of a situation, reciprocity in dyadic behaviour patterns, marital satisfaction, availability of social contacts, consensus in social stereotyping, social conscience and social adjustment. The development of published, standardised tests cannot possibly keep pace with these demands, therefore the mental health researcher must acquire two fundamental skills:

1. How to locate, compare and select measures from the published literature.
2. How to develop proper measures unique to the study at hand.

These two skills are addressed by this chapter, but there is one axiomatic statement to make at the outset; the basic principles of psychological testing are applicable to *all* forms of measurement *without exception*. It is all too convenient to forget this. For example, tens of thousands of research studies used psychiatric diagnosis as a measure before the major problems of reliability and validity were attended to, as described elegantly in an influential and scholarly book by Kendell (1975).

The basic principles of psychological testing alluded to above are discussed in the following sections. Why it is convenient to forget them will become obvious as to acknowledge them can significantly add to the complexity of research and to the time and resource necessary to allocate to a good study.

TYPES OF MEASURE: SCALING

At the simplest level, to measure is to assign a number to the properties or qualities of people (situations, objects or whatever) for the dual purposes of *description* and *analysis*.

Some description is fairly crude and merely indicates the presence of a quality or feature. This comprises assigning people to categories such as paranoid versus non-paranoid schizophrenia, those who believe they have control over their lives versus those who feel they are merely blown by the winds of fate, or those children who are behind at reading versus those whose achievements are within normal limits. More refined description comprises assigning a number on some scale which enables or implies a comparison between the subject and all other persons, such as degree of extraversion, level of intelligence or strength of fear of spiders.

Measurements are usually expressed as numbers to allow for computer coding and statistical analysis—but beware! These numbers do not necessarily have the same properties from one scale to the next since the relationship between any two numbers on a scale varies according to the *type of scale*, thus influencing the type of numerical analysis that can be legitimately undertaken.

A *nominal* scale is where numbers are used merely to name or label categories rather than to indicate order or magnitude. These are not numbers in the real sense as they are entirely arbitrary. For example, if marital status were a scale or variable in our study we might have the categories 'married' 'separated' 'divorced' 'widowed' 'co-habiting' and 'single' as the scale points. For computer coding purposes these might be translated into 0, 1, 2, 3, 4, 5, or 5, 4, 3, 2, 1, 0 or 77, 9, −4, 6½, 1000, 2, or any other set of six different numbers. It would not make any sense, therefore, to perform statistical manipulations on these 'scores', such as computing the average 'score' for the subjects in the study (though this fact does not stop some people trying).

Nominal scales are most often seen as independent variables, used as ways of splitting a population into subgroups to be compared on another scale. Hence one might divide a group of children into those that are brain damaged and those that are not (the independent variable) and compare their progress in reading (the dependent variable). This is not to imply that *no* statistical analysis can be undertaken when all the information is in the form of nominal scales because it is a relatively simple matter to compute relationships or associations between them by drawing up frequency tables of how many subjects fall into which categories and undertaking a χ^2 analysis. This is described in any basic statistics book that covers the analysis of qualitative or non-parametric data such as Maxwell (1961) or Siegel (1956). A fine example of the approach and worth looking at in this light is given by Rutter, Graham and Yule (1970) who in a very large-scale study teased out some of the complex relationships between childhood handicap, intellectual and academic performance and various measures of psychological and behavioural adjustment using almost exclusively nominal scales and variants of frequency analysis.

An *ordinal* scale is one in which larger numbers indicate greater possession of the property in question. There is therefore a logical relationship between numbers, which allows subjects to be *rank-ordered*. However, no assumptions are made about the *magnitude* of the difference between any two scale points. Suppose there were ten people in a room. Their height could be recorded using an ordinal scale by assigning 1 to the shortest, 2 to the next shortest, up to 10 for the tallest, but in absolute terms the two shortest may differ by one inch and the two tallest by three inches. For this reason, one must be careful of interpreting ordinal data. For example, returning to the people in the room, half are Finnish and half are

TABLE 3.1
Height of two subgroups expressed as mean rank (1 = shortest, 10 = tallest) and mean

Nationality	Rank	Mean rank	Actual height	Mean
Finnish	10		6'6"	
Finnish	9		6'3"	
Finnish	5	5.4	5'4"	5'7.6"
Finnish	2		5'1"	
Finnish	1		5'0"	
Venezuelan	8		5'7"	
Venezuelan	7		5'6"	
Venezuelan	6	5.6	5'5"	5'4.6"
Venezuelan	4		5'3"	
Venezuelan	3		5'2"	

Venezuelan. The mean rank of Finns is 5.4 and for Venezuelans it is 5.6. Can one conclude that the mean height of the Venezuelans is also greater than that of the Finns? Not necessarily.

The data presented in Table 3.1 show an example of how the reverse can be true, by a matter of more than three inches, with the ordinal scale being unable to take into account that the two tallest Finns are very tall indeed. The 'power' of ordinal scales (the amount of information they contain) is therefore less than it might be. There are other problems. In the next room there are five more Finns and five more Venezuelans, and these are also ranked. The mean rank of the Finns is the same as in this room, 5.4. Can we conclude that the Finns in the two rooms are of the same height? No, because all those in the second room are the young offspring of those in the first room. One therefore cannot generalise ranks across populations unless one can guarantee that the two populations are perfectly matched. Another problem is that the distribution of scores on an ordinal scale can be arbitrary, depending upon the scale intervals that the experimenter chooses. Suppose that all the people in the first room are rated on a three-point scale as follows: 1 = less than 5', 2 = 5' to 5' 11" and 3 = 6' or more, giving a distribution of 0, 8, 2. A three-point scale but with different intervals (1 = less than 5' 6", 2 = 5' 6" to 5' 11", 3 = 6' or more) will yield a distribution of 5, 3, 2, which looks quite different to the first and neither is a nice smooth curve of known mathematical properties.

For these reasons and others, ordinal data can only be subjected to *non-parametric* statistical analysis, which makes the absolute minimum of assumption about intervals and distributions (Leach, 1979). Although as mentioned these analyses are less powerful than they might be, the loss of power has a *conservative* effect, i.e. a non-parametric analysis *may* fail to find the significant differences in means or significant correlations that actually exist. Further, non-parametric analysis has progressed a great deal over recent years and offers a very wide range of techniques; it is no longer a second-class citizen and is frequently not just the only way but the best way both to obtain and to analyse data.

Finally, we have the *interval* scale, in which each scale point is a fixed distance from the next; height, speed, temperature, age and so on. Many tests and measures in psychology are taken to be interval scales such as Neuroticism scores on the Eysenck Personality Questionnaire or on the Beck Depression Inventory, or ratings on a 'Fear Thermometer' during exposure to snakes during studies of phobias, or ratings of relaxation during certain therapies. In fact, this is often just an assumption: no one has ever shown, for example, that a change of one unit on a relaxation scale, whether it occurs at the 'relaxed' end or 'panic' end, always equals a certain change in heart rate or GSR or power in the alpha band of the EEG; and does it make any psychological sense to say that someone who scores 20 on Extraversion is 'twice' as Extraverted as someone who scores 10? If I ask teachers to rate the children in their class on a scale of naughtiness from 1 to 10, am I entitled to treat it as equal interval data without further investigation?

There are three points to make. First, interval scales have to be designed and their interval properties empirically evaluated using special scaling techniques as developed, for example, by Lickert, Thurstone and Guttman (Aiken, 1985). *Ad hoc*, superficially appealing methods such as the mere use of whole integers does not constitute interval scaling. Second, it is debatable whether the concept of the equal interval scale is fully applicable to all psychological dimensions. Third, psychologists outside of the field of psychometrics and specialist scale construction (e.g. Aiken, 1980) have largely ignored these problems. Fourth, this is the right decision—although by choice one would always employ the most adequately scaled measure available, for pure practical reasons reasonable or sensible approximations to equal interval scaling will usually have to suffice unless the proof of perfect scaling is absolutely essential to or integral with the validity of the findings. Interval scales allow the most sophisticated of *parametric* statistical analyses, which require one to be able to make certain assumptions about interval and distribution.

To conclude this brief discussion of the meaning of numbers in measurement, one might recommend that the researcher aspire to interval measurement because of the statistical power it affords, but to fall back graciously to ordinal measurement and non-parametric statistics if one cannot reasonably support the claim that one's measure is truly an interval scale or if one cannot devise a method to construct such a scale. To pose a concrete problem, one of the most widely used measures of the long-term effects of cerebral trauma is the Glasgow Outcome Scale. It has four points 'Vegetative State' 'Severe disability' 'Moderate disability' and 'Good recovery'. In the absence of any scaling data (there is none) would you treat it as an ordinal or interval measure? The published literature reports it both ways, but one might feel that those taking an interval stance were being somewhat liberal.

TYPES OF MEASURE: TECHNIQUES

Thus far we have covered the nature of a scale without defining how one actually obtains the number pertaining to the subject. Here we are concerned with measures as techniques rather than abstractions. Each type of technique has a different range of convenience (i.e. is capable of measuring only certain properties) and each has various advantages and limitations.

The *rating scale* in its numerous guises is the commonest form of psychological measurement. The subject may rate him- or herself on the scale (self-report) or be rated on it by someone else (observer report). The scale always has a number of points; too few and it may lack sensitivity; too many and it may become arbitrary as to which of two or three points is indicated. Let us suppose that a five-point scale is used to measure current anxiety. The scale can come in various forms. The scale may be unipolar using a numbering system:

'Place a number in the box from 1 to 5 according to how anxious you feel at this moment, where 1 is not anxious and 5 is very anxious.
ANXIOUS $\boxed{4}$'

or unipolar using a horizontal scale:

'Place a cross in one of the five spaces to indicate how anxious you feel at this moment
NOT ANXIOUS ___X_ ANXIOUS'

or bipolar using one of these scales:

'Place a cross in one of the five spaces to indicate how you feel at this moment
RELAXED ___X_ ANXIOUS'

or may have each point explicitly described (or 'anchored'):

'Put a circle around the statement which most applies to you at this moment:
1. I feel very relaxed.
2. I feel relaxed.

3. I feel neither relaxed nor tense.
4. I feel anxious.
5. I feel very anxious.'

or may do away with all points and simply have a straight line for a mark which will later be measured by the experimenter:

'Place a cross on the line to indicate how anxious you feel at this moment
NOT ANXIOUS _____ X_ ANXIOUS'

These scales have the advantage of great flexibility, wide range of convenience and ease of administration but they are subject to various biases. The *halo effect* is when the score on a previous scale influences scores on a subsequent scale ('I rated myself as "CONFIDENT" on the last scale so shouldn't rate myself as "ANXIOUS" on this one'). The *experimenter effect* is when the subject consciously or unconsciously tries to please the test administrator ('He's trying so hard to put me at my ease I can't let him know he's making me quite anxious with all these questions'). The *leniency error* is shown by many subjects who resist assigning negative qualities to themselves or others. *Central tendency* is shown by some subjects who over-use the neutral category, which can be contrasted with *extreme responding*, a tendency to use just the extreme points of a scale in an all-or-none fashion.

There are many techniques related to the basic rating scale. There are *check lists*, for example, in which the subject is given a list of feelings (CONFIDENT, ANXIOUS, SLEEPY . . .) and requested to tick those that apply (which is really a series of two-point unipolar rating scales). There are also *card sorts* where the subject may have a pack of cards on each of which is a statement (e.g. 'I feel anxious')—each card in turn is placed on one of five piles or into one of five boxes labelled in terms of applicability ('I strongly agree with this statement', 'I slightly agree with this statement', etc.). *Grid* measures can also be mentioned here (see Chapter 13). The subject rates a number of people ('My sister', 'a famous sporting figure', 'the person I most dislike', etc.) on a series of scales ('confident' 'anxious' 'energetic' 'like myself', 'like I want to be', etc.). Here, the correlation between ratings on 'anxious' with ratings on 'like myself' becomes the measure of anxiety.

The *questionnaire* (measuring personality, attitudes, interests, etc.) is also in many cases just a thinly disguised collection of two or three point rating scales, and their verbal equivalent is the *interview*, although the interview does have an extra dimension, in that often information is elicited from the subject but interpreted in relation to points on various scales by a 'judge', usually the interviewer.

Alternatively, the subjective element can be largely removed and the data collected straight from the subject without interpretation either by the subject or the judge. Here we have *direct observation* (See Chapter 13) of behaviour, *performance* measures such as cognitive tests (See Chapter 9), and *psychophysiological* tests such as skin conductance (Martin and Venables, 1980).

But before we move on from techniques, let us preface the following sections by assuming that all of these tests aim to measure a real quantity— a person's real height, real intelligence or real social anxiety. This fabrication (i.e. real quantity) is known in Classical Test Theory as the 'true score'. This theory assumes that the score obtained on a measure (the 'observed score') is comprised of two portions, that is the true score plus an error score. If a test were ideal there would be no error component and the observed score would in fact be the true score. But no test is ideal and the problems posed by this error component have to be squarely faced.

PROPERTIES OF MEASURES: RELIABILITY

Reliability is to do with whether one gets the same answer if two measurements are taken of the same thing. For example, a wooden ruler marked out in inches would give a pretty reliable measure of the width of this page. I could measure it on two occasions and get the same answer, or my colleague from the next office could also take the measurement and get an answer very close to my own. But the same scale marked out on something slightly stretchy, let's say a length of elastic to use an extreme example, would not necessarily always give the same results across either time or persons; the answer obtained would crucially depend upon the exact tension placed on the elastic ruler as it was drawn across the page. In research, then, it is important to be sure that the measures we use are as stable as the wooden ruler. There is little point in putting a lot of effort into a research study if inaccuracies in measurement are likely to obscure the findings by generating a lot of 'noise' in the data. This analogy to radio reception is quite apt—for if the effects we are looking for are delicate (i.e. a weak signal) then it is even more important that noise and crackle be kept to a minimum, or we will miss them altogether.

Reliability is succinctly described by Aiken (1985, p. 84) as a test's 'relative freedom from unsystematic errors of measurement'. Under specified conditions the test should always yield the same results; they should not vary randomly or unpredictably. There are several ways of assessing reliability and these will be described in turn.

Test–retest reliability is when the same test is administered to the same group of subjects on two different occasions separated by a specified time interval. Scores on the first occasion are then correlated with scores on the second. If there were no errors in the measurement subjects would maintain exactly the same distance from each other (or rank order if we were using non-parametric statistics) which would result in a correlation (now called a reliability coefficient) of exactly 1.0. If the test measured nothing but error then the correlation would be zero. The reliability of psychological measures in practice never reaches 1.0 because of fluctuations in many variables such as a subject's mood or level of fatigue.

Note, though, that the *mean* score might well change because of practice effects on the specific test items. This change in means does *not* affect the computation of the correlation coefficient which is independent of the mean score. *Systematic* errors then, such as practice effects, do not affect reliability.

Parallel form reliability takes into account the fact that the state of subjects varies upredictably from the first to second testing, and assesses reliability during a single test session by giving all subjects two versions of the test. These should be equivalent or parallel, and usually the order of test-taking is organised such that half of the subjects take version A first and a half take version B first. The reliability coefficient will fall short of 1.0, depending upon short-term fluctuations in the subjects' state and upon the degree to which the forms are truly identical.

Often one can neither arrange to see subjects on two occasions nor obtain two parallel forms, in which case one can resort to *split-half* reliability. The test is split into two (e.g. odd versus even items) and the scores on the halves is correlated. A slight adjustment is made to the obtained correlation to take into account the fact that a shorter test is less reliable; this is called the Spearman–Brown formula. For obvious reasons this type of reliability coefficient is often called a coefficient of Internal Consistency. In fact there are many ways of dividing a test into two halves which would give a whole range of reliability coefficients; therefore, the natural thing to do is to compute the mean of all possible split-half coefficients using the Kuder–Richardson formula 20 (Aiken, 1985, p. 87; Anastasi, 1976, p. 114). This formula itself is only a specific instance of the general Alpha Coefficient (Cronbach, 1951) which considers the relationship of each item to every other item.

Scorer reliability must be estimated whenever scoring is fallible. At a basic level scorer mistakes can be made when entering or adding up numbers on an IQ test, say, but at a more general and subtle level most tests demand that the scorer make *judgements* during both administration and scoring which are subject to personal biases. Degree of judgement is least on those tests with an extensive and explicit administration manual and with similarly explicit scoring criteria. Such is the case with most of the commonly used intelligence tests. The degree of judgement that has to be exercised is greatest when questions are allowed to be asked in slightly different ways and when only broad guidelines can be given for scoring—this is the case in regard to interviewing. To obtain an estimate of scorer reliability two or more judges score the same subjects. The correlation (or alpha coefficient if there are more than two scores) should approach 1.0. If not, the administration and scoring criteria have to be tightened up and/or the training of the judges improved.

Having described reliability, we must be clear as to why it is important and should in general be maximised. Because every test has an error component the observed score is only an estimate of the true score. If a test were repeated many times a distribution of scores would be obtained that would cluster around the true score. Like the distribution of any variable, the distribution of observed scores would have a mean and standard deviation. The mean, as stated, would be the true score and the standard deviation (SD) is known as the *standard error of measurement*, or SEM. There is a relationship between SEM and reliability (r_{11}) as follows:

$$SEM = SD \sqrt{1 - r_{11}}$$

This simple formula tells us why reliability is so important. If reliability is perfect ($r_{11} = 1.0$) then the SEM will be zero (i.e. SEM = SD $\sqrt{1 - 1} = 0$). This would mean one had a perfect test in which repeat measures on the same subject would always be the same (because as just shown their distribution would have zero standard deviation) and would all equal the true score. Conversely, if reliability were zero ($r_{11} = 0$) then the SEM will be equal to the standard deviation of observed scores (i.e. SEM = SD $\sqrt{1 - 0}$ = SD). This would mean that all the variation in observed scores across different subjects would be due to unsystematic error and nothing whatever to do with qualities purported to be measured by the test. The test, then, would be perfectly useless. However, a test invariably *does* contain error, and so one must try to define an acceptable reliability. Acceptability in this instance is more than just the statistical significance of the particular reliability coefficient. It would be very easy, especially with a large group of subjects, to obtain a significant test–retest correlation of, say, 0.3. But if one worked through the mathematics one could show that this meant that only 30% of the variance in test scores was due to the subjects and 70% would be error variance. Broadly speaking, a reliability much less than 0.9 would be disappointing and call into question the point of using the test.

But having said this, one must also say that the search for high reliability is not the be-and-end-all of the exercises for it must be tempered with thoughtful commonsense. There are many examples of this. If the alpha of a test were unity, with all items correlating perfectly with each other, then it would mean that all items measured exactly the same thing so that all except one could be dropped.If the test–retest reliability of a trait were unity then would this not inhibit the measure from detecting genuine changes on that trait? If one tries to improve the reliability of a test one can drop individual items with the lowest reliability; but would one not reach the point where the gain in test reliability resulting from dropping an unreliable item is matched or outstripped by a *loss* in reliability caused by having a shorter test? Further, we can drop items to make a test more reliable but we must also take into account what we want the test to measure. Suppose we want a test of Extraversion (E) and that E is a trait combining elements of two things, impulsivity (I) and sociability (S). Our test of E therefore comprises I items and S items. But suppose I items were less reliable. If, in an effort to increase reliability we rejected the lowest reliability items we would in effect be rejecting I items so that our test would no longer be measuring Extraversion but only one component of it, namely sociability. Some of these issues and many others are well discussed by Levy (1973).

PROPERTIES OF MEASURES: VALIDITY

Should a measure prove to have acceptable reliability of the type needed, then it is worth pursuing its psychometric properties to see if it is also a *valid* measure of that which it is supposed to be measuring.

To return to the example of the wooden ruler marked out in inches, we can be sure that it will give the same answer twice, but is the inch as marked out on the ruler precisely what we think it is? Not necessarily. This is why in England, we have Trading Standards Authorities checking all measures of length, weight and volume used in commercial dealing, to make sure that customers are not taken advantage of through deliberate or accidental tampering with the measuring devices, making sure that scales are accurate, that pint glasses in pubs indeed contain one pint, and so on. Our ruler, then, might be compared with some accepted criterion. Further, thinking of the elastic ruler this time, we can say exactly why it is potentially not a valid measure of length, because any one reading is in fact the product of *two* constructs, both length and tension.

Validity is affected by both systematic and unsystematic error, unlike reliability which is only attenuated by unsystematic error. Consider the test–retest reliability of an IQ test. It was noted earlier that practice effects would cause scores to increase across the two occasions but that this would not affect reliability. However, the second test is clearly in some sense a *less* valid measure of IQ as it will be an over-estimate. There are several types of validity to consider.

Face Validity

Face validity concerns the fact that when confronted with a new test one automatically makes a subjective judgement as to whether it *appears* to be measuring what it is meant to. If a test of extraversion consists of questions about going to parties and cracking jokes it has 'face validity'. But if a test of extraversion comprises looking at a black spiral spinning on its axis it might seem a 'stupid' test, even though both the sensible and 'ridiculous' test might both predict certain features of extraversion quite well and correlate with each other to a significant degree. Face validity is not then a statistical concept but merely a subjective evaluation and as such is not a true measure of validity, although lack of face validity is not something to ignore as it can foster a negative attitude in the subject.

Content Validity

Content validity concerns whether a test samples from the entire domain of that which is to be measured. Suppose one wanted to measure the amount of friction in a marriage. It would not be sufficient, say, to enquire about arguments over money. One would also have to examine for conflict over child-rearing, habits, lifestyle, plans for the future and so on. Once again, it can be seen that this is not a statistical concept but a question of 'expert judgement' (Aiken, 1985, p. 94).

Criterion-related Validity

Criterion-related validity is achieved when a test yields the same result as another test that is already known to be valid (this second test is known as the *criterion measure*). The circularity of this definition is obvious and can cause problems, particularly when at a later date the validity of a criterion measure is called into question. A second feature of this definition is that it suggests a 'parallel' with reliability, in that a new test in order to be valid must have parallel form reliability with a test of proven validity.

Criterion measures can take many forms, but there is one supraordinate division that is usually made depending upon the time at which the result of the criterion measure becomes available. *Concurrent* validity is when results on the criterion measure are available simultaneously (e.g. those with a neurotic psychiatric disorder, the criterion measure, are found to be higher on a new test of neuroticism). *Predictive* validity, on the other hand, is when scores on a new test are used to predict scores on a subsequent measure (e.g. 'A' level results can be validated as a measure of suitability for a university education by correlating them with final class of degree, the criterion measure). Predictive validity seldom rises above 0.6 (thereby leaving 64% of variance unexplained) because many factors will ultimately influence final outcome.

Construct Validity

Construct validity, the most important but elusive type, is concerned with the psychological meaning of test scores. With criterion validity the concept of validity can be hedged by saying that the test measures what the criterion measure does. But in construct validity a genuine attempt is made to define the 'thing' or construct that one is interested in. Aiken (1985) manages to capture this elusiveness in a few well-chosen lines: 'The construct validity of a test is not established by one successful prediction; it consists of the slow, laborious process of gathering evidence from many experiments and observations on how the test is functioning.' Among the sources of evidence that can be cited are:

1. Expert judgement that test content pertains to the construct.
2. The demonstration of internal consistency of the test (if it can be broken down into two or more unrelated groups of items it can hardly be measuring a single construct).
3. High correlations with other measures of the construct (*convergent validity*).
4. Low correlations with easures of different constructs (*divergent validity*).
5. The thoughts and comments of subjects as they undertake the test.
6. Studies of group differences.
7. Successful prediction of task performance when one would expect such task performance to relate to the construct.

The Wechsler Adult Intelligence Scale

Some of the points above will be discussed with respect to an actual test, the Wechsler Adult Intelligence Scale (WAIS), and implicit reference made to much of the work on this test reported by Matarazzo (1972).

First, the WAIS does indeed on inspection contain subtests or individual items that most would judge as pertaining to the construct of intelligence— there are tests of conceptual thought, mathematical reasoning, speed of problem solving, etc.—although critics might say that the test is not culture fair (i.e. measures a white middle-class definition of intelligence) and fails to tap other aspects of intellectual performance such as persistence.

Next, the WAIS does have internal consistency because the manual shows that all subtests intercorrelate positively as to the two main subfactors of verbal and performance IQ.

As for convergent and divergent validity, performance on the WAIS does indeed correlate with other measures of intelligence, such as its forerunner, the Wechsler–Bellevue scale, and with less formal measures of intelligence such as gaining admission to university; whereas conversely, in regard to divergent validity, although WAIS scores do correlate with some other psychological traits none of the correlations are high enough to suggest that the test measures something other than intelligence. For example, if WAIS scores were to correlate very highly with measures of, say, fear of failure, state anxiety, neuroticism and fear of negative evaluation, then one might say that it measured not intelligence but test-taking anxiety.

More detailed statements concerning construct validation can be made using a 'psychological decomposition' approach. Levy (1973) points out that when validating a test there is a great tendency to correlate it with everything else in sight in the hope that a 'meaning' emerges. The problem is that we often know even less about the tests dragged in, so that 'what starts as a problem of understanding something about one test becomes a multiple act of construct validation'.

Alternatively, using psychological decomposition, the one test is systematically varied, changing one aspect each time, and performance on these slightly different versions correlated. Levy cites Hopkins (1971), who studied the Digit-Symbol subtest of the WAIS. Holding test format, timing, scoring and so forth constant, he developed one test that measured only writing speed (i.e. only one symbol was used which was written repeatedly); one test of eye-movement (twenty five digits were used rather than the normal nine so that Ss could not simply learn digit-symbol relationships) and so on. He found that the speed of eye movement version correlated rather well (0.68) with the original version, as did the writing speed version (0.47). Therefore, one can say that the Digit Symbol subtest of the WAIS in part measures speed of eye movement and speed of writing.

PROPERTIES OF MEASURES: GENERALISABILITY

A bridge between the concepts of reliability and validity is generalisability theory (Cronbach, Gleser, Nanda & Rajaratnam, 1972; Levy, 1974; Shavelson and Webb, 1981). This concerns the broader problem of how to make a general statement from a specific test score: that is, how to generalise from one observation to other classes of observation often known as the *dependability* of a score or test. One might wish to generalise from:

1. Scores obtained from one judge to those derived from other judges.
2. Scores on one test of, say, depression, to scores on other tests of depression.
3. Scores at this particular moment to scores at some time in the future.

4. Scores from one sample of possible items to scores from other samples.
5. Scores obtained under one set of motivational conditions to those obtained under others.

In looking at the above examples it can readily be seen that the traditional division between reliability and validity becomes quite deliberately blurred. In fact the concept of there being *one* true score is swept away as described by Wiggins (1973) to be replaced by the notion of the *universe score*, the mean of all possible observations under all 'conditions'. (The assumptions this definition requires are listed in Wiggins, 1973, p. 286.)

Cronbach, Gleser, Nanda and Rajaratnam (1972) state the problem thus:

> The score on which the decision is to be based is only one of many scores that might serve the same purpose. The decision maker is almost never interested in the response given to the particular stimulus objects or questions, to the particular tester, at the particular moment of testing. Some, at least, of these conditions of measurement could be altered without making the score any less acceptable to the decision maker. This is to say, there is a universe of observations, any of which would have yielded a usable basis for the decision. The ideal datum on which to base the decision would be something like the person's mean score over all acceptable observations, which we shall call his 'universe score'. The investigator uses the observed score or some function of it as if it were the universe score. That is, he generalizes from sample to universe.

In a generalisability study a whole range of observations is made under the different conditions that interest the experimenter. The basic data matrix for a generalisability design is given in Table 3.2, taken from Wiggins (1973). Here, conditions is a loose term that could relate to 'particular test items, test formats, stimuli, observers, occasions or situations of observation' and more. The observed score for a person in one condition is x_{pi} and the universe score is the mean of all x_{pi} over all conditions. An analysis of variance of the data will apportion the variance to persons, conditions and residual (or error). This ANOVA replaces traditional coefficients and becomes more complex as more than one set of conditions (more than one facet) is considered simultaneously.

One might measure the sociability of persons under two sets of conditions: Facet I might be different judges and Facet II different settings. Hence the study might comprise four judges rating the subjects at work, at a social gathering, with the family and with one close friend. How does one choose the range of conditions? This is a judgemental and not a statistical concept. It depends upon the type of generalisations that the experimenter

TABLE 3.2
Basic data matrix for a generalisability design (based on Wiggins, 1973)

		Conditions			
		1	2	3	---------------------- n_i
Persons	1	X_{11}	X_{12}	X_{13}	---------------------- X_{1ni}
	2		X_{22}	X_{23}	---------------------- X_{2ni}
	3			X_{33}	---------------------- X_{3ni}
	np			X_{np3}	---------------------- X_{npni}

sees as being demanded of the test: if different judges will be using it then it is necessary to gauge variance due to judges; if observations are made in a psychiatric ward but will be used in practice in hostels and out patient departments as well, then having specified the universe to which observations must generalise the researcher must 'provide empirical evidence of such generalizability in the form of generalizability coefficients or estimates of the components of variants involved' (Wiggins, 1973, p. 295). Those coefficients are often in the form of inter-class correlations (somewhat like the alpha coefficient) for the universe specified.

An example of a generalisability study can be found in the work of Mariotto and Farrell (1979) who focused upon the Inpatient Multidimensional Psychiatric Scale (IMPS). This is used as a standardised instrument for measuring change in the level of functioning of psychiatric patients. It has 75 items that are scored for (a) intensity (b) frequency and (c) presence, by a trained interviewer and observer after a 40 minute interview. It can be scored for ten 'syndrome' scores and also for some higher level factor scores. Several previous studies had shown that raters could *order* patients comparably on both syndrome and higher level scores (i.e. good inter-rated reliability of around 0.90) but the comparability between raters of *absolute* level of scores was at issue. Indeed, other studies had indicated that the absolute level of scores given by a particular rater might vary with such variables as increased professional training, years of experience and age. The suggestion is, then, that non-patient factors affect judgements on the IMPS so that 'the scale may not validly reflect patient behaviour over differing times, situations, patient groups or raters'.

Mariotto and Farrell took 10 chronic schizophrenics (mean age 43 years; mean hospitalisation 7 years 5 months) in a large state psychiatric hospital and gave each one the semistructured interview developed for the IMPs. Observing the interview on a video monitor in an adjacent room were 11 graduate raters. They had received 7 hours of training. Interrater correlations between the 11 raters for the 10 syndrome scores were calculated, and the 4 'worse' raters dropped. The next analyses therefore took place on only the 7 'best' raters.

In the first place it was found that, as in previous studies, generalisability coefficients (intra-class correlations) for the scales were generally high. On only two scales, grandiosity and retardation, did the raters fail to order subjects consistently.

Next, to assess level differences, two-way analyses of variance (raters × patients) were undertaken for each IMPS score. The main effect for raters particularly concerns us. The effect was significant on an F test on all bar two of the 14 syndrome and higher level scores. Therefore, the absolute level of ratings was significantly different between raters. Indeed, the rater effect accounted for as much as 20% and 23% of the variance on the scales Cognitive Distortion and Paranoid respectively, and for 18% of the variance of the IMPS total score. Further, with Wilk's λ multivariate analysis it was shown that different raters had different biases on different scales, so that the profiles obtained from each rater across the 10 syndrome scales were not parallel.

The contribution of rater bias to IMPS scores is therefore high, especially when one takes into account that the raters were especially selected so as to be homogeneous. Mariotto and Farrell were able to conclude that IMPS cannot be used when absolute level differences are required as in outcome studies and normative comparisons across patient groups. Further, because of the contribution of rater bias to the patient profile, IMPS profiles could not be recommended for diagnostic usage.

Generalisability theory, though widely regarded as a conceptual leap, has not caught on. An excellent book on psychological testing (Kaplan & Saccuzzo, 1982) does not mention it at all. There are two reasons. First, to estimate universe scores requires a generalisability study that is complicated to design, time consuming to carry out and awkward to analyse. Second, traditional reliability and validity are not 'wrong'—rather, they are just limited aspects of generalisability (Sechrest, 1984). As long as the researcher does not abuse reliability and validity coefficients (particularly by using reliability coefficients as interchangeable) and thoughtfully and deliberately specifies the *type* or reliability and *type* of validity that is needed, they remain a credible backbone of measurement.

A PRACTITIONER APPROACH TO MEASUREMENT

Measurement within a clinical context relates to the model of the therapist as a 'scientist practitioner' (Barlow, Hayes & Nelson, 1984). The scientific practitioner takes measures mainly because it improves treatment; by measuring *problems* one gets feedback on progress and by measuring *treatment* one can ensure treatment integrity (i.e. that the client receives the treatment intended). A second reason is that interesting results can be published as single case studies to enhance clinical science in general. Third, measures provide for accountability—they can be used as indicators of the effectiveness of a service.

Barlow and his colleagues offer excellent advice about how to go about measuring with the individual client:

1. State client problems in specific terms.
2. Specify several problem areas.
3. Obtain multiple measures for each problem behaviour.
4. Select measures that are both sensitive and meaningful.
5. Collect measures early in the course of treatment.
6. Take the same measures repeatedly, at least before, during and after treatment.
7. Make comparisons within measures only if data are collected under similar conditions.
8. Graph the data.
9. Record inconvenient measures less frequently than convenient ones.
10. Select measures with appropriate psychometric properties, looking for certain types of reliability such as inter-judge agreement, and noting that some types of reliability are less appropriate. For example, test-retest reliability presupposes consistency, but usually the therapist needs a measure of *change*.
11. Obtain client consent and co-operation.

These suggestions are developed and extended in a further book by Barlow which shows how the gap between individual therapy and research study can be bridged (Barlow & Hersen, 1984).

A RESEARCH APPROACH TO MEASUREMENT

In terms of research method, the aim of measurement is to achieve an acceptable operational definition of the aims and/or hypotheses of the study. The process used to achieve this is described below step by step, using an actual study as an example to illustrate some of the operations used.

Step One: State the Aims and/or Hypotheses

This must be done decisively, almost boldly; avoiding excessively general statements on the one hand and obsessionally elaborate detail on the other. The over-broad aim does not describe the study well, and detail can for the most part be left to the Method section. The aims must flow naturally from the introduction and the method must flow naturally from the aims.

The example considered is that of a study performed by Kaiser and Pfenninger (1984). They state the aims of their investigation as follows. 'The objective of this report is to examine if the outcome of the severely head injured child is better following a neurointensive care than without it.'

This is a pretty clear statement of intent. The outcome could have been defined a little more precisely, although in the context of the introduction the reader would have readily understood that the study was concerned with 'long-range' outcome which implies consideration of many outcome variables other than survival rate.

Step Two: Content Analysis of Aims/Hypotheses

The measures must flow from the aims, so one must define the content of each aspect of the aims. The facets to be defined and measured are:

1. The subjects ('the child').
2. Severe head injury.
3. Neurointensive care.
4. Outcome.

1. *The Subjects*   Putting 'outcome' and 'severe head injury' to one side for the moment, 'the subject' has to be defined and measured for two reasons: (a) to ensure they meet inclusion criteria; and (b) to provide independent variables that may be associated with outcome (dependent) variables. The inclusion criteria chosen by the authors were:

(a) Dates of hospitalisation (March 1978–August 1981).
(b) Place of hospitalisation (Department of Paediatric Surgery, Barn).
(c) Age (0–14 years, although this was not explicitly stated).

None of these simple inclusion criteria pose any measurement problem, although others would have, such as 'premorbid IQ' or 'able to comprehend testing instructions'.

The independent variables identified were:

(a) Age.
(b) Cause of accident (e.g. falls, road accidents).
(c) Clinical signs on admission (e.g. vital functions, extracranial injury, neurological signs, Glasgow coma scale score).
(d) CT findings (e.g. haematoma, contusion, CSF bleeding).

Again, one of these pose particular measurement problems although it cannot be supposed that either a neurological exam or interpretation of a CT scan are perfectly reliable. Other independent variables that could have been chosen, such as 'premorbid behaviour adjustment' would have been awkward.

2. *Severe Head Injury*   Severe head injury is not a technical term as such and needs an operational definition, in this case having a Glasgow Coma scale (GCS) score of 7 or less. The GCS is an extremely well-known behavioural measure of depth of coma (Teasdale & Jennett, 1974, 1976; Teasdale & Mendelow, 1984) that measures three things: conditions under which the eyes open, best verbal response and best motor response, summing observations to produce a single score. Score reliability is higher than other possible measures of severity such as length of post-traumatic amnesia, which is assessed retrospectively and depends upon often patchy observations in the notes or upon the subjective report of the patient.

One must mention one more inclusion criterion here in that only 'blunt' or 'non-penetration' injuries were accepted into the trial as penetration injuries usually require different management.

3. *Neurointensive Care*   As in any experiment the treatment must be explictly defined, usually by way of a statement of principles or strategies, since treatment can rarely be specified to the level of detailed action. Neurointensive care was defined as the use of a series of medical procedures:

(a) Continuous intracranial and arterial pressure monitoring.
(b) Normalisation of intracranial pressure and cerebral perfusion pressure.
(c) Intubation.
(d) Hyperventilation.
(e) Control of body temperature.
(f) Dexamethasone.
(g) Barbiturates.
(h) Osmotic agents.

These procedures were described in detail and present no measurement problems.

4. *Outcome*   This is the tricky one, as shown by the outline of a content analysis of outcome in Table 3.3. This breakdown could be elaborated almost indefinitely to include almost everything we could possibly measure about someone. For instance, intelligence could be broken down into

TABLE 3.3
Content analysis of outcome

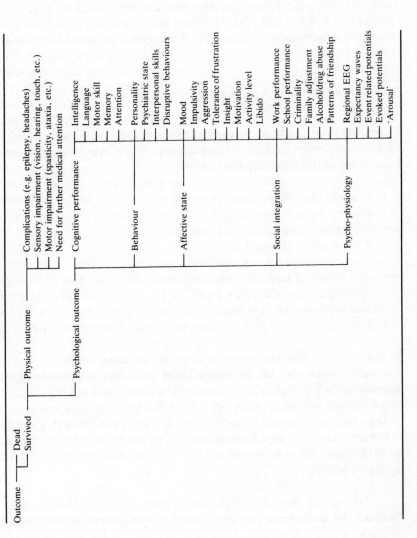

speed, persistence, verbal skill, non-verbal skill, reasoning, abstract thinking, judgement; personality could be subdivided into traits, interests,
hobbies, self-concept, self-esteem, flexibility, egocentrism, adjustment etc.

The impossibility of measuring everything in detail is self-evident.
Therefore, the next difficult decision the researcher must make is how to
limit the size of the task. At this point the accummulated experience of
other researchers needs to be sought. This is what the published literature
is for.

Step Three: Selecting from the Content Analysis and Undertaking a Literature Search

These two steps are logically distinct but in practice go hand in hand, for
the following reason. Choice of measure is a complex juggling act based on
knowledge of the following factors:

1. Content analysis of aims.
2. Priority areas of content.
3. Financial resources of the study.
4. Time-scale of the study.
5. Administration time of each test.
6. The length of time that subjects can tolerate testing.
7. Available tests of priority areas.
8. The adequacy of such tests.
9. The need for the study to relate to a larger body of research.

It can be seen that there are interactions between some of these: in
particular, what one finally selects from the content analysis in part
depends upon the analysis of alternatives available, and which alternatives
one examines in turn depends upon priorities in the content analysis.

Therefore, the examination of alternative measures through a detailed
literature search is always a compromise. One cannot possibly read around
all of the topics listed at the end of Table 3.3, therefore one *rejects* from the
literature search:

1. All aspects that one definitely cannot measure through lack of
facilities (let us suppose this takes out the psychophysiological branch of
Table 3.3).

2. All aspects in which one is confident of one's knowledge or expertise
(in Kaiser and Pfennigger's case this takes out the physical outcome
branch).

3. All aspects that are low in one's hierarchy of priorities (let us suppose
that this removes the cognitive performance branch).

This leaves the general area of psychosocial recovery; so a computer search was made on MEDLINE in March, 1986 requesting all references dating back to 1st January, 1980 which had the keyword HEAD INJUR? in combination with RECOVER? or OUTCOME? or PERSONALITY? or PSYCHOSOCIAL? (Note that a question mark indicates that the term may be followed by different endings or a second word.) An identical search was also undertaken on PSYCINFO. Together with other searches using slightly different keywords (such as BRAIN DAMAGE for HEAD INJUR?) and with a search by hand working backwards in time from the most recent issues of the relevant journals and books, 41 articles were identified, mainly 1980 or later, but including a few important articles that appeared earlier.

Step Four: Evaluation of the Measures That Have Been Used in the Literature

In evaluating the adequacy and usefulness of the specific measures employed in these 41 studies, one must keep several questions in mind that constitute broad judgemental criteria for eventual selection:

1. Are the basic psychometric properties of the measures known?

2. If known, are they adequate?

3. Are the measures generalisable to my subject population (in relation to our example, can the measure be used with children?)

4. If the measure is to be adapted (e.g. for use with children; to make it suitable for a British rather than American population; needing translation from a foreign language) then will it need re-standardising?

5. In what areas do I need only broad summary measures or first approximations?

6. In what areas do I need fine measurements that might relate to process as well as outcome?

7. Are there some papers so germane to mine that I should use some of their measures to establish a bridge for easy comparison of data and findings?

8. What resources does the study need to undertake particular measurement, such as expensive test material, equipment, access to relatives and many others?

9. What resources does the subject need in order to take the test (e.g. facility with language, demands upon concentration, motor ability required)?

10. Are there ethical problems (e.g. confidentiality of test data, the stressfulness of the test)?

To return to our example, of the studies reviewed, a large percentage (37%) just used interviews and/or simple rating scales to provide broad descriptions of psychosocial outcome, *without any knowledge whatsoever* of their psychometric properties. For example, Eggleston and Cruvant (1983) examined recovery from intracerebral haemartoma in children and adults and developed, or rather invented, a 'Patient Data Scale' which included 4 point ratings of 'Activities of daily living' 'Psychosocial Adjustment' 'Work/school adjustment; developmental progress' and 'Speech function'. Sometimes these studies also included a simple checklist of symptoms, also invariably of unknown reliability and validity, such as the 'Head injury symptom checklist' of McLean, Temkin, Dikman and Wisler (1983).

In fact only three studies (7%) ascertained the reliability of their rating or interview measures. One study in particular (Rappaport *et al*. 1982) was especially concerned with reliability and made it a focus of the study. They developed the Rappaport Disability Rating Scale and computed the inter-rater reliabilities for trained raters. These were very high at between 0.97 and 0.98, but reliability for *un*trained raters (of the type who would in practice be using the scale) was not computed.

Similarly, only three studies (7%) tried to ascertain the *validity* of their measures. One was the study of Rappaport cited above, one is as yet unpublished, and one was an older study by Shaffer, Chadwick and Rutter (1975), who validated a rating of psychiatric handicap in brain injured children against detailed questioning of the parents. They also used questionnaires of known validity such as the Teachers' Questionnaire (Rutter, Tizard & Whitmore, 1970).

Finally, 29% of the studies used ad hoc interviews and scales mixed with a few well-known, standardised tests such as the Katz Adjustment Scale (Katz & Lyerly, 1963).

This brief review makes somewhat chilling reading, especially in an area like neuropsychology which is renowned for its experimental rigor. It would be usual at this stage to draw a few conclusions about measurement within the field of interest. In this case:

1. Most of the measures in the studies reviewed provided data of dubious credibility since psychometric properties were ignored.
2. Where psychometric properties were known they were on well-known psychiatric scales not intended for use with the head injured and as such they may well have missed important features of this population.
3. Description of behaviour and cognitions were extremely broad—not to say gross, in more senses than one.
4. Data collection was never theory driven. The studies mainly aimed at obtaining a description, even then without a proper content analysis.

Clearly, if Kaiser and Pfenninger had had access to the above searches, they would *not* have found a body of tried and trusted outcome measures upon which they could draw as needed. On presumably limited resources (i.e. within the context of an on-going clinical service with no special research grant) they sensibly used measures that are readily applied to children and are widely used in other studies, notably the Glasgow Outcome Scale. It is a crude scale admittedly, compressing all features of recovery onto a four-point scale:

Vegetative state.
Severe disability.
Moderate disability.
Good recovery.

But direct comparisons can be made with many other studies, the measure usefully relates to actual performance, and it is probably sensitive enough to offer a first approximation to the question of whether intensive care is worthwhile. On the other hand, it certainly can never have construct validity since outcome is multifaceted, and as it does not relate directly to the detail of the content analysis in Table 3.3 it can never obtain information about specific patterns of mechanisms of recovery.

In general terms, what *might* have been done? General principles are considered here, as many researchers will find themselves in this position:

1. Select from previous work measures of known psychometric properties, so as to form a solid bridge with the corpus of knowledge.
2. Select from previous work interesting measures of unknown psychometric properties, but design the new study so as to assess these properties. This also forms a bridge with the corpus of knowledge, but in addition improves our understanding of the dependability of that knowledge.
3. Undertake a content analysis of areas of interest to define what other variables one needs to measure, and develop them psychometrically in the new study.
4. Be reasonable; accept that no study is perfect and that the inclusion of one or two measures of unknown properties is 'allowed'.

SUMMARY

The principles of psychometric testing should also underpin all forms of measurement whatever the metric or technique used. Therefore for every measure employed, one should be able to state the type of reliability that it should and does have, the type of validity that is required and demonstrated, and the universe of conditions to which test scores can generalise. Good measurement is a prerequisite for the scientific approach to both treatment and research. It is facilitated by a clear statement of aims, by a content analysis of these aims, and by a critical appraisal of measurement within the relevant literature. Good measurement usually demands that a portion of research resources is allocated to the development of measures.

REFERENCES

Aiken, L. R. (1980). Problems in testing the elderly. *Educational Gerontology*, 5, 119–124.
Aiken, L. R. (1985). *Psychological Testing and Assessment (5th edition)*. Boston: Allyn & Bacon.
Anastasi, A. (1976). *Psychological Testing*, 4th edn. New York: Macmillan.
Barlow, D. H., Hayes, S. C. & Nelson, R. O. (1984). *The Scientist Practitioner: Research and Accountability in Clinical and Educational Settings*. New York: Pergamon.
Barlow, D. H. & Hersen, M. (1984). *Single Case Experimental Designs: Strategies for Studying Behavior Change*. New York: Pergamon.
Cronbach, L. J. (1951). Coefficient alpha and the internal structure of tests. *Psychometrika*, 16, 296–334.
Cronbach, L. J., Gleser, G. C., Nanda, H. & Rajaratnam, N. (1972). *The Dependability of Behavioural Measurements*. New York: Wiley.
Du Bois, P. H. (1966). A test-dominated society: China 1115 BC–1905 AD. In A. Anastasia (ed.) *Testing Problems in Perspective*. Washington: American Council on Education.
Du Bois, P. H. (1970). *A History of Psychological Testing*. Boston: Allyn & Bacon.
Eggleston, C. & Cruvant, D. (1983). Review of recovery from intracerebral hematoma in children and adults. *Journal of Neurological Nursing*, 15, 128–135.
Galton, F. (1879). Psychometric experiments. *Brain*, 2, 149–162.
Hopkins, N. (1971). Unpublished observations, cited in Levy (1973).
Kaiser, G. & Pfenninger, J. (1984). Effect of neurointensive care upon outcome following severe head injuries in childhood—a preliminary report. *Neuropediatrics*, 15, 68–75.
Kaplan, R. M. & Saccuzzo, D. P. (1982). *Psychological Testing: Principles, Applications and Issues*. Monterey: Brooks/Cole.
Katz, M. M. & Lyerly, S. B. (1963). Methods for measuring adjustment and social behaviour in the community I Rationale, description, discriminative validity and scale development. *Psychological Reports*, 13, 503–535.
Kendell, R. E. (1975). *The Role of Diagnosis in Psychiatry*. Oxford: Blackwell.
Leach, C. (1979). *Introduction to Statistics: A Non-parametric Approach for the Social Sciences*. Chichester: Wiley.
Levy, P. (1973). On the relation between test theory and psychology. In P. Kline (ed.) *New Approaches in Psychological Measurement*. London: John Wiley & Sons.
Levy, P. (1974). Generalizability studies in clinical settings. *British Journal of Social and Clinical Psychology*, 13, 161–172.
Mariotto, M. J. & Farrell, A. D. (1979). Comparability of the absolute level of ratings on the Inpatient Multidimensional Psychiatric Scale within a homogeneous group of raters. *Journal of Consulting and Clinical Psychology*, 47, 59–64.
Martin, I. & Venables, P. H. (1980). *Techniques in Psychophysiology*. Chichester: Wiley.
Matarazzo, J. D. (1972). *Wechsler's Measurement and Appraisal of Adult Intelligence*, 5th edn. Baltimore: Williams & Wilkins.

Maxwell, A. E. (1961). *Analysing Qualitative Data*. London: Methuen.

McLean, A., Temkin, N. R., Dikmen, S. & Wyler, A. R. (1983). The behavioral sequelae of head injury. *Journal of Clinical Neuropsychology*, **5**, 361–376.

Rappaport, M., Hall, K. M., Hopkins, K., Belleza, T. & Cope, D. N. N. (1982). Disability rating scale for severe head trauma: coma to community. *Archives of Physical Medicine and Rehabilitation*, **63**, 118–123.

Rutter, B. M., Graham, P. & Yule, W. (1970). *A Neuropsychiatric Study of Childhood*. Clinics in Developmental Medicine. London: Heinemann.

Rutter, M., Tizard, J. & Whitmore, K. (eds) (1970.) *Education, Health and Behaviour*. London: Longman.

Sechrest, L. (1984). Reliability and validity. In A. S. Bellack & M. Hersen (eds.) *Research Methods in Clinical Psychology*.. New York: Pergamon.

Shaffer, D., Chadwick, O. & Rutter, M. (1975). Psychiatric outcome of localised head injury in children. In *CIBA, Outcome of Severe Damage to the central nervous system*. Amsterdam: Elsevier.

Shavelson, R. J. & Webb, N. B. (1981). Generalizability theory: 1973–1980. *British Journal of Mathematical and Statistical Psychology*, **34**, 133–166.

Siegel, S. (1956). *Nonparametric Statistics for the Behavioural Sciences*. New York: McGraw-Hill.

Teasdale, G. & Jennett, B. (1974). Assessment of coma and impaired consciousness. *Lancet*, **ii**, 81–84.

Teasdale, G. & Jennett, B. (1976). Assessment and prognosis of coma after head injury. *Acta Neurochirurgica*, **34**, 45–55.

Teasdale, G. & Mendelow, D. (1984). Pathophysiology of head injuries. In N. Brooks (ed.) *Closed Head Injury: Psychological, Social and Family Consequences*. Oxford University Press.

Wiggins, J. S. (1973). *Personality and Prediction: Principles of Personality Assessment*. Reading, Ma.: Addison-Wesley.

4

Analysing Data

Paul R. Jackson
MRC/ESRC Social and Applied Psychology Unit, University of Sheffield, S10 2TN.

Data analysis is impossible without presuppositions; it assumes world knowledge. The difference between statistics and arithmetic is that statistical analysis is about data and arithmetic is about numbers. Data are (usually) numbers with reference to some part of the real world. Consequently data analysis is not possible unless we ask questions of the data; about how they were gathered, what was measured, what measurement scale was used, and what choices were made in order to produce the data to hand.

The main purpose of statistical work is to derive summaries of some aspect of data, and in this way to reduce complexity in data without losing structure which is critical. Summary measures have to work hard and we cannot expect that a single index of structure will tell everything about a set of data. Summary measures are specialised tools; they capture one aspect of structure, so that it is generally necessary to produce several measures from the same data set, one for each aspect of structure. Simple examples are the arithmetic mean or median as a summary of location (or centre of gravity) and the standard deviation or interquartile range as a summary of spread around a centre.

Most data analysis is concerned with global or local structure in data. *Global structure* is concerned with the data set as a whole, and every observation contributes in some way to the summary measure. Global summaries like this gloss over variations in structure from one part of the data to another. These variations constitute the *local structure* of the data. In some circumstances the social scientist treats local structure as a nuisance (and is apt to call it 'error' variation); in other circumstances the scientist prefers to remove global structure in order to see changes in local structure more clearly.

A familiar example of the difference between the two kinds of structure comes from economic data such as unemployment statistics which are reported monthly. Variations in average unemployment from year to year (or long-term trends upwards or downwards) are *global* structure; while seasonal trends are *local* structure and reflect the weather, school-leaving dates and so on. Here it is not sensible to take one aspect of structure as 'error'; rather we prefer to consider both kinds of structure but not at the same time. When unemployment figures are reported, they are accompanied by 'seasonally adjusted' figures to tell us about long-term trend. These adjusted figures use all of the data available but then discard seasonal factors using complicated and arcane formulae in order to make aspects of global structure clearer. If we wish we can look back at the local seasonal factors more clearly against the background of long-term trend.

Here I want to draw together a number of approaches to the exploration of structure with illustrations of how they might profitably be used. The term 'exploration' is used quite deliberately for two reasons. Much of what I want to say is in the spirit of Tukey's *Exploratory Data Analysis* (1977) without the Tukeyesque obscurities. More important than this though is the fundamental point that analysing any set of data is a process of exploration; getting to know data can only be done step by step, without making unwarranted assumptions too soon.

The new procedures of Exploratory Data Analysis are of two general kinds. The first kind consists of procedures for looking at data in new ways: the development of more effective forms of display. Other procedures are for summarising data, but rely on summary measures that are cheap in assumptions. Taken together, these two classes of analytical tool can go a long way towards allowing the data to speak for themselves. The process of analysis is guided by two contradictory principles that are always in creative tension. On the one hand, data analysis is guided by what we know of the world, so that we use what we already know to make intelligent choices. On the other hand, the greatest value of data analysis comes when data show us something we never expected to see. Tukey refers to easy forms of analysis as a security blanket to reassure rather than to reveal.

ROBUST MEASURES

This section of the chapter presents a brief introduction to robust measures in data analysis. It is in three parts: what robustness is about, a short description of some types of robust measures, and some examples of robust measures in practice showing where they make a difference and where they do not (and therefore why we should care about using them). A lengthier account can be found in my chapter in Lovie (Jackson, 1986).

Statisticians argue over precise definitions of what the term robustness means. For our purposes, though, it can be taken simply as the sensitivity of a summary measure to departures from ideal assumptions. Two kinds of departures have been the subject of technical analysis in the statistical literature: throwing in small amounts of large errors (generally in a few data values), and slight alterations to all data values. The first of these can come about by missing out the decimal point in recording a data value, or by lapses in concentration in transcribing data. The second kind of problem occurs where values are rounded (either deliberately or because of limited accuracy in a measuring instrument), or where several values have been grouped together. These problems should not necessarily be considered to be errors; for they may not be accidental. Consider pulse rate data recorded in beats per minute. If the person recording the data followed normal practice and counted the number of beats in 15 seconds, then the data values must have been multiplied by 4 to get beats per minute. This procedure will lead to data values all of which are divisible by four, so that we need not concern ourselves with accuracy of less than plus or minus two.

In the presence of possible outliers several strategies have been suggested: carry on regardless (maybe even without looking to see whether outliers are present!); perform the same analyses with and without the outliers present and assess what difference it makes; discard the outliers as distracting contaminants; use methods of analysis that are known to work well even in the presence of contamination.

Influence functions have been developed in order to define the effect of each observation on a summary measure calculated from a set of data. Technical definitions vary slightly, but the commonest way of finding the influence of a data point is to calculate the summary measure from the whole data set, and then recalculate it dropping each data point in turn. The influence of a data point is the difference between the two summaries.

Consider a sample of 11 measurements in all, where 10 of them sum to zero and have fixed values. What will happen to the sample mean and median as the value of the remaining observation is allowed to change from very small to very large? Suppose that 10 of the observations have the values:

$$10, 7, 3, 3, 3, -2, -5, -5, -6, -8$$

which sum to zero (simply for convenience in the arithmetic). Because they sum to zero, the grand total including the 11th observation, x, must be x, and the sample mean is $x/11$. Thus the sample influence curve (shown in

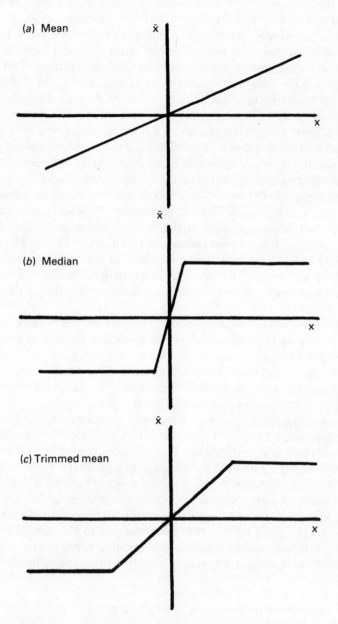

FIG. 4.1.   Influence curves for three summaries of location.

Fig. 4.1(a)) is a straight line with slope 1/11. The larger is our 11th observation, the larger will be the mean.

Now consider the median. Because the sample has an odd number of observations, the middle observation is the median. If the extra observation, x, is bigger than or equal to 3, the median is 3; if x is smaller than or equal to -2, the median is -2; and if x is between the two the median is x. Try it for yourself and see. Thus the sample influence curve for the median (Fig. 4.1(b)) is composed of three straight lines segments—the central portion reflects the changing value of x, and the two horizontal lines on each side indicate that the median is unaffected by the size of x except within a narrow range. The use of the concept of influence gives a precise way of assessing the properties of different kinds of summary and also some criteria for choosing between them.

UNIVARIATE SUMMARIES OF SHAPE

Summaries 'stand for' the data they replace. Univariate summaries describe the shape of a batch of data in terms of such features as location, spread, symmetry (or skewness). Other features of data distributions which are easy to see informally but hard to summarise are unimodality and connectedness. The commonest way to summarise a data set is in terms of location and spread; and there are lots of different measures of each which could be used.

Note that using a particular summary measure is a choice, so what criteria can we use to help us make this choice? There are three criteria that matter:

1. *Ease of calculation*—This is the first, and the least important. Doing things by hand might mean that we choose the measure that is easiest to work out; on a computer, we will probably pick what the program offers. Most of us are far too busy to spend a long time agonising over an average, but we really do have to learn to be fussy enough. Remember too that the choice depends on the data as much as on the mathematical properties of the summary measure itself. The summary 'stands for' the data.

2. *Efficiency*—summaries carry information about some aspect of the data (not every aspect, remember), whether it be location or spread or something else. Efficiency refers to the extent to which the summary measure uses all the information in the data that is relevant to the feature being summarised. The most efficient measures milk the data dry of everything that each observation has to tell about what is being summarised.

3. *Robustness*—This term has several slightly different meanings, as we saw earlier. It may refer to the vulnerability of the summary measure to

large disturbances in a small number of observations (perhaps by missing out a decimal point in recording an observation); or to small changes to a large number of observation (perhaps by rounding each data point to the nearest whole number, or by grouping into a few categories—which is the same thing). Robustness is also used as a term to describe invulnerability of a summary to incorrect assumptions being made about technical properties of a model (for example, we may incorrectly assume that our data are drawn from a population whose distribution can be modelled by the normal distribution).

In general, efficiency and robustness are opposite ends of a continuum: very robust measures are usually not efficient, and efficient measures are generally not robust. The arithmetic mean and the standard deviation are the most efficient summaries of location and spread respectively (statisticians define efficiency in terms of the standard error of an estimator—if you don't recognise the term, don't worry). They are also the least robust summaries.

There are many different types of more robust summary measures (Jackson, 1986), but the most convenient family of summaries for everyday use is the family of trimmed means. Trimmed means can be calculated quite simply (at least for small to medium-sized batches of data). All that is required is to delete a proportion of extreme observations (called the 'trim proportion') from each end of the ordered batch, and then calculate the arithmetic mean of the remaining observations. It is easy to see that the zero-percent trimmed mean (i.e. no data trimmed from either end) is the familiar arithmetic mean; and trimming 50% of the observations (half from each end) gives the median. The influence curve for the trimmed mean is shown in Fig. 4.1(c), and it is easy to see that trimming in this way gives a summary measure of location which is not unduly influenced by a small number of way-out values. Common trim percentages are 10% (one in ten deleted from each end), and 25% trim. The 25% trimmed mean has a special name, the mid-mean: it's the mean of the middle half of the data.

If we then label a dimension in terms of trim percentage, we have zero trim at one end (the mean) and 50% trim at the other (the median). Thus the trim dimension also indicates high efficiency/low robustness at the 0% end and low efficiency/high robustness at the 50% end. Statisticians have shown that 5 or 10% trim gives almost as high efficiency as the ordinary mean with a useful degree of robustness against outliers.

MAKING LOCAL STRUCTURE CLEAR—SMOOTHING

Scatterplots have been used for a long time as powerful tools for investigating the relationship between two variables. However, it can be difficult to see clearly the shape of a dependence relationship if either (a) there is a

FIG. 4.2. Learning curve for dart throwing.

great deal of scatter around the basic relationship; or (b) the density of the scatter varies in different parts of the plot. The question of density changes is a difficult one as it is perceptually difficult to disentangle variations in level from variations in spread.

One answer to this problem is to use robust summaries like those described above to give indications of level of one variable at each part of the other. (I should say that this process is harder to describe in words than to do.) Moving averages have been used for a very long time to summarise slow changes in level in a series which is also subject to short-term fluctuations (remember seasonal and annual trends?).

The basic idea can be grasped by using a simple three point moving median for the data shown in Fig. 4.2, taken from an unpublished study described by Watson (1930). The study investigated adults throwing a dart at a target from a distance of 20 ft (6 m). Each of ten people threw a dart every 2 minutes for 20 hours, with food (a cold meal with tea or coffee, taken between the throws) every 6 hours. After each throw, the distance from the target was measured and this is the index of accuracy used. The data points in the figure are averages for each hour over 30 throws from ten people (300 throws in all, then). The purpose of the study was to examine the process of extended learning.

Take the three data points with the lowest scores on the horizontal axis (the ones farthest to the left of the plot), and replace the second point with the median accuracy value on the vertical axis. Now move on by one data point and do the same thing with the second, third and fourth points: replace the accuracy score of the third observation with the middle of the three values. And so on. The result is a smoothed sequence which is less spikey than the original. I call this an analysis of local structure because each of the summaries (the median values) applies only to values that are local to it. If you were to draw this smoothed sequence onto a plot of the original data, what you see is a picture of changes in local dependence of *y* on *x* through the levels of the *x* variable.

There are many variations on this theme. We could use running medians of 5 instead of 3, for instance. Can you see that a 20% trimmed mean of 5 is the average of the middle three observations? My trials with this data were done in less than half an hour using a spreadsheet program, Supercalc; but they could also be done by hand without too much problem. Velleman and Hoaglin (1981) described some sophisticated variations on the same principle they call compound smoothers, which involve applying several smoothing procedures one after the other. The results can be most impressive: Fig. 4.3 shows the application of their 3RSSH smoothing to the data in Fig. 4.2. The method first involves repeated running medians of 3 (hence the 3R). This tends to flatten out peaks and troughs but leaves flat sequences with jagged 'cliffs' between them. These jumps in the sequence are smoothed by a procedure called 'splitting' (the S of the name). Finally, a

FIG. 4.3.   Smoothed learning curve for dart throwing.

procedure called 'Hanning' is used which is a weighted running average rather than a running median. Because the computer is doing the leg-work, we can afford to run the whole thing twice.

There are two main reasons for applying smoothing techniques like these. The first is to see changes in local structure clearly. The second reason is to *remove* this long-term change in order to see better another aspect of structure in the same data. Tukey (1977) gives the following simple but profound formula to describe the way in which a data set consists of systematic 'smooth' structure together with local variation:

$$Data = Smooth + Rough$$

In our example, the smooth is a moving summary of level of the accuracy scores across time (Fig. 4.3); while the rough is what is left when the smooth is subtracted from the original data. Plotting the rough (often also called residuals) without the smooth as in Fig. 4.4 shows much more clearly any extra structure that may be present in the data. In particular, it is possible to see whether the intake of food at the times marked on the plot has had any systematic effect of accuracy (it isn't very obvious that it does).

FIG. 4.4 Residuals from smoothed learning curve.

HYPOTHESIS TESTING

~ The logic of significance testing can be described quite simply, although the implications of each step are often subtle and non-trivial in their implications (good accounts are given by Leach, 1979; and Box, Hunter & Hunter, 1978). Suppose that you have been pursuing a testing programme for a number of months in a health centre as well as in an out-patients clinic of the local hospital. The same test is used in each site, and you also have a file of test results from your predecessor at the same clinic. You notice that the results from the health centre seem to be different from those obtained at the hospital clinic and you begin to wonder whether there really is a difference.

First, define a *null hypothesis*, namely that the two sites generate the same results. If we can discredit this hypothesis then we can say that there is a statistically significant difference between the two sites. To do this we need more information, either in the form of extra data or in the form of assumptions about the data.

The second step is to calculate a summary measure for the test scores from each site (this might be a mean or a median). If the null hypothesis is true than we would expect the summaries to be similar, and the difference between them to be small. How small small actually is can only be assessed from a reference distribution which shows what the distribution of differences would be if the null hypothesis were true. By using an appropriate reference distribution, we can calculate the probability that a difference at least as large as the one observed would occur by chance if the null hypothesis were true. If this probability is sufficiently small, then we can reject the null hypothesis in favour of an alternative that the two sites are different.

There are many different kinds of significance test developed specifically for particular jobs, but the essential logic of all tests is as outlined above.

Earlier, I said that discrediting the null hypothesis (or not!) depends either on extra information or extra assumptions. These are needed in order to define the reference distribution. One procedure that is described by Box, Hunter & Hunter (1978, Chapter 2) is to use existing data. In our example, we could use the archive of test scores left by the predecessor to draw up a reference distribution against which to compare the results from your own observations. This has the advantage that it uses past data from the same setting which should be relevant to the present task; but the disadvantage that the reference distribution can sometime be tedious to calculate. (The details are not given here; see Box *et al.* 1978, Chapter 2.)

A second alternative for a reference distribution is to choose one of the standard theoretical distributions that statisticians have developed. In our example, the Gaussian distribution (sometime wrongly called the normal distribution, as if it were the normal thing to be distributed this way) or the t-distribution might be appropriate. These alternatives give relatively simple calculations, even by hand, although they sometimes make stringent and unwarranted assumptions about the process that generated the data. Most introductory statistics texts describe how to use these standard reference distributions to perform hypothesis test.

In the rest of this section, two more ways of defining a reference distribution are described in detail. The first is based upon ranks, and the second is the bootstrap which takes advantage of the mindless number crunching that computers (but not people) are good at.

Permutation Tests

The principle behind permutation tests is the simple one that the observed outcome in a sample of data is only one of a number of possible orderings of the observations. Taking a null hypothesis that all possible ways of ordering the data are equally likely, then it is possible to draw up a reference distribution for a test statistic against which to compare that for the observed outcome.

The data in Table 4.1 are taken from a study by Fryer and Payne (1984) of the relationship between aggregate unemployment levels in parts of South Yorkshire and the average number of books borrowed per day from local libraries. The data used here are just for the years 1975–1979 for Sheffield Central. The hypothesis of interest is whether book borrowing declines as unemployment levels rise; and we will use an index S which summarises the extent to which the two variables are ranked similarly (see Leach, 1979, for a readable account of the S-statistic generally).

If we order the pairs of values according to the unemployment level then we find that the book borrowing scores are ranked thus: 1, 3, 4, and 2. The question at issue is how likely this ranking is on the assumption that the two variables are independent of each other. If we reject the null hypothesis,

TABLE 4.1
Book borrowing and unemployment rates in Sheffield
Central area between 1975 and 1979

Registered unemployed		Daily book borrowing	
No.	Rank	No.	Rank
5,542	1	17,909	1
9,872	2	19,017	3
10,539	3	19,354	4
10,730	4	18,817	2

S statistic = 2

TABLE 4.2
All possible alternative rankings and their associated
S statistics

Ordering				S		Ordering				S
1	2	3	4	6		2	3	4	1	0
1	3	2	4	4		3	1	4	2	0
2	1	3	4	4		4	1	2	3	0
1	2	4	3	4		2	4	3	1	-2
2	3	1	4	2		3	4	1	2	-2
3	1	2	4	2		3	2	4	1	-2
1	4	2	3	2		4	1	3	2	-2
1	3	4	2	2		4	2	1	3	-2
2	1	4	3	2		3	4	2	1	-4
3	2	1	4	0		4	2	3	1	-4
1	4	3	2	0		4	3	1	2	-4
2	4	1	3	0		4	3	2	1	-6

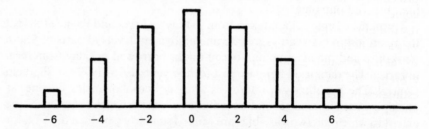

FIG. 4.5. Permutation distribution of the S statistic for sample size of four pairs of observations.

then we can say that there is a significant correlation between the two variables. The S statistic for these data is 2, and Table 4.2 lists all 24 possible alternative rankings of 4 data points with their associated S values. Figure 4.5 shows the histogram of the permutation distribution for the S statistic. As you can see, 9 of the 24 possibilities generate an S value as high or higher than the value from the sample. The significance level associated with our S values is thus $9/24 = 0.375$. Taking a conventional significance level of 0.05 for rejecting the null hypothesis, we can say that there is no evidence for a correlation between unemployment level and book borrowing.

The Bootstrap

The bootstrap is a recently developed method for assessing the variability of an estimate derived from a sample; and it does so without making any assumptions at all about the form of the parent distribution. The basic

TABLE 4.3
Stem and leaf plot of Zung depression scores
for married and single unemployed men

Single (n = 22)		Married (n = 45)
	1.	888
30	2*	1133444
9865	2.	5577889
400	3*	00012344
986	3.	5567889
32210	4*	112224
9877	4.	55689
	5*	02
7	5.	

principle is that all the evidence we have about the parent distribution comes from the shape of the sample data itself. If we take this empirical distribution as an approximation to the unknown parent distribution then we can generate what is known as the *bootstrap distribution* of our estimate by taking repeated samples from the empirical distribution. The standard error of our estimate is then simply the standard deviation of all the estimates in the bootstrap distribution. Efron and Gong (1983) give a relatively non-technical exposition of the theoretical derivation of the bootstrap as well as some practical applications; I have used one of their examples in the chapter on robust methods (Jackson, 1986).

Here the data given in Table 4.3 are used to demonstrate the bootstrap in action. The table reports data on the Zung Self-rated Depression Scale for 67 men who were interviewed when they had been unemployed for just over one year. The first 45 observations were from married men and the second set of 22 observations were from single men. The hypothesis to be tested here is that the mean depression scores for the two groups are different. Conventional methods would involve using a t-test here: this shows that married men have a mean of 33.38, while single men have a mean of 37.00—a difference that gives a t-value of 1.46 with 65 degrees of freedom.

Applying the bootstrap to these data comprises a number of steps. First, choose a sample size for each bootstrap sample; this will usually be the same as the number of observations in the sample data, but either larger or smaller values are possible. In this example bootstrap samples of size 45 from the married group and 22 from the single group were drawn—the same size as the data set.

Next, select observations for inclusion in a bootstrap sample by drawing random numbers in the range 1 to n (in this case 45 from the first group and

TABLE 4.4

Two bootstrap samples drawn from the data of Table 4.3—sequence numbers in each group

---

Sample 1
Married group: 1,3,5,5,8,9,10,11,11,11,11,11,13,13,15,16,16,18,18,20,21,21,24,25,26,26,
                26,29,29,29,32,33,34,35,36,37,38,39,40,41,42,42,43,44,45

Single group: 3,6,6,11,11,11,11,11,11,11,12,13,15,15,15,16,17,19,20,20,21,22

Sample 2
Married group: 2,2,2,4,5,6,7,8,8,8,9,10,13,14,15,15,18,19,22,24,24,24,25,26,27,27,28,29,
                29,30,30,32,34,34,34,35,36,37,38,41,42,42,44,44,45,

Single group: 1,2,2,2,2,3,4,4,4,7,9,10,11,11,12,13,13,13,14,17,19,19

---

22 from the second group). Note that this gives sampling with replacement, so that the bootstrap sample may contain an element of the empirical data more than once. Table 4.4 shows just 2 bootstrap samples out of 100 in all, each selected using a random number generator. Not all observations appear every time, and each bootstrap sample contains duplicated observations.

The next step is to calculate the summary estimate of interest, in this case a difference between means, from each bootstrap sample in turn. This is done quite simply by calculating the average scores for the groups of 45 and 22 chosen at random from the original data. If a data point is chosen more than once, it is added in as many times as it is chosen. The bootstrap

2	2	05
5	1	157
9	+0	0111
17	−0	23447899
30	−1	2345566677899
44	−2	01122334568899
(7)	−3	0124447
49	−4	11234667788
38	−5	00012333355666789
21	−6	112456677999
9	−7	00029
4	−8	01
2	−9	48

Mean = −3.65
Standard deviation = 2.64

FIG. 4.6.   Stem and leaf plot of bootstrap distribution.

estimate of the standard error of our test statistic is simply the standard deviation of all differences calculated from lots of bootstrap samples. Figure 4.6 shows the histogram of 100 bootstrap samples for the data in Table 4.4. For this example, the bootstrap estimate of the standard error is 2.64, compared with the t-distribution estimate of 2.47, both significant at the 2% level. The bootstrap method gives a slightly more conservative test of the hypothesis of no difference between the groups; but applying the bootstrap involves no distribution assumptions at all about the normality of the population from which the two samples were drawn. Here, we have paid only a small price for not having to buy assumptions which in everyday work may often be questionable.

REGRESSION—GLOBAL SUMMARIES OF DEPENDENCE

Correlation coefficients are often used as global summaries of the joint shape of a distribution, and their key feature is that they indicate a symmetric relationship–co–relationships. Often though, interest focuses on how to summarise *asymmetric* relationships—dependence of one variable on another. Dependence may reflect causal precedence, or simply be a matter of the convenience of using something that is easy to measure to stand for something else that is difficult or expensive to measure. Either way, regression relationships like this call for indices of global structure rather different from the indices of local structure; though they retain the essential features of summaries. (Remember that a summary *stands for* an aspect of the data, and an efficient summary is one that retains everything in the data that is related to the aspect being summarised.) At the same time, a good summary is simple, requiring fewer numbers than the original data.

This part of the chapter describes the general characteristics of a regression model as a summary of dependence and a number of techniques available to fit a regression model. The same steps apply, from the simplest model for two variables and a few observations to many variables and thousands of observations.

Characteristics of regression models

The purpose of a regression model is to summarise the dependence of one variable on at least one other: how the dependent variable behaves at different levels of the predictor variable. (Note in passing that we cannot expect to make valid inferences about the effects on one variable of *change* in another without actually changing the predictor variable.) How can we seek a summary of such dependence? One way is shown in Fig. 4.7

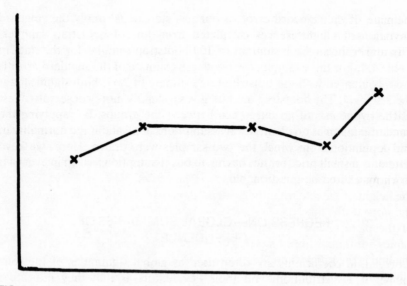

FIG. 4.7. Example of how to describe a dependence relationship exactly but not parsimoniously.

where each point is joined to the next from left to right. We can see quite clearly in this plot that the dependent variable (shown on the vertical axis) tends to increase as the predictor variable scores (on the horizontal axis) increase.

Note some features of this figure:

1. The lines joining the points describe the relationship exactly—no information is lost—but at the same time we cannot say that we have a summary. It takes as much to present the lines as to present the points they join, so we have not reduced the information load at all.

2. Figure 4.7 does not really show a regression summary because we could reverse the two axes and draw exactly the same lines between points.

3. We can say exactly what is happening for two adjacent points but very little in a formal or precise way about the two variables as a whole. In fact we see *local* structure but not *global* structure.

The most complex model describing two variables has almost as many lines as there are points available; the simplest model has just a single line which may or may not coincide with the recorded observations. Now defining a straight line requires very little information: to cross the Sahara Desert, start from *here* and go in *that* direction. All that is needed to draw a straight line on a page like this one is a starting point that fixes the level, top to bottom, and an angle that determines direction relative to the bottom of the page. Try it for yourself, by starting a line six inches from the bottom of the page at an angle of 45 degrees to the bottom of the sheet.

In algebraic language, statisticians often describe straight lines like this:

$$Y = a + bX$$

Each symbol in this language stands for something (it's the Pitman short-hand of mathematics), Y stands for the dependent variable (lots of values), and X stands for the predictor variable (again, lots of values). The small letters, a and b, stand for the two pieces of information that are all we need to know where the line goes. The letter a tells about the *level* of the line, the height of the line from the bottom of the picture; the letter b tells about the *slope* of the line, the angle relative to the horizontal axis or the bottom of the picture. For any particular line, the letters a and b have single values—different lines have different values. This means that the slope of the line is the same wherever we start to look at it—not like those slides at adventure parks which have bumps and hollows in them to increase the excitement!

A straight line then has two characteristics that we value in a summary: it is simple (only two items of information needed to describe it) and it is global (the same two items describe the summary *here* and also *there*). We cannot say yet of course whether any particular straight line has the other two features of a good summary; does it summarise the proper pattern of dependence (maybe the line should be gently curving), and does it stand for the data adequately?

Fitting a regression line

There are many different procedures developed by statisticians for fitting a line. The differences between methods is nothing to do with the finished line—its properties as described above are intrinsic to its being a line, not to how we calculate where to put it. Rather, the methods differ in terms of:

1. Simplicity of calculation (often these days by computer).
2. Efficiency in using the information in the data.
3. Robustness, or invulnerability to the kinds of problems data are heir to.

By way of example, we will use again the data from unemployed men from the previous section. Among the variables measured in addition to the Zung Depression Scale was a shortened form of the Beck Hopelessness Scale, and here we will examine whether depression scores can be used to predict scores on the hopelessness scale. A scatterplot of the two variables produced using SPSS-X is shown in Fig. 4.8.

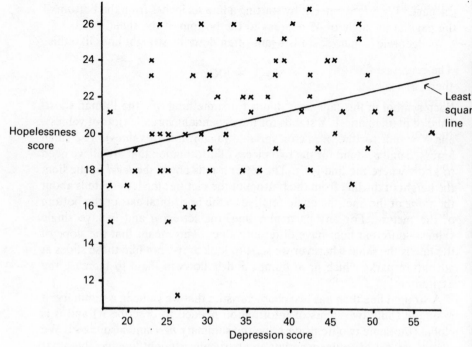

FIG. 4.8. Scatterplot of hopelessness and depression scores with least squares line.

Least squares. The commonest, and often the worst, method is the method of least squares; indeed many people think that least squares fitting is the only kind there is. This method is within the same mathematical tradition as means, standard deviations and product–moment correlation coefficients as summaries of centre, spread and co-spread respectively: mathematically elegant, highly efficient in idealised situations, and intuitively tough on the understanding.

The method of least squares makes maximum use of all the information within the data that is relevant to assessing dependence of one variable on the other (that's what the statistical term 'efficiency' means). However, in the process, it accepts every data point at face value, and gives greatest influence to those observations that are a long way from the regression line itself. In the language used earlier, the influence curve describing what happens by this method is similar to that shown in Fig. 4.1 for the mean. Thus the single data point at the bottom of Fig. 4. 8 with scores of (11.26) has more influence on the positioning of the regression line than those in the centre of the plot.

The regression equation given by SPSS-X using the method of least squares gives the following results:

$$\text{Hopelessness} = 16.95 + 0.110 \times \text{Depression}$$

The regression line is superimposed upon the scatterplot in Fig. 4.8, and there is a modest difference in hopelessness scores for individuals who differ in depression scores. We can't tell from this plot alone how much the fitted line has been affected by the extreme observation at the bottom of the plot. When I played about with the data by changing this observation to (1,26) in order to see the result of moving it further away from the rest of the data, the least squares fit was affected considerably. The level of the line was pulled down closer to the outlying observation, while the slope value was larger, falsely overestimating the degree of relationship between the two variables. Alternative methods have been proposed by statisticians to get around this problem of the vulnerability of the least squares method. We will use two which have very different characteristics but share the feature that they are resistant to the influence of outlying values which may be rogue observations.

The three-point resistant line. The first method gives what has come to be known as the three-point resistant line, and it has a long but little known history within statistics. There are many refinements on the basic method but the principle is quite straightforward. The line required is one that goes through the data, so we divide the data into thirds using the ordering on the x variable; work out the middle of the points in the left-most third of the data and the middle of the right-most third of the data. 'Middle' is defined as follows. Using a ruler, start at the left of the picture with the ruler parallel to the vertical axis. Move the ruler in to the right until it meets the middle data point, and draw a line. Now do the same the other way, moving the ruler upwards. Where this second line cuts the first one defines the middle of that part of the data. In other words, to find the summary points in the outer thirds is to find first the median x-value, and then, separately, the median y-value. These x- and y-values define the coordinates of the summary points for each data third. None of the summary points needs to coincide with a data point because the medians for x- and y-values are calculated separately. It is the use of the median for the summary points that makes this method resistant to wild values in either variable (because the median is much less vulnerable than the mean to extreme values).

Joining the two summary points together with a line allows calculation of the slope, which is one of the two summary values needed. Finally, we need to look at all of the data points (those in the middle third as well). If we take 'throughness' to mean as many points above the line as below it, then we need to shift the line up or down using a ruler until we get the kind of symmetry required. This last step needs a little care to keep the line parallel to the one we started with. The end result is our regression line.

A useful quick test of whether a straight line is adequate to summarise dependence of Y on X is to calculate the summary point for the middle of the centre third of the data. If our fitted lines runs close to this summary point than a straight line will do.

That is the method in outline; now we need to consider some points in detail to see exactly how it works out. Forming three groups based on the X-values depends on whether the number of observations is divisible by three. If not, then aim to make the outer two groups equal in size: thus, for 9 points we get (3,3,3), for 10 points we get (3,4,3), and for 11 points we get (4,3,4). If there are ties in the X-values then additional complications arise (see Velleman and Hoaglin, 1981 for how to cope here).

The literature contains several variants on the basic method, including iterative procedures for 'polishing' the estimates of level and slope. The underlying principle is the same though. The computer program of Velleman and Hoaglin (1981) gives the following regression equation:

$$\text{Hopelessness} = 16.00 + 0.143 \times \text{depression}$$

Robust regression by M-estimation. A more efficient as well as a more general method of fitting regression models is given by the group of procedures known as M-estimators. These methods combine the range of applicability of least squares regression fitting with the in-built protection against departures from ideal assumptions that the resistant line technique possesses.

The way in which M-estimation provides this protection is by applying to each observation a weight which depends on the distance of the observation from the fitted line. In least squares regression by contrast, every observation has the same weight. The effect of this equal weighting is that the observations furthest away from the fitted line have the greatest influence on where the line is located. This pays most attention to those observations least likely to be typical of the data set as a whole; and M-estimators down-weight such observations in order to reduce their influence. In extreme cases one or more observations may be given zero weight—they are ignored in defining the fitted line.

The simplest way to use robust regression is by repeated application of a weighted least squares algorithm (such as that offered by the Glim package), with the weights separately calculated at each step. Huynh (1982) describes how to do this using the SAS package. Taking the data shown in Fig. 4.8, robust M-estimates of level and slope were calculated using an

M-estimator named after Huber, the statistician who developed it. The influence curve for this M-estimator is very similar to that for the trimmed mean shown in Fig. 4.1(c).

The resulting regression equations is:

$$\text{Hopelessness} = 17.02 + 0.109 \times \text{depression}$$

Comparing the results from the three methods of fitting a line shows close agreement between the non-robust least squares method and the two robust methods for these data. Interestingly, M-estimation has given the lowest observation in Fig. 4.8 a weight of 0.55 compared with a weight of 1.0 for most other observations, so that there is some suggestion that this observation, with scores of (11,26), should be given some special attention. The modified data set, with a gross error added to one observation, produced different values for both parameters in the model fitted by least squares. However, the robust regression model was identical with that reported above. The only difference was in the weight given to the offending observation: now given a weight of 0.25, rather than 0.55.

ANALYSIS OF INTERACTIONS

Many of the most interesting findings in applied work show up as interactions between predictor variables. For instance, Bolton and Oakley (1987) looked at the relationship between perceived social support and employment status in a study of the antecedents of depression. Unemployed men reporting low levels of social support had higher depression scores than unemployed men with high support scores; there was no corresponding difference for employed men. The authors concluded that there was an interaction between the two variables. This type of design is known as a *between-groups* design because each cell contains independent sub-groups of the total sample.

In many circumstances analysis of variance can be used to give appropriate tests of hypotheses of interest (see Keppel, 1973, for a lucid account of how to do this), though interpretation of the results it gives can sometimes be a problem. Consider for example what would happen in the Bolton and Oakley study if the sub-groups being compared also differ on some other variable which the researchers ignore or don't know about. Suppose that the low social support unemployed group were mostly single men, while the other groups were mostly married. In that case what looks like an interaction effect could equally be interpreted as a main effect of marital status showing lower depression scores for married men. This kind of confounding can make life very difficult in the interpretation of observational studies. You can see that the significance tests for interactions rely on the groups being *equivalent* on all other relevant variables.

It is this issue of the equivalence or non-equivalence of groups that has led many researchers to prefer designs where the same people appear in more than one cell of the design. These types of design are known as *within-groups*, or repeated measures designs, and they solve some of the problems inherent in between-groups designs (see Chapter 8). Looking at interactions in these designs involves the relationship between a group classification variable and time as a second explanatory variable: the dependent variable is measured on several occasions for two or more groups.

To illustrate some of the issues that arise with designs like these, let us look at a recent study by Milne (1984). He tested the efficacy of a course designed to train psychiatric nurses in elements of behaviour therapy. Two groups were selected from different hospitals; and individuals in the two groups were matched on a number of background variables. One group served as a control group and were simply tested on three occasions; while the experimental group received the training programme and measures were taken at the start of the course, after it finished and again as a long-term follow-up. Two key tasks are required of the researcher in a study like this. First, she needs to assess whether the treatment and control groups were in fact equivalent on salient variables at the start of the study. The second task is to decide whether the treatment group has improved on relevant criteria by comparison with whatever changes may have occurred in the control group. The control group is needed to allow for the possibility of change brought about either by the process of measurement itself or as a result of external influences on both groups (such as organisational changes or a strike among workers). How should we make decisions on these questions?

There are a number of different types of analysis which can be used for this type of problem. Some of them are equivalent to each other, some are very complicated, and some are specifically tailored for tricky problems. One approach (in fact the one adopted by Milne himself) is to perform a series of comparisons using simple tests applied to data from different parts of the design. Table 4.5 shows part of the data from the original report, scores for the Knowledge of Behavioural Principles Questionnaire (KBPQ). He found no difference (using non-parametric tests throughout) between the two groups on the baseline test (column 1 of the table), and a significant difference at post-test (column 2). Furthermore, the control group showed no change over time (row 2) while the treatment group changed significantly (row 1). This seems clear then, but there are some worrisome aspects of the table. First, the control group started higher, and *did* improve over time. Second, we cannot infer from the tests reported

TABLE 4.5

Scores on Knowledge of Behavioural Principles Questionnaire for control and behaviour groups, from Milne (1984)

	Baseline	Post-test
Treatment group (n = 41)	34%	56%
Control group (n = 18)	40%	45%

that the change in the treatment group is significantly bigger than the change in the control group: all we are told is that change in one group was significant while change in the other group was not.

Milne's approach has the merit of keeping each bit of the analysis simple but has two damning drawbacks. It can be very hard to pull together lots of simple tests to give a clear overall picture; and the results so obtained can often be very misleading. My own strong preference is for procedures which, though more complicated, match the requirements of the design and deal effectively with the main threats to valid inference.

Two very common techniques are the two-way analysis of variance and the repeated measures t-test, and these will give identical results when applied to the same data. The interaction term in the analysis of variance indicates whether the time effect is the same for the two groups; and this is also what the t-test does using the difference score as the dependent variable. The technical term that statisticians use to describe these tests is that they focus on *unconditional* models: that is, we take the change score as it stands and ignore the individual's initial score. There are lots of settings where this gives sound results but also many occasions where it would be a foolhardy thing to do. For example, if our control and experimental groups were intact groups selected from very different organisations then aspects of the environments they work in could interact in important (but unknown) ways with the variables we focus on for study.

Interpreting comparisons of the absolute change in two groups depends a great deal therefore on the process whereby individuals were assigned to the groups in the first place. The unconditional approach makes sense if groups really are equivalent at the start of the study, and it is generally only safe to assume this if individuals are assigned randomly (and also if there is no differential loss of subjects from groups—for example, the healthier people in a control group refusing to continue, and the least healthy people in an environmental group being removed from the study for clinical treatment elsewhere). In quasi-experimental studies where random allocation is not possible or not desirable then unconditional models produce questionable and often misleading results.

Very often absolute change is much less meaningful than change which is *relative* to the individual's starting level—this might be recorded as percentage change or proportional change. When they want to look at relative rather than absolute change, statisticians turn to what they call *conditional* models. These are fundamentally different from the unconditional models already discussed in that they take measures on the first occasion as fixed, and then explore change over time conditional on the initial values of the dependent variable. In essence, the conditional model asks the question: if the groups had been alike on all relevant explanatory variables, then what difference would there have been between the groups at time two? The simplest way to do this is to use analysis of covariance with the time-2 score as the dependent variable and the equivalent time-1 score as a covariate. Any initial differences between the groups are thus held constant statistically. An extended and very lucid account of the problems of analysing and interpreting change data is given in the book by Plewis (1985) which should be consulted by those who face such problems. An example taken from my own research on the consequences of change in employment status is reported in Jackson, Stafford, Banks and Warr (1983).

CONCLUSIONS

This chapter has covered a large number of issues in only a little detail. I have tried to give a flavour of how modern statistical procedures are being used on real data to address practical problems. Perhaps what has been included here, as well as what has been left out, is surprising. I have not tried to explain analytic procedures such as multivariate analysis or time series—these may be found in other specialist texts such as Everitt and Dunn (1983) and Plewis (1985). My purpose has been to focus on principles rather than on cookbook recipes, to increase statistical numeracy rather than number-crunching capacity. Behind it all is the conviction that data analysis is an enterprise involving the user and the computer jointly. The distribution of effort is that the user does the thinking while the computer does the easy bit—the calculation. Your job in analysing data is to ask intelligent questions of your data to understand part of the world better. If data analysis confuses rather than illuminates then something has gone wrong.

REFERENCES

Bolton, W. & Oakley, K. (1987). A longitudinal study of social support and depression in unemployed men. *Psychological Medicine*, **17**, 453–460.

Box, G. E. P., Hunter, W. G. & Hunter, J. S. (1978). *Statistics for Experimenters*. Chichester: Wiley.

Efron, E. & Gong, G. (1983). A leisurely look at the bootstrap, the jackknife and cross validation. *The American Statistician*, **37**, 36–48.

Everitt, B. S. & Dunn, G. (1983). *Advanced Methods of Data Exploration and Modelling.* London: Heinemann Educational.

Fryer, D. M. & Payne, R. L. (1984). Book borrowing and unemployment. *Library Review,* **32**, 196–206.

Huynh, H. (1982). A comparison of four approaches to robust regression. *Psychological Bulletin,* **92**, 505–512.

Jackson, P. R. (1986). Robust statistics. In A. D. Lovie (ed.). *New Developments in Statistics for the Social Sciences.* London: Methuen and British Psychological Society.

Jackson, P. R., Stafford, E. M., Banks, M. H. & Warr, P. B. (1983). Unemployment and psychological distress in young people: The moderating role of employment commitment. *Journal of Applied Psychology,* **68**, 525–535.

Keppel, G. (1973). *Design and Analysis: A Researcher's Handbook.* Englewood Cliffs, N.J.: Prentice Hall.

Leach, C. (1979). *Introduction to Statistics.* Chichester: Wiley.

Milne, D. (1984). The development and evaluation of a structured learning format introduction to behaviour therapy for psychiatric nurses. *British Journal of Clinical Psychology,* **23**, 175–185.

Plewis, I. (1985). *Analysing Change. Measurement and Explanation using Longitudinal Data.* Chichester: Wiley.

Tukey, J. W. (1977). *Exploratory Data Analysis.* Reading, Ma.: Addison-Wesley.

Velleman, P. F. & Hoaglin, D. C. (1981). *A,B,Cs of EDA.* Boston, Ma.: Duxbury Press.

Watson, J. B. (1930). *Behaviorism.* Chicago: University of Chicago Press (revised edition).

5 Using Computers

Christopher J. Colbourn
Department of Psychology, University of Southampton, SO9 5NH.

My aim is to provide busy clinicians and researchers with a relatively jargon-free introduction to using 'new technology'. You may think that wasted learning time outweighs potential benefits. Hopefully, this guide will clarify the issues, demonstrating potential uses and benefits.

I start with an overview of the core uses of computers in research, framed by the central concept of the 'personal workstation'. Then each area will be considered to show how using a computer can assist you. Details of actual computer programs are not possible here, but selected references and information sources are provided for you to follow-up. Finally, there is some practical advice on acquiring computing skills, and selecting suitable equipment. There is also a short glossary which attempts to explain basic computer jargon, which often baffles readers. Fuller descriptions of computing terms can be obtained from specialised dictionaries (e.g. British Computer Society, 1984; Chandor, Graham & Williamson, 1985).

1. COMPUTERS IN THE RESEARCH PROCESS: AN OVERVIEW

1.1. Range of Applications

My comments are directed at clinical researchers as a specialist group, although there is considerable overlap in the ways professionals use computers. I shall concentrate on the equipment's functions and use, rather than specific products.

First, let's specify the main type of 'office' functions where computer assistance is valuable:

1. Document and report production (including audio-visual presentations).
2. Small-scale numerical data manipulation.
3. Storing and retrieving textual and numerical information.
4. Mail and document communication.
5. Planning.

Second, some researchers require computers for extensive handling of numerical information, including complex statistical analyses.

Third, many psychologists have developed computer techniques to control experimental procedures. These include 'automated clinical testing' which some clinicians use regularly in assessing patients.

Finally, I refer to the computer tools called 'expert systems' which are intended to provide 'expert' advice and, possibly, instruction in fields like medical diagnosis, or psychological assessment.

1.2. 'Personal Workstation'

The 'personal workstation', a kind of electronically enhanced office desk, has built-in facilities for researchers to tackle most of their daily work independently of a large, and commonly inaccessible, office infrastructure. A 'business-type' microcomputer-based personal workstation offers considerable local processing power, and when connected to networks (via hardwiring or telephone), can access the greater facilities on larger, remote computers. Ongoing microcomputer and network developments will offer even greater 'power'. Figure 5.1 outlines the main current functions of personal workstations as appearing on many academic and business desks.

The basic minimum hardware consists of a microcomputer with two floppy-disk drives (or one floppy-disk and one hard-disk drive), and a dot-matrix printer. A computer network offering data storage and printing facilities would reduce these requirements.

A local area network (LAN) based within a department or office building/complex, enables colleagues to share expensive computing resources (secure disk storage of documents, etc; high-quality printers; devices for telephone and direct-line communications to other computers and networks), and communicate with one another via 'electronic mail' (E-Mail) systems. Many commercially available LANs for microcomputers are reviewed by Bridges (1986) and Moody, Malone and Stobie (1986). Wide area networks enable use of distant computers when local software or databases are not available. They also facilitate access to national and

FIG. 5.1   The functions of a 'personal workstation'.

global E-Mail systems (Fig. 5.1). Stokes (1984) gives a readable general account of computer networks.

2.   MAIN FUNCTIONS: A MORE DETAILED LOOK

2.1. 'Electronic Office'

There is already heavy and beneficial computer use in many office tasks although, as yet, no 'paperless' office. A personal secretary's services (not widely available) cannot be replaced; but the workstation provides facilities impossible to command otherwise, and can pay handsome dividends in saved time and efficiency in everyday working lives.

You probably envisage users continually at their workstations, perhaps both suffering the posited health hazards of long exposure to the computer screen—although evidence for these, and the conditions of occurrence, are presently unclear (Hammond, 1986; Pearce, 1984); and missing essential social interaction (see Oborne, 1985 for a review of this aspect of 'computerisation'). The intention and purpose of office computer-use is reducing the time spent on many routine tasks, thus increasing the time for other, more central, aspects of one's profession.

The electronic office's major functions are document preparation and production using 'wordprocessing'/text-editing software and graphics editors/processors; manipulating small sets of numerical data (e.g. departmental/project accounts, research data, etc.) using 'spreadsheet' software; storing and retrieving information (e.g. patients records/reports, research findings, bibliographical references, etc.) with 'database management' software (DBMS); E-Mail preparation and transmission involving text editors and 'communications' software; and time and resource management (appointments calendar, project planning, etc.). Johnson (1984) gives a general account of such facilities. An important principle is 'integrated' software allowing easy transferral of information between functions, e.g. references stored in a database can be retrieved and inserted into a paper you are writing on the wordprocessor.

2.2. Document Preparation and Production

2.2.1. *Wordprocessing*.

Many people's familiarity with computers is via document production. The idea of 'wordprocessing' (WP) has become very general. Much more than a clever form of typewriter, the WP function of a computer generally allows the user to design and control the format of documents simply and flexibly. The modification of text or formats is straightforward and advantageous whether a letter or a book is produced. The WP concept now extends to 'desk-top publishing', where a combination of powerful desktop-sized hardware (e.g. 'laser' printers using photocopier technology) and software enables production of documents almost indistinguishable from conventionally produced typeset material. Some WP software can produce computer files of your paper or book that will directly drive a printing press! However, these evolving products are still expensive.

Conventional WP software abounds and most can produce a wide variety of documents. Differences mainly lie in: the relative ease of achieving different formats; how the user gives commands to the computer; the range of sophisticated features like merging a mailing list and other specific information with a standard letter to produce 'personalised' letters ('mail-merge' facility)—useful in research involving outpatient treatment where patients must be circulated with new information intermittently. There are built-in or add-on 'spelling checkers' (mainly using American spelling). Other facilities allow graphs and diagrams, produced using a graphics-editing program, to be incorporated into the wordprocessed text.

Seeing the exact printed form of the document on the microcomputer screen is valued by many and labelled 'what you see is what you get' (WYSIWYG; pronounced 'wizzywig'!).

Useful references here are Lawrence (1984), Madron, Tate and Brookshire (1985), Schrodt (1984), and McWilliams (1984), who provides an amusing WP guide.

Notable developments include 'outliners' (stand-alone or within WPs), containing facilities for developing papers, talks, etc. You can expand headings or 'ideas' with annotated sub-headings, text and graphics; and powerful versions allow you to zoom in or out, viewing any level of structure, etc. Making 'instant' overhead-projection slides from any part is another valuable feature. Recently, a WP package incorporating automatic production of a document in the editorial style of the American Psychological Association journals (Pergamon Press's *Manuscript Manager*^{TM} *APA Style*) was announced. Two new journals concentrating on computer use by psychologists are also to be launched. Such developments are potentially valuable to mental health researchers.

2.2.2. Text Editing. The compatibility between different types of hardware and software in terms of stored information is often queried. The transfer of information or data between computers (see Section 2.4) may be necessary for processing that your own machine cannot carry out, or transferring your existing files to a new, more powerful microcomputer. 'Pure text files', i.e. containing nothing but alphanumeric and punctuation characters, can be readily transferred between any two computers. However, formatted material like manuscripts, databases etc. requires special 'translation' software, or their text re-formatted on the new machine. Such software is available for transfer between many of the standard software packages, but not necessarily for the combinations that you require. Most WP packages can generate 'pure text files' (ASCII files).

2.2.3. Graphics Editing/Processing. Besides text for reports and publications, research can demand graphical representations of data, ideas, and theories. If you cannot draw well, the computer can assist you. Graphics-editing packages exist for mere doodlers to industrial designers. A good general-purpose 'drawing' program meets most researchers' needs. A range of on-screen tools facilitates the production of geometrical shapes, shading, and labelling. A package for creating various forms of graphs (i.e. histograms, line graphs, etc.) from an input of data and design specification (i.e. axes, labels, etc.) can also be helpful.

I utilise such packages (Fig. 5.2) to produce diagrams, graphs, and high-quality transparencies for overhead projection. Some packages include facilities to present 'pictures' to an audience via a suitably-sized

FIG. 5.2 Screen shot of a graphics-editor in action. (Full Paint™ on the Apple Macintosh computer.)

screen, or video-projector often available in lecture theatres and conference centres. However, unless you need only to transport your floppy disk containing the 'slides', this is rarely worth the effort and overhead projection slides produced from your computer graphics are preferable.

2.3. Information Handling

Computers are invaluable in other research activities, such as handling both numerical and textual information so that desired aspects are easily retrievable.

Various software packages offer painless dealings with numbers and structured textual material, providing a powerful automated version of the pocket calculator (i.e. the spreadsheet-type program), and the filing cabinet or card index (i.e. the database-type). Truly portable ('lap-top') battery-powered computers can be used almost anywhere, so data gathering from fieldwork can be enhanced using conventional WP packages or purpose-designed data recording software (see Ager, 1985 for a review of this in mental handicap research). Using 'communications' software (see Section 2.4), such a machine could 'telephone in' your collected data to a laboratory/office-based computer for processing.

Portable computer use in fieldwork is specialised, but the information-handling packages are potentially valuable to most researchers.

2.3.1. *Spreadsheets.* VisiCalc™, the first spreadsheet program, of Seventies vintage, supposedly started the trend towards microcomputers in business, where they are called personal computers (PCs; originally a specific machine manufactured by IBM, now widely copied).

A spreadsheet is an electronic data sheet based on the 'squared paper' used to set out research data at the first stage of analysis. Each row and column is labelled so individual squares can be cross-referenced, as on a graph or map. Each 'cell' contains a data item (number or text). The advantage is that cells can alternatively contain a formula, which automatically calculates the cell's contents, usually from values held in other cells. Formulae can be defined once then replicated across a specific row or column with automatic adjustment of the cell references.

Many of the original programs were designed for financial analysts, hence the formula entries could include various specialised operators. Now that it is realised that others could find spreadsheets useful, many current programs also offer various mathematical and statistical functions. Modern spreadsheets can calculate means, standard deviations, and be configured for exploratory data analysis, analysis of variance (ANOVA), etc., often required in mental health research. Once drawn up, such spreadsheets with their formulae can be saved for use with different data sets. Most packages can convert the sheet to a text/WP file allowing transferral of data to a mainframe for more extensive analysis, or direct incorporation of financial planning into a grant proposal.

Researchers working on financial aspects of grant proposals will find these programs' facilities useful. Advantageous here is the ease of assessing 'what if' planning. Changing one or two cell entries representing salaries of research assistants, or project duration, provides an immediate outcome. Various options for project parameters could be entered and all the outcomes calculated together for you to choose the optimum.

Further details of spreadsheet use in research, including examples, are given by Brownell (1985), Madron *et al.* (1985), and Schrodt (1984). Day and Rees (1985) give a well-illustrated description of some standard commercially-produced spreadsheet packages.

2.3.2. *Database Management Systems.* Mental health research, and the social and behavioural sciences deal with textual information almost as much as with numerical data. Software to organise and structure such information is called a 'database management system' (DBMS). Almost any set of structured textual information can be considered a database: maintaining and searching a large file or conventional card index for literature sources, patient records, etc. is a daunting and time-consuming task where computer assistance can be invaluable.

DBMS packages come in basically two types:

1. 'File management systems': providing an electronic card index, with facilities for generating reports using database information; overall, a good text editor is almost as powerful.
2. 'Relational databases': contain flexible advanced features for information searches using both logical and mathematical operations on several database files at once. Facilities for creating new files from current ones exist, and a specialised programming language for writing complete information management applications is embedded in the package. Mastery of the awesome facilities of the most popular DBMSs used on PCs and mainframes is very time consuming.

Researchers commonly use a DBMS for computerised bibliographies. Several clinicians (notably Kapur, 1984; Ager, 1985, who mentions purpose-built systems for 'record keeping' and 'curriculum management' tasks in the area of mental handicap; Norris, Skilbeck, Hayward & Torpy, 1985; Sellu, 1986) have reported a DBMS of great value. Kapur (1984) noted the value of DBMSs in clinical decision-making, by cross-referencing patient and 'reference files' built up of particular diagnostic category information. Patient data records are an obvious choice, and useful for later adding an 'expert system' front-end (see Section 2.8) to aid diagnosis. Many complain of the time-consuming nature of database work, and suggest as a prerequisite a secretary or research assistant to set up and maintain the DBMS. Schrodt (1984) explains how to choose a suitable DBMS, while Lawrence (1984) and Madron et al. (1985) provide examples of typical packages.

2.4. Inter-computer Communications

There are many tasks for which microcomputers, especially 'smaller' models, are not really suitable, i.e. analysing large sets of data (1000 data points or more) with complex numerical computations, and maintaining large bibliographic databases. However, most microcomputers communicate marvellously with computers capable of such tasks.

2.4.1. *Necessities for Computer Communications*. Inter-computer communication ('comms') requires your microcomputer to be equipped with a serial interface to RS-232-C or RS422/3/4 standards. Access is needed to the target computer system (see Section 1.2), possibly via a 'modem', which links your computer to the telephone (assuming the 'target' computer is 'on' the telephone). The necessary 'communications' software will emulate 'standard' forms of inter-computer communications protocols ('terminal emulation'), and provide facilities for transferring files to and from other computers.

For details, see Cornwall (1986), Hammond (1984) or Knox (1985). Connecting your microcomputer to a mainframe via LANs, telephone, etc, is comprehensively discussed by Durr and Walker (1985).

2.4.2. Why Communicate with Other Computers?   The main reasons have already been mentioned: statistical analysis (see Section 2.6); literature searches; file and mail transfers (discussed below). Of value in the mental health context, possibly forming part of a research project, are on-line information systems ('bulletin board systems', BBSs, or 'computer conferencing systems').

2.4.3. Bibliographic Searches.   Literature searches by computer are probably familiar indirectly via library services. Most on-line bibliographic databases are not designed for individual researchers but for information specialists, i.e. librarians (Baker, 1984). Using services like the giant California-based DIALOG system (containing behavioural, social and medical science databases) have confirmed Baker's point; even with the recommended expert guidance some test searches are necessary using well-known literature. Many databases are not archival i.e. containing information on sources more than 10 years old. Examples of such searches are demonstrated by Lawrence (1984) and Madron *et al.* (1985).

Online library catalogue systems (called 'online public access catalogues', OPACs; see Miter, 1986) promise a useful facility for busy researchers: from your workstation, you can check whether a particular book or periodical is in your institution's library, if it is on loan, etc.

2.4.4. Bulletin Boards.   BBSs are another type of on-line information resource whose size varies from national information and E-Mail services to smaller scale privately-run facilities based around a particular theme (commonly microcomputers). Most systems offer news, advice, even software, and are acessible by telephone. Several London boroughs have BBSs with information on local health services, and microcomputer-based terminals to the BBSs in local libraries. The 'viewdata' or 'videotex' standard (screens of colourful text and/or primitive graphics accessed via on-screen menus) has been adopted by many, including British Telecom's national Prestel information service. Cornwall (1986) and Hammond (1984) further describe BBSs. Raitt (1984) gives a general account of videotex use; while McBride (1985) provides an in-depth account of viewdata systems, including how to run them.

An easily-updated on-line information system for local mental health services, including an E-Mail facility, could simply be based on a microcomputer.

2.4.5. *File Transfer and Electronic Mail (E-Mail).*   I have already mentioned most important uses of file transfer between computers, but the following may be less apparent. In the co-operative writing of books or papers between physically remote individuals, speedy electronic exchange of text documents can greatly facilitate the process (although conventionally mailed disks containing the text can have advantages if colleagues use the same WP). Cotton (1984) pointed out that 70% of the life cycle of a document transmitted by letter post is spent in the actual mail. E-Mail and the file transfer is now easy in the academic and research community since the advent of the 'joint academic network' (JANET) linking all university and major research sites in the UK, with links to similar networks in the USA, Europe, etc. Thus from your personal workstation you can send and receive mail, chapter, and paper drafts and submit final copy to publishers.

2.5. Work Management

As the personal workstation provides a focus for one's work much 'work management' software has been produced. Some, in the form of small applications that can run simultaneously or over the top of major applications like WPs, etc., enable one to switch from entering data or writing a research paper to an electronic diary, calendar, notebook, or phonebook (which can even dial a voice call), etc., and then switch back to the main task. Martin (1985; Chapter 11) describes some of these 'desk accessories' on computers using the desktop metaphor in screen displays. Some people feel these tasks are better done conventionally, but it is surprising how habits can change.

Complex time and project management could benefit from specialised packages especially where there are deadlines. For example, when planning a one-year project, you break down the separate stages and estimate both time and the resources required. These packages work like spreadsheets although using 'critical path analysis' as their underlying technique, and 'grid' or 'network' displays show how the project stages and resources dovetail. Similarly, sophisticated time management software when configured with your current appointments and other commitments, can quickly inform you of free time for extra appointments, etc. Some typical packages are reviewed by Jackson, Chamberlain, Sanders and Tyler (1986).

However, the amount of usage and the time taken to learn the use of such software must be balanced. Researchers are not always planning projects, and revisions are probably more complicated than many software packages can handle. Researchers should, however, be aware of them and consider their use as the need arises.

2.6. Statistical Analysis

Given the familiar ground and substantial literature on statistical computing I attempt only an overview and address the question of microcomputer versus mainframe computer for running actual analyses.

The large integrated statistical packages for mainframes like SPSS-X (SPSS Inc., 1983), BMDP (Dixon, 1985), GENSTAT (Alvey, Galwey & Lane, 1982; Weekes, 1986), Minitab (Ryan, Joiner & Ryan, 1985) and SAS (e.g. Kleiger, 1984), and specialised packages for particular forms of analysis like GLIM (General Linear Modeller), CLUSTAN (CLUSTer ANalysis), ECTA (Extended Contingency Table Analysis), MULTIVAR-IANCE (MULTIvariate analysis of VARIANCE), etc, have long been the researchers' first choice. These packages offer considerable flexibility in manipulating, organising, and recoding research data, and an extensive range of statistical analyses. Being very large, they require powerful mainframe computers. Recently, versions of SPSS, BMDP, Minitab, and GLIM have been implemented on certain PCs. Usually a large subset of the original package, the expensive 'micro' versions require large, expensive PCs to run. A key advantage is that these packages are well tried and tested, and continually maintained and improved by a team of statistical programmers. Thus you can depend on the results, provided you input your data and specify the analyses correctly and accurately. They can almost certainly handle any size of data set. But they are complicated, so familiarising yourself with them requires time, although comprehensive manuals are readily available. The SPSS package is particularly good, with a substantial user guide (SPSS Inc., 1983), and statistical handbooks (Norusis, 1983, 1985) providing examples of different types of data analysis. Also, the computing services at university and research establishments often run courses in their use.

For mainframe use, create the data and command files (which instruct the statistical software how to handle your data) using your microcomputer's WP/text editor. Using your microcomputer as a terminal to a mainframe, you can transfer these files and initiate the analysis (see Sections 2.3.2 and 2.4). Results are presented as printed output, or a text file which can be downloaded into your machine for perusal and/or printing.

Clinical researchers without access to mainframe-based statistical software may rely upon what can be achieved by a workstation. By virtue of design and capacity, the microcomputer is no match for a large mainframe when 'number crunching'; but, given relatively small data sets and modest demands for type of analysis, the microcomputer is invaluable. Many PCs can run sophisticated statistical software with good graphical facilities (often lacking in mainframe packages) and can cope with substantial data sets. Although microcomputers are slower than their 'bigger brothers', when the mainframe's many simultaneous users are considered, results can take as long or longer to obtain than on the single-user microcomputer for the equivalent type of analysis.

Schrodt (1984) discussed the problems of statistical software on a microcomputer, and highlighted accuracy in particular. Microcomputers can represent numbers as accurately as mainframes, but need more storage resources to do so and hence longer processing times. However, statistical software must be carefully written for microcomputers to avoid rounding errors causing an erroneous result especially when test statistics are near to a critical value. One should always carefully check results from microcomputer-based statistics or numerical packages. Versions of mainframe packages specially designed for micros (e.g. SPSS-PC) need at least 512K of RAM and a hard disk, but they are sophisticatd and accurate. They run fast enough for the average user, and much faster when a math co-processor is fitted, or when 'add-on' RAM is available for use as a 'virtual' disk. Unfortunately, they are also expensive.

Running 'micro' versions of mainframe packages will not be cost effective, relative to using a mainframe service, for many small research groups. But smaller-scale statistical packages are available for modest equipment (e.g. Norris et al., 1985, discuss parametric statistical techniques; and Meddis, 1984, describes an 'omnibus' approach to rank statistics).

Some micro-based packages can be relatively fragile, i.e. the novice can easily 'crash' them (a program or system failure) so data are lost and have to be re-entered. Also, menu-driven packages, where the computer constantly prompts you for the required inputs, can be irritating. The facility to bypass the menus or prompts and input direct commands is an advantage. Similarly, the possibility of inputting data via a text file (earlier, this section) is another advantage. Then if errors occur, there is no need to type all the data in again—having to re-type 20 data points in a menu-driven system can drive researchers to distraction!! Before buying try to find another user of the package to get both their opinion and some 'hands on' experience with some of your own data.

Small microcomputer-based statistics packages are rarely entirely satisfactory and data exploration is often best achieved with a spreadsheet (see Section 2.3.1; Lee & Soper, 1986) or software designed for carrying out exploratory data analysis (Velleman & Hoaglin, 1981).

Finally, it should be remembered, as Lovie (1986) aptly indicates, that statistical packages should not and cannot be used instead of a knowledge of data analysis techniques and their interpretation. In Lovie's words, 'The computer is an aid to thought not a substitute for it' (p. 171).

2.7. Automated Testing and Experimental Control

For over 20 years psychologists have used computers to control experimental apparatus and procedures and record behavioural and physiological data (e.g. Cacioppo, Marshall-Goodell & Gormezano, 1983; Norris *et al.*, 1985, Chapter 8; Coles, Gratton, Kramer & Miller, 1986). Recent widespread availability of cheap microcomputers pushed these techniques beyond the research laboratory into both undergraduate education and clinical practice. Burton (1985) observed that 97% of the 38 British university Psychology Departments answering his survey used computers for experimental control. Automating various psychological test and assessment procedures essentially developed from computer control of psychological experiments.

The key advantages of transferring standard psychological tests to a computer are improved standardisation in presentation, and time-saving for busy clinicians, enabling them to focus on understanding patient's problems and planning suitable treatments. Morris (1985) and Norris *et al.* (1985) suggest that computer-driven initial screening interviews could help the clinician pinpoint problems and are generally accepted by patients, who sometimes find it easier to disclose sensitive details to the impersonal computer. The main rationale for computer use here is to utilise the clinician's time more efficiently.

Both The British Psychological Society and the American Psychological Association have issued cautionary statements on 'test' computerisation (see Standing Committee on Test Standards, 1984). Concern mainly relates to possible effects on the construct validity (although Morris, 1985, disagrees), and the possible use of untrained personnel. Specifically developed tests for the new medium may solve such problems.

Excellent reviews of automated clinical assessment appear in Morris (1985), Norris *et al.* (1985; Chapter 8), and Simpson and Linney (1985).

2.8. Expert Systems and Artificial Intelligence

The construction and application of 'expert systems' (ES) is an increasingly important clinical research use of computers.

ESs are computer programs which offer the advice and reasoning of a human expert. Popular domains are medicine, geology, financial investment, etc. Originally used experimentally, this software has only recently been commercially produced (Forsyth, 1984; Harmon & King, 1985; Jackson, 1986), and assessing whether it is routinely used is difficult. The techniques for building ESs were developed from 'artificial intelligence' (AI) research, aimed at building computer models of cognitive behaviour (e.g. see Boden, 1977 for an overview; Winston, 1984, for a survey of techniques).

AI techniques are valuable in psychological theorising (Colbourn, 1984); and Colby's research provides an example applied to mental health (Boden, 1977, Chapter 3; Colby, 1981).

Earlier I cited Kapur's (1984) work (see Section 2.2.2), using a reference database, gradually constructed from patient data, to help assess new patients. ESs can now be 'bolted-on' to certain DBMSs and the system itself will develop the 'rules' for determining particular diagnoses from an established database of patient information, or allowing a clinician to input such rules directly. These are usually expressed in 'IF . . . THEN' form. A simple example from work that Kapur and I are carrying out is:

IF   memory-impairment mild
AND   pattern-of-memory-performance atypical
THEN diagnosis depression/anxiety-state

These ESs are called 'knowledge-based systems' because they depend on encapsulating the expert's knowledge in the program (called an ES 'shell') in the form of rules and 'facts', e.g. a simplified 'fact' might be:

CEREBRAL TUMOUR–SYMPTOM–HEADACHE

representing that a symptom of a cerebral tumour is headache. In contrast there are probability systems using Bayesian statistical inference on a substantial database of symptom-diagnosis probability relations (see Norris *et al.*, 1985, Chapter 10). Each type of ES has advantages and disadvantages (see Ramsey, Reggia, Nau, and Ferrentino, 1986), but a particular virtue of the knowledge-based approach is the 'explanation' facilities. The user can ask 'why?' such a conclusion was reached and the ES will backtrack and provide a trace of each stage of reasoning and the rules used to make particular inferences. Increasingly, ESs are written in flexible high-level programming languages like LISP and PROLOG. The latter is particularly favoured, and interested researchers can familiarise themselves via de Sarum's (1985) painless introduction, or Bratko's (1986) thorough treatment.

The necessary software has been implemented recently on microcomputers. Simons (1985) references microcomputer-based ESs and Vaghi (1986) demonstrated an elementary type of ES simply using one of the standard microcomputer operating systems (i.e. PC-DOS). Although there are considerable problems, there is much scope for experiment.

'Computer assisted learning' (CAL) in the context of the rehabilitation of neurological and psychiatric patients must be mentioned. Although CAL exists for all levels of education, developments in 'authoring languages', allowing clinicians or therapists to write their own training packages, and AI developments re-awakened interest. There are reviews by Hartley [1980], Barker and Yeates (1985), and O'Shea and Self (1983), while Norris *et al.* (1985, Chapter 10) and Ager (1985) describe specific applications to mental health.

3. PRACTICAL ADVICE ON ACQUIRING COMPUTING SKILLS AND CHOOSING APPROPRIATE HARDWARE AND SOFTWARE

3.1. Acquiring Computing Skills

Learning computing skills seems unattainable to those whose education finished before its widespread introduction. But this is not true.

Various strategies exist for the computer-naïve. My emphasis here is on *use*, because learning programming can take a considerable time, especially for producing useful software. The following requirements arise in learning to use computers:

1. A conviction that time spent learning computer use is well spent because it may not be especially productive in terms of your research and/or clinical work.

2. For a busy researcher or clinician, concentration on learning to use the computer only for those tasks of clear benefit to you is the best strategy. Having appreciated that, you may later feel confident enough to explore other potentially beneficial uses.

3. The realisation that you need know nothing about how the hardware works. A functional knowledge of the various components is sufficient (e.g. floppy and hard disks are for 'filing' your data, text, programs, etc.). Some computer systems get this message across clearly (e.g. O'Malley, 1986; Martin, 1985).

The two main strategies for acquiring skills are:

1. Attend some intensive courses run by many university computing centres, often in an inexpensive adult education programme. These courses (2–5 full days) are generally better than a weekly hour or two for getting you using a machine; avoid expensive commercial courses inapplicable to the experience required in research or clinical applications. Any course must include actual use of a computer.

2. Obtain or borrow a microcomputer system fitting your requirements (see below); sit down with its tutorial and reference manuals and work through them alone, with a colleague also wishing to learn, or one knowledgeable about the hardware and software (preferably *not* a 'computer buff'). Many people prefer to master a machine alone, and consult

others only when really stuck. That way you work at your own pace, with your own data, documents, etc. Mistakes will happen, but remember that the computer only does what you ask, and you cannot damage it just by typing. Mistakes can be frustrating, especially if you erase a whole day's work. If you unfortunately encounter a software 'bug' (possible even in commercial software) which corrupts the data on your disk making it unreadable, the ensuing frustration encourages learning to make backup copies of important disks or files.

The second strategy is usually followed by academics and clinicians, owing to time constraints, and despite notoriously poor computer documentation (although standards are improving). There is a publishing boom in guides to particular microcomputers and in standard software packages. The level and helpfulness of these varies: many only re-work the manufacturer-supplied manuals. As when choosing hardware and software, advice and comments from experienced colleagues and various BBSs (Section 2.4.4), reviews in computer magazines, newspapers, etc. are still the main information sources. Dealers can be very helpful, but they are salesmen of specific products which they will be biased towards!

Finally, many potential users worry about unfamiliarity with the QWERTY keyboard used on microcomputers. Touch-typing is not a prerequisite for effective computer use but it may be more efficient in the long term. Many systems use a 'mouse' for some input. This device, attached to the computer by a lead, is moved around the desk to control an on-screen pointer. Using this to point to command words or small pictures, called 'icons', displayed on the screen, the computer can be made to execute various tasks. This is simpler than typing command words (see Martin, 1985 for a good example).

3.2. Choosing Appropriate Hardware and Software

Owing to continuous developments in the personal computer industry it is difficult to give firm advice on choosing particular products. Demonstrations of hardware and software can be misleading. You must be allowed to 'test drive' any product and see demonstrations of it solving the kind of problems you intend it to handle.

However, these additional points are important:

1. Hardware and software must be chosen together, since not all machines may have the applications you require. Perhaps you need a wordprocessor and a statistics package now; and later a communications package which is not a feature of your initial system. Do ensure that a system will cater for possible future needs as well.

2. Standardisation is always a weak point: the only real standard in portable software is the IBM PC one. Non-IBM manufactured PCs are

described as 'IBM compatible', meaning that the machine can run the considerable software that an IBM PC can. Unfortunately, the standard includes the PC-DOS/MS-DOS 'command-driven' operating system, which is not easy to use unlike later developments using iconic desktop representations on screen selected via a 'mouse' on the desk, the so-called 'Windows, Icons, Mouse and Pull-down menus' (WIMP) environment (e.g. Martin, 1985). Choice should be determined by existing microcomputing equipment in your institution, which could determine the level of assistance obtainable; the suitability of the equipment; and its relative ease of use. Having said that, however, any system can be learned with time, but busy researchers and clinicians may prefer the faster learning curve, which seems more frequent with WIMP systems.

3. Purchasing hardware and software from a local dealer can often pay dividends despite a higher initial cost. Microcomputers are very reliable, but if things go wrong then a good relationship with a local dealer should get them rectified quickly. You will find that the machine rapidly becomes integrated into your work and is therefore difficult to be without.

I trust that these brief comments will be useful to readers now wishing to become computer users.

CONCLUSIONS

I hope this chapter has shown the computer to be a valuable tool, assisting researchers and clinicians, and that time spent acquiring the few necessary skills is well worth it. If you are not already a computer user, I hope you will be encouraged to become one. You won't regret it, but take care that the machine doesn't become an end in itself (e.g. Burton's 1985 comments). If you are already a computer user, I trust that I may have helped you realise more potential application to your work and provided some guide to further information. I'm sure the future holds even more helpful information technology!

ACKNOWLEDGEMENTS

During the writing of this chapter, I have had much valuable advice and comment from many people, especially Tony Hasemer, Tony Gale, Narinder Kapur and Isobel Colbourn.

GLOSSARY OF SOME COMMONLY USED COMPUTING TERMS

Terms given in italics are also defined in this glossary.

ASCII: 'American Standard Code for Information Interchange'; standard code using a *byte* to represent all alphanumeric and special control characters. A standard that allows just about *all* computers to intercommunicate.

BASIC: 'Beginners' All-purpose Symbolic Instruction Code'; easy to learn *high-level programming language* available on most computers.

BYTE: Commonly accepted measurement of computer storage. Used as a parameter for describing *RAM, ROM, Floppy disks, Hard disks*, etc. Equivalent to eight bits (binary digits) of information, the minimum required to represent alphanumeric characters, etc. using a standard code (e.g. *ASCII*).

CP/M: 'Control Program for Microcomputers' or 'Control Program Monitor'; Early *operating system* designed for 8-bit *microcomputers*. Still available on some *personal computers* (i.e. C/PM-86).

CPU: 'Central Processing Unit'; nerve centre of a digital computer. CPU coordinates and controls the activities of all other parts of the complete machine; carries out all the arithmetic and logical processes applied to data by following a program. CPUs are commonly implemented using *microprocessors*.

DOT MATRIX PRINTER: 'Hardcopy' peripheral device producing printed output via a printing head made up of a matrix of wires. Each character formed by pre-programmed combinations of these wires striking a typewriter-like ribbon onto paper. Contrast with a 'daisy-wheel printer' which uses typewriter-style 'hammers' to mark the paper.

FIRMWARE: *Software* which is stored within a *ROM*; available immediately without recourse to loading from disk.

FLOPPY DISKS: Commonest form of 'backing' storage, consisting of a lightweight flexible magnetic disk inside a protective square-shape sleeve. When rotated rapidly inside a computer disk drive, it behaves as if rigid allowing information to be written and read from it, providing a fairly permanent record. Two main types of floppy disk: the 5.25 in. size protected by a cardboard sleeve and relatively easily damaged; and the 3.25 in. type housed in a more robust hard plastic shell. Storage capacity depends on the computer system; generally ranges from $300K$ to $1.2Mb$. Disks are rarely interchangeable across machines using different *operating systems*. Due to flimsiness, 'backup' copies should always be kept.

HARD DISK: or 'Winchester disk'. Another form of backing storage, consisting of a rigid magnetic disk usually permanently housed with the associated drive components. Advantages are considerably faster read and write access to a greater quantity of stored information (typically between 10 and $40Mb$). More reliable than floppies but important to make backup copies of stored information. Devices called 'tape streamers' offer a relatively high speed economical form of backup.

HARDWARE: Computer system's electronic and mechanical components, i.e. the physical parts like the system units, monitor, keyboard, disk drives, etc.

HIGH-LEVEL PROGRAMMING LANGUAGE: Means of instructing a computer to carry out specific functions using a 'natural' or 'scientific' type of specialised language. There are many high-level programming languages like *BASIC*, FORTRAN (FORmula TRANslation), ALGOL (ALGOrithmic Language), LISP (LISt Processing), PROLOG (PROgramming in LOGic), etc., making the task of programming easier than using 'low-level' or 'assembler' languages, a mnemonic form of instruction codes used by the *microprocessor*.

ICON: Pictorial or ideographic representation of a computer function shown on the *VDU*. A *mouse* device is used to point to an icon to initiate the function. Seen as a way of making computers easier and more 'friendly' to use.

INTERFACE: Usually a hardware device, internally fitted to pieces of computer equipment, enabling a computer to 'talk' to its printer, modem, disk drive, etc. Also used for important software interface between the computer and the human user, known as the 'human-computer interface' (HCI).

KILOBYTE (K): Literally a thousand *bytes* but actually 1024 bytes because of the base two arithmetic. *Kilobyte* has become the standard unit for specifying computer storage.

MAINFRAME: Large fast computers with substantial memory, and backing store capacity, offering multi-user fully managed services. Contrast with *microcomputers* and *minicomputers*.

MEGABYTE (Mb); One million bytes.

MICROCOMPUTER: Generally small desk-top computers often housed within a single case containing electronic circuit boards and a keyboard. Originally based around 8-bit *microprocessors* with relatively small memories, now much more powerful microcomputers are available and often called *personal computers*.

MICROPROCESSOR: Heart of *microcomputers*, *personal computers*, and even some *minicomputers*. Consists of a *CPU* encapsulated in a single microelectronic device or 'silicon chip'. Microprocessors are usually referred to in terms of size of 'word' or basic unit of processing that they use, e.g. 8-bit, 16-bit or 32-bit being the current range. 'Word' size indicates the largest number that the microprocessor can represent without resort to sophisticated processing routines, so related to the maximum number of bytes of memory (*RAM*) theoretically addressed. An 8-bit microprocessor can only address a maximum of 64K bytes *RAM*.

MINICOMPUTER: Somewhat inexact term referring to machines somewhere in size and facilities between a *microcomputer* and a *mainframe*. Often have extensive *interface* facilities for use in laboratories, but computing power similar to *personal computers*.

MODEM:'MOdulator/DEModulator'; device to connect a computer to telephone lines for communication with another computer.

MOUSE: Device whose movements around a desktop are reflected by a pointer on a *VDU*. Used in a *software* environment with *icons* and menus to give commands to the computer; invention often credited to psychologists.

MS-DOS: 'MicroSoft (major American software company) Disk Operating System'. Almost a *de facto* standard *operating system* for *personal computers*. IBM has even adopted a version (called PC-DOS) for its PCs.

NLQ: 'Near Letter Quality'; standard of printer output for *dot-matrix printers* emulating, with varied success, the print quality of a good typewriter.

OPERATING SYSTEM (OS): Program supervising the running of other programs, commonly incorporating facilities for managing disk files and other resources. First program run when a computer is started up. When an application program finishes, control usually passed back to the OS (e.g. *MS-DOS*, *PC-DOS* and *CP/M*).

PERSONAL COMPUTER (PC): *Microcomputers* with sufficient memory and processing performance for 'business applications' (i.e. large or integrated software packages for wordprocessing, spreadsheets, databases, etc.). This somewhat fuzzy concept usually defined in terms of requiring a minimum of a 16-bit *microprocessor* addressing at least 256*K* of *RAM*. But 'smaller' machines can be used for business applications.

PC-DOS: The IBM variant of the *MS-DOS operating system*.

RAM: 'Random Access Memory'; memory available for storing programs and data while they are being processed by the machine. Rapidly accessed for either read or write operations by *CPU*, but contents are lost when the power supply is turned off. Computers often described in terms of RAM capacity, e.g. 512*K RAM*, giving an indication of size, and therefore sophistication, of programs and data files that can be handled.

ROM: 'Read Only Memory'; contrasts with *RAM* in that information can only be read and not altered. ROMs are usually chips installed inside computers, containing application programs termed *firmware*. Most *micro* and *personal computers* have some *ROM*-based software.

SOFTWARE: General term for computer programs, contrasted with *hardware*. Distinction between 'applications software', i.e. task-specific programs for wordprocessing, statistical analysis, etc., and 'system software', i.e. the *operating system, high-level programming languages*, etc.

VDU: 'Visual Display Unit'; screen where computer presents information that is input to and output from it.

REFERENCES

Ager, A. (1985). Recent developments in the use of microcomputers in the field of mental handicap: Implications for psychological practice. *Bulletin of The British Psychological Society*, **38**, 142–145.

Alvey, N., Galwey, N. & Lane, P. (1982). *An Introduction to Genstat*. London: Academic Press.

Baker, C. (1984). Human aspects of online information retrieval. In A. Burns (ed.) *New Information Technology*. Chichester: Ellis Horwood, pp. 122–133.

Barker, P. & Yeates, H. (1985). *Introducing Computer Assisted Learning*. London: Prentice-Hall International.

Boden, M. A. (1977). *Artificial Intelligence and Natural Man*. Hassocks, Sussex: Harvester Press.

Bratko, I. (1986). *Prolog Programming for Artificial Intelligence*. Wokingham, England: Addison-Wesley.

Bridges, S. P. M. (1986). *Low Cost Local Area Networks*. Wilmslow, Cheshire: Sigma Press/Wiley.

British Computer Society. (1984). *A Glossary of Computing Terms: An Introduction*, 4th edn. Cambridge University Press.

Brownell, B. A. (1985). *Using Microcomputers: A Guide Book for Writers, Teachers and Researchers*. Beverley Hills, C. Sage.

Burns, A. (ed.). (1984). *New Information Technology*. Chichester: Ellis Horwood.

Burton, A. M. (1985). Computer use in British university departments of psychology. *Bulletin of The British Psychological Society*, **38**, 1–5.

Cacioppo, J. T., Marshall-Goodell, B. S. & Gormezano, I. (1983). Social psychophysiology: Bioelectrical measurement, experimental control, and analog-to-digital data acquisition. In J. T. Cacioppo, and R. E. Petty (eds). *Social Psychophysiology: A Sourcebook*. New York: The Guildford Press, pp. 666–690.

Chandor, A., Graham, J., & Williamson, R. (1985). *The Penguin Dictionary of Computers*. Harmondsworth: Penguin.

Colbourn, C. J. (1984). Moulding minds with modern machines. *Educational and Child Psychology*, **1**, 40–46.

Colby, K. M. (1981). Modeling the paranoid mind. *The Behavioural and Brain Sciences*, **4**, 515–560.

Coles, M. G. H., Gratton, G., Kramer, A. F. & Miller, G. A. (1986). Principles of signal acquisition and analysis. In M. G. H. Coles, E. Donchin and S. W. Porges (eds). *Psychophysiology: Systems, Processes and Applications*. New York: The Guilford Press, pp. 183–221.

Cornwall, H. (1986). *The New Hacker's Handbook*. London: Century Communications.

Cotton, K. (1984). Electronic mail. In A. Burns (ed.) *New Information Technology*. Chichester: Ellis Horwood, pp. 47–54.

Day, N. & Rees, O. (1985). *Computer Spreadsheets*. London: British Broadcasting Corporation.

de Sarum, H. (1985). *Programming in micro-PROLOG*. Chichester: Ellis Horwood.

Dixon, W. J. (ed.) (1985). *BMDP Statistical Software*. Berkeley: University of California Press.

Durr, M. & Walker, D. (1985). *Micro to Mainframe: Creating an Integrated Environment*. Reading, Ma.: Addison-Wesley.

Forsyth, R. S. (ed.) (1984). *Expert Systems: Principles and Case Studies*. London: Chapman & Hall.

Hammond, C. (1986). The hazards of VDUs. *Practical Computing*, June, 73–75

Hammond, R. (1984). *The On-line Handbook*. London: Fontana.

Harmon, P. & King, D. (1985). *Expert Systems: Artificial Intelligence in Business*. Chichester: Wiley.

Hartley, J. R. (1980). Computer assisted learning. In H. T. Smith and T. R. G. Green (eds), *Human Interaction with Computers*. London: Academic Press.

Jackson, D., Chamberlain, S., Sanders, J. & Tyler, T. (1986). Of mice and managers. *MacUser*, **March/April**, 29–34;36;38–40.

Jackson, P. (1986). *Introduction to Expert Systems*. Wokingham, Addison-Wesley.

Johnson, R. (1984). The office workstation. In A. Burns (ed.) *New Information Technology*. Chichester: Ellis Horwood, pp. 40–46.

Kapur, N. (1984). Using a microcomputer-based data management system for neuropsychological record filing, report generation, and as a clinical decision aid. *Bulletin of The British Psychological Society*, **37**, 413–415.

Kleiger, D. M. (1984). *Computer Usage for Social Scientists*. Boston: Allyn & Bacon.

Knox, B. (1985). *Hotline: Personal Guide to Computers*. London: Century Communications.

Lawrence, J. S. (1984). *The Electronic Scholar: A guide to Academic Microcomputing*. Norwood, N.J.: Ablex.

Lee, M. P. & Soper, J. B. (1986). Using spreadsheets to teach statistics in psychology. *Bulletin of The British Psychological Society*, **39**, 365–367.

Lovie, A. D. (1986). Getting new statistics into today's crowded curriculum. In A. D. Lovie (ed.) *New Developments in Statistics for Psychology and the social Sciences*. London: The British Psychological Society/Methuen, pp. 163–172.

Madron, T. W. M., Tate, L. N. & Brookshire, R. G. (1985). Using Microcomputers in Research. *Sage University Paper Series on Quantitative Applications in the Social Sciences*, Series no. 07-052. Beverly Hills & London: Sage.

Martin, J. and The Arben Group, Inc. (1985). *A Breakthrough in Making Computers Friendly*: The Macintosh Computer. Englewood Cliffs, N.J.: Prentice-Hall. (A review of the design philosophy underlying a very user-oriented computer system together with a practical introduction to its use in sufficient detail to allow an evaluation by a potential user.)

McBride, J. (1985). *Instant Access: The Videotex Approach to Information Management*. London: Marathon Videotex.

McWilliams, P. A. (1984). *The Wordprocessing Book*. New York: Doubleday.

Meddis, R. (1984). *Statistics Using Ranks: A Unified Approach*. Oxford: Blackwell.

Miter, N. N. (1986). Users and ease of use: Online catalogues' raison d'etre. *Program*, **202**, 111–119.

Moody, G., Malone, S. and Stobie, I. (1986). Time to connect (MS-Net; Appletalk; Mix and Match). *Practical Computing*, **June**, 91–93; 96–98; 100–101; 103; 105. (A review of LANs available in the UK and how to approach choosing one.)

Morris, R. G. (1985). Automated clinical assessment. In F. N. Watts (ed) *New Developments in Clinical Psychology*. Chichester: The British Psychological Society/Wiley, pp. 121–138.

Norris, D. E., Skilbeck, C. E., Hayward, A. E. & Torpy, D. M. (1985). *Microcomputers in Clinical Practice*. Chichester: Wiley.

Norusis, M. J. (1985). *SPSS-X Advanced Statistics Guide*. New York: McGraw-Hill.

Norusis, M. J. (1983). *SPSS-X Introductory Statistics Guide*. New York: McGraw-Hill.

Oborne, D. J. (1985). *Computers at Work: A Behavioural Approach*. Chichester: Wiley.

O'Malley, C. E. (1986). Helping users help themselves. In D. A. Norman and S. W. Draper (eds.) *User Centred System Design: New Perspectives in Human-Computer Interaction*. Hillsdale, N.J.: Lawrence Erlbaum,

O'Shea, T. & Self, J. (1983). *Learning and Teaching with Computers: Artificial Intelligence in Education*. Brighton: Harvester.

Pearce, B. (ed.) (1984). *Health Hazards of VDTs?* Chichester: Wiley, 1984. (To get to the most relevant aspects of this topic for researchers, the following chapters are recommended: 2: Health hazards in perspective; 10: Issues in vision and lighting for users of VDUs; 13: Postural loads at VDT work-stations; 16: Optimal presentation mode and colours of symbols on VDUs.)

Raitt, D. (1984). Videotex its use and users. In A. Burns (ed.) *New Information Technology*. Chichester: Ellis Horwood, pp. 133–147.

Ramsey, C. L., Reggia, J. A., Nau, D. S. & Ferrentino, A. (1986). A comparative analysis of methods for expert systems. *International Journal of Man-Machine Studies*, **24**, 475–499.

Ryan, D. R., Joiner, B. L. & Ryan, T. A. Jr. (1985) *Minitab Handbook* (2nd edn.). Boston: Duxbury Press.

Schrodt, P. A. (1984). *Microcomputer Methods for Social Scientists*. Sage University Paper series on Quantitative Applications in the Social Sciences, series no. 07-040. Beverly Hills & London: Sage.

Sellu, D. P. (1986). A comprehensive bibliography database using a microcomputer. *British Medical Journal*, **292**, 1643–1645.

Simons, G. L. (1985). *Expert Systems and Micros*. Manchester: NCC Publications.

Simpson, J. M. & Linney, A. D. (1985). Use of computer automated psychological tests to assess mentally impaired old people. In H. P. von Hahn (ed.). *Modern Approaches to the Dementias*. Basel: Karger.

SPSS Inc (1983). *SPSS-X User's Guide*. New York: McGraw-Hill.

Standing Committee on Test Standards (1984). Note on the computerization of printed psychological tests and questionnaires. *Bulletin of The British Psychological Society*, **37**, 416–417.

Stokes, A. (1984). Computer networks. In A. Burns (ed.). *New Information Technology*. Chichester: Ellis Horwood, pp. 111–122.

Vaghi, S. (1986). Come out of your shell. *Personal Computer World*, **April**, 182–185; 187–188.

Velleman, P. F. & Hoaglin, D. C. (1981). *Applications, Basics, and Computing of Exploratory Data Analysis*. Boston: Duxbury Press.

Weekes, A. J. (1986). *A Genstat Primer*. London: Edward Arnold.

Winston, P. H. (1984). *Artificial Intelligence*, 2nd edn. Reading, Ma.: Addison-Wesley.

6 Writing a Research Report

Glenys Parry
Department of Psychiatry, University of Southampton.
Department of Psychotherapy, Royal South Hants Hospital,
Southampton SO9 4PE.

It is surprising how many people undertake a piece of research and carry it almost to completion, but fail to take the final steps of writing about it in a formal paper and seeing it through to publication. Many of us have some results lying in a drawer which we intend to write up—one day—or an idea for a paper which has not been written—yet. There are a number of reasons for this. Sometimes, having embarked on a project, one can become disillusioned with it, believing it not to be worth publishing. This may be true, but until you have written at least a draft of a possible paper, it is difficult to be sure. A much more common reason is that people lack confidence in writing and find it difficult. We sometimes forget that to write successfully needs practice, as with any skilled behaviour. Unfortunately it is a skill often neglected during clinical and research training, and many people do not have anyone to help them acquire it. This chapter aims to help the relatively inexperienced researcher at every stage of writing a research report. I shall focus on writing an empirical paper for publication in a journal, but many of the points apply equally to other forms of writing, such as a case report, a review article or a dissertation for examination.

HOW TO START

Getting Ready

Before you sit down to write, there is some important work to do in preparation. This time is well spent and will save a lot of problems later. The first question to mull over is 'What do I want to say?'. Writing is much easier if you have something you want to say. It is quite likely that there is no one clear idea in your mind. Perhaps your study addressed a range of questions which, in hindsight, are not closely related, or there may be some meaningless or negative results. These may be due to design flaws or measurement problems and cannot be interpreted. Despite this, I shall assume that you have some results which you find interesting and which are worth communicating. This is the purpose of the paper, to communicate your findings.

The same principle applies to writing a dissertation or a thesis. Here you have more room and more excuse to list your negative findings, but be careful. It has been remarked that there are many reasons for negative findings, but most of them are trivial. Do not spend pages over-interpreting the reasons why you did not find what you expected to; it is better to focus on what you did find. The quality of the dissertation will be enhanced by thinking carefully about what you found and presenting it as clearly as possible.

When writing up a case study or a piece of qualitative research, there are no numerical 'results' to present. The general importance of thinking through the purpose and the message of the paper is, if anything, even more important in language based research. In a case study, for example, it is easy for the reader to become lost in a mass of clinical detail. The case study is at its best when making a theoretical point. The clinical material, having previously been analysed by the author, can be used selectively to illustrate the argument, and, above all, presented in a logical sequence. There is some discussion of presenting findings from qualitative research in Chapter 11.

Having decided what it is you want to say, the next question, just as important, is 'Who wants to know about it?'. Even at this preliminary stage you should be thinking about the readers. The research paper is a communication from you to someone else. Imagine you were asked to give a talk about your work. You would find it disconcerting if the person who invited you refused to tell you who the audience was. American psychiatrists? Health visitors? Behaviour therapists? The same thing applies to writing a formal research report. You are not writing in a social vacuum, although it can feel like it sometimes. Think about which journal you are writing for, and what kind of readership it has. Study other articles published by the journal of your choice to get an idea of the style.

If you are writing with co-authors, you will need to allocate tasks and, just as important, decide in which order your names will appear. This can be a source of much bitterness to junior researchers who discover, when the paper reporting their research is nearly ready for submission, that a senior colleague expects to have his or her name first. Alphabetical ordering does not solve this problem, especially for people called Zug.

There are, unfortunately, no hard and fast rules about author precedence. It seems fair that the person who did most work should be the senior author, but of course this is often not clear cut. Sometimes the person who planned the research or who wrote it up is not the one who carried it out or analysed the data. In any case, get the rules straight at the beginning, before starting to write—it will prevent acrimony later.

The next stage is to gather together all the ingredients for the paper. In empirical research, the results are the heart of the paper. Sort out all the findings you want to present and get them into a form you can work with. This means creating rough tables, graphs and figures rather than leaving it all on computer printout or scribbled on the backs of envelopes.

You will also need your notes on relevant articles. Ideally, you would have made notes on other papers at the time you first read them; a succinct but informative summary of each paper complete with a full reference. Alas, it is more likely that you have a few photocopies, a few references and several memories of interesting articles you read 6 months ago but cannot now remember—was it Bruddle and Dakey or Brobble and Daly? Was it 1985 or 1984? You can remember the journal had a green cover! Now is the time to spend some hours in the library searching out relevant articles. But beware! It is very easy to fall into the hands of the arch-enemy of academic writers—procrastination. This devious opponent can take many forms, and if you catch yourself, 3 weeks later, saying 'I can't possibly start to write my paper until I've managed to get hold of so-and-so's article', you must take this as an urgent signal to start writing, immediately.

The Right Conditions

By now you have some idea of what you want to say and to whom you wish to say it. You have gathered all your materials, or at least enough to be going on with. Now you must find the right conditions in which to work. This is a very individual thing. Different people have different strategies, from the well-known psychologist who is reputed to tackle the first draft walking along a towpath with a Dictaphone, to a colleague who can only write at the kitchen table surrounded by the tea things with the radio on. You must find your own style, and this is one area where you can be entirely self-indulgent. If you like to write in 2B pencil on yellow paper and only in your garden shed—so be it.

There are some groundrules, though, which you ignore at your peril. The two most important are solitude and uninterrupted time. It's amazing how we expect to be able to dash off a quick paper between telephone calls, meetings and seeing patients, and then seem puzzled and disheartened when nothing happens. The single most common reason for failure to write is the lack of adequate clear time in which to do it. The longer you have the better, the more frequent and regular your sessions the better. You also need a refreshed, clear mind. Writing demands your highest cognitive functions, so it's a good idea to find your own best time of the day, when you have most energy. For many people that is first thing in the morning, so it seems a shame to waste this prime time opening the post or chatting to colleagues. Others like an evening session. Very few people can give their best at four-thirty in the afternoon at the end of a day in the clinic, or during the lunch hour. You also need support and encouragement.

Many would-be researchers working in health service jobs find their writing is not valued and can even be seen as an indulgence. You need to find someone, somewhere, who believes in you and will support you. This support can take many forms, for example shielding you from phone calls when you're writing, or reading and commenting on drafts. You are in the best position to know what kind of support you need and you should take yourself seriously enough to get it.

The final prerequisite for successful writing is having the right tools. A good dictionary is just as essential as pen and paper. Many people find word-processors invaluable as you can draft and re-draft, cut text or move it around on screen so easily. They are particularly liberating for those who are blocked by a perfectionist need to draft the perfect sentence on that blank sheet of paper.

So here you are, sitting in your locked room with the morning ahead of you, notes and results easily to hand and writing tools at the ready. It's time to start writing!

THE OUTLINE

The first thing to write is definitely not the introductory paragraph, but an outline, a plan of your paper. There are many excellent reasons for this. It is absolutely essential that the material you are presenting is organised so that there is a logical flow of ideas from beginning to end. There is nothing more frustrating for the reader than a muddled, formless paper which gets off to a few false starts, fails to explain why the study was undertaken, presents results in the method section and then describes previously unmentioned measures in the results. Taking the time to think through the content and structure is part of a genuine desire to communicate, since you are trying to help the reader. The outline is also a very good way of getting ideas down—you learn to tolerate partly formed ideas by sketching them in at an early stage under the appropriate heading. Gradually the structure of the paper takes shape without your getting bogged down in the minutiae of the method or results. A good outline also helps you to write the first draft.

Example 1

What the chapter is about
People undertake a piece of research but do not report it in a formal paper.
People lack confidencs in writing and find it difficult.
Chapter aims to help the inexperienced.
Focus is on writing an empirical paper for publication in a journal. Mention case reports, review articles and dissertations for examination.

How to start
Getting ready
    What do you want to say? To whom do you want to say it?
    Gathering your results. Background reading and notes on other articles.
The right conditions
    Quiet solitude and uninterrupted time.
    A refreshed clear mind—support—the right tools.
What to do if you can't get started
    Why it is difficult.
    How to recognise procrastination.
    Getting into the habit.
    Some techniques to overcome a block.

The outline
Why bother?
    The supreme importance of a clear structure.
    If you can't write on outline the paper will be muddled.
    Good ways of getting ideas down—learning to tolerate partly formed ideas.
The main headings
Rough notes

The first draft
Using the outline.
What to write first—how much at a time.
The method—results—the introduction—the discussion.
Getting feedback.

Subsequent drafts
Redrafting and revising for major changes.
Re-analysing results.
Correcting for style.
Reading more articles—knowing when to stop.

Preparing the manuscript for submission
Tables and figures.
References.
The title and abstract.
Authors and addresses.
Acknowledgements.

The editorial process
The covering letter—packaging it.
Reviewers—how long to wait for the decision.
The decision and what to do about it.

The Main Headings

In an empirical paper, the standard headings are Introduction, Method, Results and Discussion. This format allows a logical and economic exposition of why you conducted the study, what you did, what you found and what it means. It is not meant to be a realistic account in chronological order of what you thought before you started, the whole story of the fieldwork, every piece of data you collected or how you changed the design twice in the middle. It is a formal, public account. It is scrupulously honest, but it is constructed. There may, for some purposes, be a better set of main headings, but convince someone else as well as yourself.

Under each main heading, sketch out subheadings. Don't worry if they are not all at the same level of detail. You may have quite a good idea of how your method and results will be written but be more hazy on the introduction and discussion. The aim is to have a working model of the paper, an overview of the whole thing. Under each subheading you can then sketch in rough notes of material you wish to include. There is no need to write in detail. An example might help—there is an initial outline of a paper in Example 1. This is as far as you need to take it before starting writing. The final paper will be rather different from the outline, but that is to be expected, since the paper develops in the process of being drafted and redrafted. The outline is your starting point. It is useful at this stage to make a list of all the tables and figures you want to present.

THE FIRST DRAFT

Now you are ready to write the first draft of the paper. It is best to do this quickly. Some authorities advise us to complete the first draft at one sitting, but I have always found this impossible. Getting started is the most difficult part, as a law of inertia seems to apply. The basic principle is to work intensively on the paper over a short period, so that you can be completely immersed in it. One or two hours a week are useless for this, since you have to begin painfully each time; much better to clear a day or two completely. This enables you to build up a momentum where you can become preoccupied with what you are writing. If you do this, you will be surprised and pleased by how much you achieve. When you do stop work, leave your draft at a point in the middle of a section or paragraph where you know exactly what you want to write next. It will be much easier to start writing at the next session than if you had to start thinking afresh about a new section.

The first draft can be written as an expansion of the outline, taking a section at a time. People sometimes wonder which section to write first. The books in the bibliography give a variety of opinion on this matter. Most authors are agreed, though, that it is unwise to start at the beginning and write through to the end. The introduction is often best left in outline form until the results and method sections are drafted. The method is often the easiest section to write, and on the principle that getting started is the most difficult thing, many people make life a little easier by beginning there. On the other hand, the whole reason for the paper is the findings, so it also makes sense to begin by examining these carefully and writing the results section first. Do not imagine that this will necessarily be the final set of results. In the course of writing a paper, gaps in the analysis are often revealed and extra analyses may be needed. The process is reiterative!

As you write the first draft, do not worry too much about niceties of style and grammar, just concentrate on getting it down. There will be ample time for revision later.

Method

In the method section you should aim to explain fully, but concisely, the procedures you used that yielded the data. There should be enough detail for a conscientious specialist to repeat your investigation. This would include the nature of the sample, how it was obtained, the context of the data collection, the procedures used, the measures used and the form of statistical analysis. Where measures are fully described elsewhere, a brief summary description should be given together with the reference. Never mention a measure without the reference, however familiar it may be. If you have included measures of your own devising, give fuller details, including some indication of the measure's psychometric properties (for example, internal consistency, test–retest or inter-rater reliability, validity estimates) and one or two sample items.

Results

The results section should also have a logical order. Methodological checks need to be reported first, for example you may expect certain measures to correlate highly with each other, whereas others should be unassociated. Other checks might include an analysis to determine whether one group within the sample differs systematically from another group (such as where the sample consists of patients from different sites), or you may wish to check that two equivalent groups are well matched on crucial variables.

As a general rule, descriptive statistics precede exploratory data analysis which precedes confirmatory data analysis. If you are discussing the results in a separate section, simply report them here. On the other hand, do not refrain from comment if it helps to organise and structure the section. When reporting significance levels, use two-tailed tests. Don't use a one-tailed test simply because you had a hypothesis which predicted a particular direction. It is really only safe to do so if a result in the other direction would have no meaning. Do not report a p value without the statistic from which it was derived. Give enough information for someone else to check it (for example, an F ratio needs both degrees of freedom). A golden rule is not to report any statistical procedures which you don't understand. This sounds obvious, but the rule is often violated. Ideally you will have analysed your own data. If someone else carried out the analyses, you must know exactly what was done and why. It is much better to report simple procedures clearly and appropriately than complex ones which are muddled or, worse still, non-sensical.

Do not repeat in the text what is already clear from the tables or figures. These should be thought through very carefully. Do not include too much material in any one table or clarity suffers. Often it is better to have two smaller tables than one massive one, unless there is a good reason why the results must be presented together. Always make sure that each table and figure makes sense on its own without the reader having to refer to the text. This means it should have an explanatory title. Make sure you don't call a table a figure or vice versa. Avoid abbreviations if you can, but if you must use them, make sure they are explained on the table (and if used in more than one, on each table) rather than in the text. In graphs, all axes must be clearly labelled. In general, editors prefer tables to figures because they convey more information in a smaller space. Reserve figures for results that need them. In Example 2a, the information in Fig. 6.1 does not need a graphical presentation. It would be better presented as in Table 6.1. Figure 6.2 (in Example 2b) is useful, however, because the crucial point is communicated better visually. Having said all this, don't worry about perfection at this stage, so long as you have a 'working version' of all your tables and figures.

Introduction

The introduction should 'set up' the paper. You are trying to explain as economically as possible why you undertook the investigation, and why you approached it in the way you did. There is no point in writing a 2000 word literature review simply to demonstrate that you have read a lot! One hallmark of a badly written paper is a verbose and muddled introduction. The literature reviewed should be apposite, enabling you to make a series of points. If you find this difficult, imagine you are having a conversation

Example 2a

FIG. 6.1 Comparison between single and married mothers on measures of psychiatric symptoms and psychological distress.

TABLE 6.1

Single (n = 21) and married (n = 172) mothers: Comparison between groups on measures of psychiatric symptomatology and psychological distress

		PSE	Beck	Anxiety	Zung
Single	mean	6.76	9.95	3.50	5.67
n = 21	(SD)	(7.06)	(9.72)	(2.39)	(4.10)
Married	mean	5.32	7.81	2.63	4.84
	(SD)	(6.27)	(7.12)	(2.48)	(3.78)
t-value (191 df)		<1	1.25	1.48	<1
Significance		ns	ns	ns	ns

Example 2b

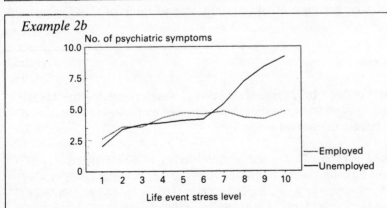

FIG. 6.2 Moving average of psychiatric symptom score in employed and unemployed groups across increasing life stress.

with an interested and intelligent colleague (this may be quite a feat of imagination but try it anyway). You are asked a series of questions, such as 'Why was it important to do this investigation? Have other people examined this in the past? How might your study add to existing knowledge? Why did you choose this design? Did you have any special reasons for using these particular measures?'. Answer the questions in normal conversational English and you have the basis for your first draft. When you do describe someone else's study, be specific about the major details without being verbose. For example, compare the two descriptions of the same study in Example 3. The second is only a few words longer than the first, but it is much more informative. It is essential to be accurate when describing other people's results. Misreported findings have a habit of slipping into future papers by authors who don't bother to check them. Remember the reviewers of your paper may be the authors of the papers you cite, or are likely to be familiar with them. Your notes will be helpful here; but if you are in any doubt, check.

Discussion

The discussion should not reiterate the results but should do what it says, discuss them. You are trying to explain what your results mean and to relate them to other people's work. Often you are pointing out the implications of the results. You can refer to material from the introduction in the light of your findings, but do not simply repeat it. You are taking it further now you have reported your results. It is appropriate in the discussion to take a sceptical view of your findings. If there are any design flaws (and there will be), this is the place to discuss how they might have affected your results. It is also the place to consider alternative explanations of your findings. If you are not able to think of these, wait until

---

Example 3

First Version In a large-scale survey, Kessler and McRae (1982) found a significant relationship between employment status and self-esteem in married women.

Second version In a questionnaire survey of 532 married women whose husbands were employed, Kessler and McRae (1982) found paid employment was correlated ($p < 0.05$) with self-esteem measured by a short form of Rosenberg's (1965) scale.

someone else has read and commented on the paper. Try to end the paper on a positive, interesting point. Do not finish it with any variant of the tedious cliche 'more research is needed to investigate this further'. We can take that for granted!

SUBSEQUENT DRAFTS

Your first draft is a major achievement. The good news is that everything gets easier from now on. The bad news is that you are only half-way there, is that. Many inexperienced researchers assume that the first draft needs only tinkering with before it is submitted. Not at all. Many authors go through two or three major revisions before they are satisfied with the paper. Some do more. The first draft is the basis of your paper, not the paper itself. You can do the first revision yourself by reading through carefully, putting yourself in the reader's shoes. Is it clear? Are there any parts which are particularly muddled or clumsy? Do you stay in the same tense or oscillate between past and present? Have you overused a particular word or phrase? Iron out the worst faults and get it typed—now, as always, double-spaced with wide margins. This is the point at which the word-processor comes into its own, since it is so easy to print out new drafts—as many as you want. Typists (including yourself) are neither so tireless nor uncomplaining.

Next, give the paper to at least one other person to read and comment on. Encourage them to write all over the draft. Tell them if there is something you particularly want them to do; for example, check that the results make sense, think of alternative explanations for the findings, spot unbuttressed assertions. One of these people could be a specialist who understands the field, but it is also useful for a non-specialist, even a layperson, to read the paper. They will be less tolerant of obscurities and the use of jargon. Remember that although your paper must be useful to the specialists, most of the journal's readers will not be; be considerate of them.

Your 'reader' may come up with a major problem, finding an error in your results or showing your argument is based on a fundamental misunderstanding. Don't be discouraged, however negative the feedback seems, since the value of writing the paper is to sort out these problems and to get it right. Having written the first draft you can more easily spot gaps in the argument or the analysis, and new ideas will occur to you. Again, this is one of the ways your work is improved, so don't shy away from new analyses at this stage, or a major redraft. Your adviser may also mention other research that you have missed but which bears on your paper. Again, it is worth checking this out and including new material, but don't fall prey to procrastination. At this stage you will probably find that the paper is far too long and diffuse. You may have to rethink the central point of the paper and omit results that are not essential in order to provide a clear focus.

When you have redrafted the article to a point where you are happy with what it says, turn your attention to how you have said it; go through the paper carefully and correct the style. There are many useful guides to writing style, some are mentioned in the reference section at the end of this chapter, but the golden rule is to write as simply and clearly as you can. Ruthlessly cut out all the waffle, the redundant and circumlocutory phrases; fearlessly replace the passive verb forms with active ones, the cliches with fresh images, the 70-word, eight-clause sentences with two or more smaller ones (see Example 4). As well as trying your best to write in plain English, you must also observe the house-style of the journal. For example, the American Psychological Association publishes a guidebook on style (*The Publication Manual of the American Psychological Association*) which includes everything from whether to use single or double inverted commas to how to avoid sexist use of language.

PREPARING THE MANUSCRIPT FOR SUBMISSION

References, Acknowledgements, Abstract

You will find the reference list a time-consuming and frustrating job, but so does everyone else and there's no way round it. Write the references on cards or a word-processor so that the odd one can be popped in the right place without having to re-write the lot. The references must be complete and accurate. This sounds easy but isn't and you will have to take trouble over it. Follow the style of the chosen journal obsessionally, down to the

---

Example 4—Correcting for style

First draft   It is of interest to note that the approach employed by the present author is somewhat similar to that of Jones (1985) in terms of the assessment of individuals' conceptual structure, with the exception of the number of items included, where, in the present paper, ten is considered to be a sufficient number, as will be seen by examination of Table 3.

Second draft   I used a ten item version of Jones' (1985) method to measure conceptual structure (see Table 3).

last full-stop. Check that every reference you cite is in the reference list and that every reference in the list is cited in the paper.

The acknowledgements should include those who gave substantial help in supporting you, collecting data, advising on statistics, reading and revising the manuscript. On the other hand, do not mention absolutely everyone with whom you had a coffee-time conversation about the research. Always tell someone if you intend to acknowledge their help.

The abstract should be a very brief summary of the paper, written with the non-specialist in mind. Try to include the main findings rather than the uninformative 'Results are reported of a comparison of two matched groups of outpatients'. It is better, for example, to say 'A group of depressed outpatients were found to have significantly smaller social networks than a matched group of anxious patients'. The journal will give a word limit for the abstract in the instructions to authors. Keep to it. You will have to draft and re-draft the abstract to whittle away every unnecessary word.

Tables and Figures

When preparing the final version of the tables and figures, always double check that every number is correct. An error that creeps in at this stage has every chance of remaining undetected until after publication—an embarrassment so intense it is not worth risking. Eventually, you should have the figures professionally produced by a graphic illustrator, who will produce high-quality glossy prints suitable for reproduction. It is safer to wait until the paper is accepted, and the definitive version of the figures is known, before committing yourself to the expense.

The Title Page

Now you have to worry about the title of the paper. You have probably been using a working title, but think about it again now. The title should be as concise as possible, but should accurately describe the paper's concerns. Your own and any co-authors' names and affiliations should also appear on the title page, but nowhere else. This enables the editor to send your manuscript for blind review.

The Final Manuscript

Take loving care over the final manuscript, so that it looks really professional. This means that if you do use a word-processor, learn to use it properly. The life of an editor or an examiner is made miserable by poorly formatted manuscripts littered with misspelt words, produced by misguided authors who have prematurely dispensed with the services of a professional typist. If you cannot find the time or take the trouble to get a really good result yourself, you could use the word-processor for all but the final draft, then get that properly typed. The typing should be perfect, double-spaced (that means everything, including the references), with wide margins. Show in the text where each table and figure belongs (Fig. 6.3). Make a final check that all the references in the text are in the reference list (and vice versa) and that the names and dates are identical in both places. Similarly, make sure that all the tables are referred to in the text and that any table you mention does indeed exist. Read the manuscript for typing errors, checking every word. Preferably, persuade someone else to proof-read it too, to pick up the mistakes you missed. The order in which the paper should be compiled is as follows:

1. Title page; includes title and authors' names and addresses.
Some journals need index keywords here and a short title which will be used as a heading for subsequent pages (running head).
   2. Abstract.
   3. Text.

When the sample was split into 'cases' and 'non-cases', all the measures showed a significant difference between the two groups (see Table 1).

TABLE ONE ABOUT HERE

The two self-esteem measures most clearly reflected differences between respondents. It is likely that even for these measures, there is considerable overlap between the distributions of scores of cases and non-cases. The breakdown of means of the two self esteem measures across the eight ID levels is presented graphically in Figure 1.

FIGURE ONE ABOUT HERE

There does appear to be a discontinuity in the linear relationship between ID level and self esteem, occuring at ID5.

FIG. 6.3   An example of typed manuscript. (Originally on A4 paper; reduced to 55% on reproduction.)

4. Acknowledgements.
5. References.
6. Tables (each on a fresh page).
7. Figure legends.
8. Figures.

Before sending it off, check that all the pages are there, numbered and in the correct order. Send the top copy and two good photocopies, accompanied by a short, formal letter to the editor.

THE EDITORIAL PROCESS

The process of sending papers out for independent review does not only benefit the journal's editor, but gives you useful feedback on your paper and the research itself. The most frustrating thing is when you have no reply, save a postcard acknowledgement, for months on end. How long should you leave it before writing again to enquire about the decision? I think that 3 months is long enough, because if you have heard nothing by then your paper is probably sitting in the in-tray of one of the reviewers who needs to be reminded about it.

The decision you receive will be one of four—accept, accept subject to amendment, revise and re-submit, or reject. It is unusual to have a paper accepted outright, so please don't expect this. If it is accepted subject to amendment, you have done very well. After a celebratory night out, start the new version, so that the paper can be off your desk and back to the editor as soon as possible.

If you have been advised to revise and resubmit the paper, it will probably be sent to the reviewers again and there is no guarantee that it will be accepted. On the other hand, most revisions that are conscientiously undertaken do get accepted in the end. Don't think you can get away with a superficial readjustment of a few words; you must address the points raised by the reviewers and do everything you can to meet them. Read what they say carefully before deciding whether to attempt the revision or submit the paper as it stands to another journal. If you do revise the paper, an important part of the resubmission is the letter to the editor. Here you should list the points raised by reviewers, explaining how you have altered the paper, or what new analyses are included, corresponding to each point. A reviewer may suggest something with which you honestly disagree. If so, after the list of amendments you have made, explain why you have not made that particular change. Such a letter, if carefully written, can be very helpful to the editor and hence to your paper's chances of acceptance.

Rejection

The 'rejection' is a narcissistic blow and you will almost certainly feel bad about it. Read the reviewers' comments as objectively as possible and ask someone else to read them too.

If the editor advises you that the paper's subject matter is outside the scope of the journal, start to think where else you can resubmit it which would be more appropriate. Also submit it to another journal if the reviewers make a number of points which can be incorporated into the text, thus improving the paper and making it more likely to be accepted the second time. If the editor advises you that the results are unsound, do not submit it to another journal until you have thought how to improve the evidence in the paper.

If you are convinced that the editor's letter and the reviews are of poor quality, superficial, have missed the point or are just plain wrong, put the whole thing aside for a few days before reading them again. If you still feel unfairly treated, you are quite entitled to write to the editor explaining why and asking for the decision to be reconsidered. If you do this, take care that your letter is based on sound argument; avoid a shrill and acrimonious tone. Never telephone, and only write after thinking it over very carefully.

If you have taken care over the research and the earlier drafts of the paper, you should not be disheartened in the face of one rejection. Remember that there are very few academic writers, however distinguished, who have not had a paper rejected. Many good papers were rejected by the first journal to which they were submitted. Some journals are much more difficult to be published in than others, so you can patiently work your way down the hierarchy until you succeed. One important point though—always get the paper retyped in the style of the journal to which you are submitting. A dog-eared manuscript clearly intended for a different journal will be at a big disadvantage from the start.

COMMON PROBLEMS

You Can't Get Started

I have already said that the most difficult thing is beginning. For some people this is so difficult that they never do, putting off the fateful day for months on end. Procrastination is probably a response to anxiety about whether one is good enough; a fear of falling short of one's ideal, of failing, of being exposed, criticised, judged, vulnerable or lonely. It can sometimes feel as if something in you is actively blocking the work, rebelling against getting on with it. Successful avoidance (which includes a range of displacement behaviours like taking on too much clinical work, getting drunk, suddenly deciding the house needs redecorating) does have a pay-off because one's anxiety level goes down. Alas, this only serves to reinforce the procrastination, which has you ever more firmly in its grip. Eventually, if you have someone else policing a deadline, there is an anguished and undignified last-minute scuffle in which, amazingly, the paper gets written. Unfortunately, for most research papers intended for publication there is no deadline at all; it is entirely your own affair. Procrastination is so deadly to productivity and so painful for the sufferer (and I speak from personal experience) that one wonders why it is so hard to relinquish. Perhaps it is because, as well as reducing anxiety in the short term, it also provides a ready-made attribution, an insurance policy against failure or criticism: 'Well, I know it isn't much good, but I only had two days to write it in'. Thus one can keep unsullied the fantasy of the perfect paper one might have written, given enough time.

The first step is to recognise these processes in oneself. The way out is to get into the habit of writing, doing it regularly. It is often helpful to set up a plan of the week's work, setting realistic goals and building in rewards for when they are achieved. What seems like an enormous task can be tackled by slicing it into small pieces and doing one at a time. Simply to put an end to the avoidance is useful. Set the time aside, find the right conditions and sit there. If you really can't get on with the paper itself, write something else—rough notes, ideas, notes on other people's papers—anything. The important thing is to be in the habit of setting pen to paper (or fingers to keyboard), to get practice at forming sentences, working with words. Even if you sit for the whole of your designated session staring at the wall, you are breaking the pattern of avoidance, starting to face the anxiety that freezes you. Since procrastination depends on self-deception, the next session will not be so difficult.

Isolation

The other major problem you are likely to face is being a lone researcher, trying single handed to carry your project to completion. Do not struggle on alone if you are getting nowhere. Find someone else with whom you can share your work, on the basis that you give them the same kind of research support. This kind of reciprocal help can include a regular meeting to talk about research issues, how the writing progresses, to set deadlines. You can read and criticise each other's papers and help with boring jobs like checking the accuracy of references and proof-reading. You then also have someone with whom you can discuss the editor's letter, someone who will congratulate or commiserate as needed.

You will find more detailed guidance about the technical issues in writing a paper by reading the books in the reference section. I hope this chapter is a springboard to them and to achieving what is, in the end, a profoundly satisfying experience; seeing your own research paper published.

REFERENCES

Barzun, J. & Graff, H. F. (1977). *The Modern Researcher*. New York: Harcourt Brace Jovanovich, Chapters 11, 12 and 13.

Bausell, R. B. (1986). Evaluating and communicating the results. In *A Practical Guide to Conducting Empirical Research*. New York: Harper and Row, Chapter 17.

Day, R. A. (1979). *How to Write and Publish a Scientific Paper*. Philadelphia: ISI Press.

Fowler, H. W. (1978). *A Dictionary of Modern English Usage*, 2nd edn. Oxford University Press.

Gowers, E. (1986). *The Complete Plain Words*, 3rd edn. London: HMSO. (Also (1987) Harmondsworth: Penguin.)

O'Connor, M. & Woodford, F. P. (1978). *Writing Scientific Papers in English*. Tunbridge Wells: Pitman Medical Publishing.

7

Writing a Grant Application

Neil Brooks
Department of Psychological Medicine, University of Glasgow.

Obtaining research grants has never been easy. With the continuing heavy decline in the Government funding for biomedical research, the situation concerning Government monies (the British Medical Research Council, DHSS, etc.) has become ever more difficult. Nevertheless, although the picture is gloomy for Government funded research, this is not the case for Charitable research. Indeed, the recent compilation of British Charities Funding Neuroscience Research (1986), identifies 24 Charities disbursing amounts from £300 to £20,000, and some Charities (e.g. the Wellcome Trust) are major rivals to Government sources of research funding.

Whatever the amount and range of sources of research money available, the fundamental exercise is one of competition. Inevitably, any researcher seeking limited funds is competing with others equally keen to obtain those same funds. While it is rare that one can identify a direct competitor—'direct' in the sense that they are seeking similar money for an identical project, there are often a number of projects in a similar area, and a deciding factor will then be quite simply the quality of the research application. The better the application the more likely it is to get funded.

Although the 'bottom line' is one of quality of research application, any experienced obtainer of research monies will admit that the process of research application is at least partly a gamble, with an element of luck. The prudent applicant is the one who reduces the odds in his/her favour, and this can be achieved by a variety of means. This chapter is essentially about ways of reducing those odds. There are some very simple strategies that are worth describing at the outset, and then the chapter will discuss a series of more detailed procedures to assist in an application.

Whatever the source of research money, an application involves a series of discrete processes. Firstly, the Officers of the funding body will check that the grant application matches the formal requirements and funding policies of that body (length of application, total amount of money requested, duration of grant, etc.). Secondly, the application will usually go to referees who will concern themselves with the quality of the science, the adequacy of the case made for the amount of money requested, and the practicalities of the application (is it possible to complete the research in the time proposed, etc.). The referees will then report back to the awarding body with the recommendation for funding or not. Some bodies add an extra stage at which requests for clarification made by referees can be fed back to applicants for their comments prior to a final decision about funding. Finally, some bodies in the event of an unsuccessful application will give feedback of varying degrees of length and detail.

Any research application must address a range of issues. For the major grant awarding bodies (in the UK, the Medical Research Council, Department of Health & Social Security, Scottish Home & Health Department, Mental Health Foundation, Wellcome Trust, etc.), these may be addressed by means of the detailed application form with its clear guidelines for submitting the proposal. The guidelines are crucial, and the applicant who fails to conform to them will quite simply not get past the first round. The exact information sought by the different fund awarding bodies varies, but a number of headings appear so consistently on the application forms that they are worth using to structure much of the rest of the chapter. Even if the applicant is applying to a body that does not have clearly specified application procedures, the headings about to be described are worth using in order to impose maximum structure and clarity on the application.

THE RESEARCH APPLICATION—HOW TO FILL IT IN

Introduction

Obviously the purpose of an application is to obtain research funding, but bearing in mind that the applicant is competing with others for limited resources, it is worth considering the different justifications which need to be made. Any applicant must justify tackling a particular problem, in a particular department, using a particular method, with a particular group of patients/subjects in a particular amount of time. Applicants will have to indicate why they themselves and those whom they hire are so crucial to the project, and must justify why the research will cost the amount of money which is being requested.

Before even beginning to submit an application, applicants must ensure that the appropriate preliminary work has been carried out. A literature review should have been done, and the applicant should know enough about the population to be studied to avoid elementary blunders. This point is a particularly important one where experimentalists are attempting to study a clinical population. Lack of experience with that population can result in the submission of an inappropriate project simply because of failure to appreciate the constraints imposed by the condition (e.g. examining higher visual processing in Alzheimer's disease without examining visual acuity first, etc.). At this early stage it is well worth discussing ideas and tentative proposals with as many colleagues as possible. This is the stage at which the clinician seeks the views of the theoretician and vice versa, and detailed and honest discussion here can prevent future disasters. As a result of these discussions it may become obvious that the first stage of the research is to carry out a small pilot study to identify problems and propose solutions. Pilot studies are seldom wasted, and many research referees expect to see evidence that methods and procedures have indeed been piloted.

Often during this early stage the researcher is not sure whether the research topic fits within the ambit of a particular grant awarding body. In addition, there may be problems in understanding exactly what is required in the application, and this is the stage at which to seek advice from the officers of the body awarding funds. A telephone call here may save hours of needless work in the future. The call may identify that the resources of the grant awarding body are too small for the project. It may indicate that the research area being proposed is one that the body does not wish to support, or alternatively, that it is one that has a high priority. It may result in helpful advice about 'marketing' a particular application. If in doubt, telephone.

Before considering detailed headings for the application, there are a number of other points to bear in mind in attempting to make the strongest application. Referees will need to know details about the applicants themselves, the Institution from which they are working, and the justification for the timing of the application.

It goes without saying that applicants must state who they are and what their relevant qualifications are. However, applicants should go beyond this. They shoud be able to communicate to the referees a sense of why it is that the applicants and *only* those applicants are so uniquely well qualified to obtain the research award. Applicants should not hesitate to spell out details of particular qualifications or particular past or current experience that bear on the current application. In addition, they should identify any research collaborators. Many referees and many sources of research funding are keen to develop collaborative interdisciplinary research. Indeed, research that marries the skills of a theoretician and clinician can be particularly valuable, and conversely, failure of a theoretician to secure access to a clinical population can simply prevent research being carried out. Similarly, failure to secure access to a computer or to data processing expertise can equally prevent research succeeding. Access to high-quality enthusiastic help can tip the balance in favour of funding an application. The wise applicant chooses his/her collaborators with care.

Not only must applicants state who they are and with whom they are co-operating, but they will also need to spell out the nature of their institution. The referees will want to know where the research is to be based (university, clinical service department, etc.), and will need to be assured that the base is an ideal one for the proposed research. Relevant links with other institutions can with benefit be spelt out here, and letters of support from other institutions can always be included in an appendix. As a practical point, the awarding body will need to be assured that the host institution will administer financial aspects of the research (salaries, purchasing, etc.), and it is increasingly the case that institutions are charging for such a service. Does the host institution charge, and if so, will the grant awarding body meet such a charge?

There is a further point to bear in mind here. With performance indicators assuming ever greater importance in the public sector, it has recently become known that in the UK the University Grants Committee block grant to universities will be based at least in part on the value of Research Council and similar peer-review funded awards obtained by the researchers within the university. Quite obviously some institutions and departments may suffer gravely as a result of this, but others may benefit considerably. Assuming that this system does indeed happen and continues for some time, then the scope for negotiation within universities is obvious. The research worker who brings in a substantial grant is directly benefiting his/her university, and may reasonably expect the university to benefit the researcher in turn. It will no longer be enough for universities to tell enthusiastic researchers that equipment purchase or laboratory refur- bishing or hiring of extra staff is simply not possible. It is very likely that the whole process of accepting major awards will change, with researchers who have obtained a major grant, delaying formal acceptance of that grant until bargains have been struck with Finance Officers in the universities.

There are two aspects of timing that are important. The first is the total amount of time for which the grant will be held, and the second is the amount of time that the applicant him/herself will be able to devote specifically to the project. Obviously the longer the project, the more expensive, so referees are particularly careful to scrutinise the justification for the length of time involved. If applicants are requesting funding for 3 years, but have not made a good case for this period, then referees are likely to advise that the research simply not be funded, or that funding be awarded for a 2- rather than 3-year period.

Referees will also be interested to know how much time the applicant will be able to devote specifically to the actual research, or to supervision of researchers employed on the award. Experienced referees are well aware that active researchers manage to find 25 hours in every 24, but if it is obvious that the nature of the applicant's other duties mean that he/she simply cannot spend the proposed amount of time on the grant, then this may well count against them in deciding on an award.

A thorny problem in deciding on the length of the award is the amount of time that should be devoted specifically and exclusively to data analysis and writing up the results. Grant awarding bodies differ in the extent to which they see these activities as crucial parts of the research, or as addenda which can be dealt with after funding has stopped. A careful reading of the guidelines for submission, and if necessary a telephone call to Officers of the body awarding the money can be invaluable here.

Headings For The Application

Abstract.   Many bodies demand a simple abstract of the research, and this is usually the first thing that referees read. It gives the applicant an early opportunity to communicate clear thinking and excitement at pursuing an interesting project. The abstract should be brief, it should not over-run the number of words allowed in the guidelines for submission. It should be clear and informative, and should give a flavour of what is intended and why. An example of such an abstract is given below:

'Although anecdotal evidence that . . . exists, there is little empirical support for this. Our research proposes to investigate . . . by means of . . . in . . . patients. Our results should provide evidence that . . . .'

Background and Purpose of Research.   This substantial section is where the applicant addresses the main conceptual and clinical issues, and communicates the sense of excitement and commitment which in its turn will excite referees. It incorporates the relevant literature review, and allows applicants to make the case that there is a crucial gap in knowledge that is important enough to be filled, and that only the applicant with his/her techniques and ideas can fill it. The background should be written with the knowledge that the application will be read by referees who may be as knowledgeable as the applicant, and will be able to detect major omissions, padding, incorrect citing of references, and inappropriate conclusions. Bearing this in mind, the background should be as brief as possible, consistent with the guidelines for applicants, and with the need to communicate effectively. There is often a temptation to stray into areas that are not relevant, but which signal some aspects of the applicant's knowledge. This can only detract from the main central case.

This section of the application is one which referees often find very difficult to read. Applicants in their enthusiasm may present a closely argued and densely written case which is difficult for referees to follow. Applicants should try to help referees as much as possible by using a clear and logical structure to this section, with headings and subheadings, and a clear flow of ideas. At the end of the section, the applicant should be able to state a series of simple aims or questions or hypotheses, and ideally the background should have been so well structured that the knowledgeable referee should almost be able to complete the end of this section him/herself.

Plan of Investigation. In this section, the applicant can spell out in detail the precise methods and procedures to be used, and the population of subjects or cases under investigation. Referees will expect the applicant to specify the exact procedures that are to be used, and to justify why these rather than other related and apparently equally appropriate procedures are not to be used. Applicants should try to be honest in identifying procedures that are up and running, and those that are being developed or have yet to be developed. If development work is required, then estimates of the likely timescale of this development should be included. Inevitably and quite appropriately, the methods will often incorporate novel procedures which have not been used before, or not with the specific population to be studied. The fact that procedures are novel may be very positive, but it also means that problems such as reliability and validity of procedures become important. A procedure that is appropriate for a 4-year-old child may not be appropriate for a mentally handicapped adult, etc. If very novel procedures are to be used, applicants must consider how reliable they are likely to be in the new population, and how accurately they are likely to measure the underlying processes being addressed in the application. When such novel procedures are being used, it is always worth including some conventional laboratory or clinical procedures which are known to work, and which would then act as 'marker variables' for the new procedures.

Precise details of the population under study should be given. Referees need to know how many subjects are to be studied, and will often expect a justification for the number chosen. Applicants, before writing this section, should ask themselves exactly how they arrived at the number of cases they proposed to study. Was it simply a convenient figure; a figure based on the size of the population; a figure based on statistical theory, etc? Not only should numbers be given, but the defining features of the population must be described. Ages, volunteer status, diagnostic categories and criteria, chronicity, etc., are all important. Applicants should also spell out how often and over what duration the subjects will be seen, and by whom. For example, is the researcher him/herself going to carry out the studies, or will it be wholly or partly in the hands of a research assistant? If the latter, is the assistant already competent, or will specific training be given?

Finally, in clinical studies, the researcher often identifies clinical problems that have been missed in the routine clinical follow-up of patients. This faces the applicants with ethical and practical questions, and the wise applicant will have a policy for dealing with hitherto undetected clinical problems. If a decision is made to try to deal with the problems by the applicants themselves, then they must consider the extent to which this is ethically appropriate (is the applicant qualified, etc?); practically appropriate (are there others able and willing and competent to undertake clinical management?); and conceptually appropriate (will intervention by the researchers compromise the research design?). As a general rule, it is unwise for the researchers themselves to take on the management of clinical problems, and at the outset they should open lines of communication with clinical colleagues to enable patients to receive appropriate management wherever necessary.

Data analysis.   Whenever a research design involves very straightforward data analysis, this section can be dealt with very briefly. If, however, the researcher is going to generate a substantial data base involving more than simple univariate analyses, applicants may have to spell out in some considerable detail how they propose to set up and manage the data base. If statistical help is going to be needed, applicants have to show that this is available, and that is is either free of charge, or can be paid for out of the research grant. If the results are to be analysed by means of a mainframe computer, applicants should demonstrate that they have ready access to the machine, and will have to budget appropriately for the cost of computing time. Some grant-giving bodies are reluctant to pay for computing costs, and applicants should ascertain the policy of the body before preparing the computing budget.

Frequently, research applicants make a common error in this section of the application. The effor is to deal very sweepingly with data analysis, saying rather grandly that 'data analysis will be by means of multivariate analysis'. Such a reference to multivariate analysis is unrevealing, and may raise suspicions in the minds of the referee that applicants have not in fact thought at all clearly about how they propose to handle the mass of data collected. It is rarely the case that multivariate analysis is the initial approach of choice, although with large data bases it will inevitably be *one* of the appropriate approaches to be employed.

Ethical and legal considerations.   Any study carried out from a university or clinical base and involving patients will need to go through some form of ethical vetting. Clinically based submissions will need to have been cleared by the relevant hospital or unit Ethical Committee, and university and similar applications by the relevant departmental ethical committee. Such processes can take time, and ideally, ethical permission should be obtained in the very preliminary stages of the research application.

Although it is rare for experiments involving volunteer adults to pose ethical problems, problems do arise as soon as the researcher studies groups who cannot readily give informed consent (children, handicapped, confused elderly, etc.). In these situations the researcher has to show that procedures are available to deal with ethical problems that may arise. Such procedures, together with approval from the relevant Ethical Committee, should always be appended with an application.

Recently in the UK, a further problem has arisen, and this is the Data Protection Act which is designed to protect personal data held in information repositories. Clinical data collected for research purposes may well come within the restrictions imposed by the Act, and may demand two separate registrations (one from within the University, and one from within the Health Service). Institutions such as hospital and universities will almost certainly have a Data Protection Officer from whom advice can be sought, and if applicants have any doubts about the restrictions and obligations placed upon them by the Act, they should seek advice early in the research application. A formal statement of how applicants will deal with their obligations under the Act can only enhance an application.

Financial Aspects.   The application is designed to obtain money, and the money will be used mainly for hiring staff and purchasing equipment. Some bodies will only fund salaries; others only equipment. Some may have special schemes for purchasing a specific piece of equipment for a specific research project. Applicants should ascertain the policy of the body on funding. Both staff and equipment need to be justified in detail to show that without the exact staff and exact equipment proposed, the research could not be carried out. Applicants have to make a case for the type of staff they wish to employ (postgraduate or postdoctoral researchers, etc.), and also, the level within the particular salary scale. Applicants frequently try to save money by quoting a starting salary for research staff which is at the bottom of a scale. As soon as they interview staff they find that the ones they want to hire will have to be paid some increments up the scale, but the money is simply not available. A case for extra funding has to be made, and this takes time and may not always be successful. A realistic appraisal of the needs of the research (in terms of level of staff, etc.) at the outset can prevent problems of this type later on.

Obviously, applicants should aim to pare costs down as much as possible, but to do so without making the research impossible to carry out. For example, if medically qualified staff are to be hired, this may well need an extra justification, as such staff tend to be more expensive than non-clinical. In situations in which two or three staff are to be hired, it may be worth phasing their hiring over a period rather than hiring all at once. Often there is not enough work for all staff members at the beginning, and the volume of work increases steadily as the grant gets underway. In this situation, phased hiring of staff may be advantageous scientifically as well as financially prudent. Wherever it is possible to save money, applicants should do so, but *without* jeopardising the scientific quality of the research.

Similarly with equipment, the aim is to cut costs as much as possible, while still allowing the research to take place. Equipment must be described and justified, and the case made to say why a specific piece of equipment is necessary rather than a cheaper alternative. In the UK there is a continuing decline in UGC funding for buildings and equipment (although see earlier comments about the block grant). This results in a temptation for applicants to use a research grant as an opportunity to re-equip a laboratory, or to buy top quality equipment when a simpler and cheaper version would do perfectly well. Referees invariably scrutinise equipment requests very carefully, and often suggest pruning in this area to allow applicants to buy equipment that is sufficient for the research, but no more than that.

DISCUSSION

Inevitably, many applicants will fail to obtain research funding, and often there is a very simple reason for this. The first reason is that the research was not good enough. The second is that although the research is fully up to standard, there was not enough money available. The third is that the research topic does not fall within the ambit of the grant awarding body, and the fourth is that the research, while good enough, cheap enough, and appropriate to the awarding body, was presented in such a way that it failed to communicate adequately.

While these may be concrete reasons for failure to receive a grant, rejected applicants may consider themselves hard done by, and console themselves with a variety of common defences. Two are particularly frequent. The first is that the referees simply did not take the trouble to read the research carefully enough. Obviously there are occasions when the referees have been incompetent; but usually referees take their job seriously, and referee applications with care. The second common defence is to say that referees had a personal bias against the applicant or his/her particular area of research. Only the foolish would deny that this never happens, but the system regarding the larger grant awarding bodies builds in a range of checks and balances. For example, in the UK the Medical

Research Council uses both external and internal referees. The external referees are drawn from a very large panel, while the internal referees comprise members of the relevant Grants Committee, and membership of such Committees is public information which applicants should obtain. In this sort of situation of internal and external refereeing, personal or professional bias soon becomes obvious, and the biased referee is unlikely to be asked for an opinion in the future.

If an application has been submitted and rejected, it is obviously disappointing for the applicant, but the situation can be helped by means of feedback. Differing grant awarding bodies have very different policies about feedback, ranging from absolutely no information at all other than a statement of failure, to detailed summaries of referee's comments, or indeed copies of the comments themselves. There is a natural tendency for rejected applicants to argue against such comments, or to use them as a basis for a dialogue of the 'he said I did—I say I did not' variety, but this is likely to be counterproductive. If at all possible, applicants should read and listen to critical comments dispassionately and positively, and try to use such comments as a basis for a strategy for submission of a considerably strengthened application elsewhere.

SOURCES OF FUNDING

Major grant awarding bodies are well known. These include the British Research Councils (MRC, ESRC), the American Institutes (e.g. Health, Mental Health, etc.) various Government Departments or Government sponsored organisations (DHSS, SHHD), and Charities and the like. The first two sources of money have clearly specified procedures, detailed application forms, officers who are informed and helpful, and an understanding of the problems in setting up and running a research study. The charities range enormously from medical charities, such as the Wellcome Trust, which functions in a manner very similar to the Medical Research Council, to those that may be disbursing small amounts of money on an irregular basis. It is impossible to give a detailed list of grant awarding bodies in a chapter like this (see Appendix 1 for a range of possible sources of funding) but a very useful directory has been complipled by Villemur (1983), and a very recent up-to-date list of UK Charities funding specifically neuroscience research has been published (British Charities Funding Neuroscience Research, 1986). These are two particularly valuable sources of information. A further very helpful publication is by Burcham and Rutherfurd (1985) which discusses successful grant obtaining strategies, and gives examples of successful applications. This is highly recommended.

Despite problems with shrinking funds for research, it is important to be aware that psychological research is still being carried out, and successful applicants are being awarded substantial sums of money. A brief letter in the *Bulletin of the British Psychological Society* asking researchers to supply details of research monies held resulted in replies from six researchers giving details about projects attracting support ranging from £2000 to £75,000. The sources of funding included the conventional Research Councils, the Wellcome Trust, the Mental Health Foundation, the Leverhume Trust, DHSS, SHHD, the Parkinson's Disease Society, NATO, and Sainsburys. For the right projects directed to the right body, money is still available.

REFERENCES

British Charities Funding Neuroscience Research (1986). *Trends in The Neurosciences*, **9**, viii–ix.

Burcham, W. E. & Rutherford, R. J. D. (1985). *Writing Applications for Research Grants.* Educational Development Advisory Committee Occasional Publication, No. 3. University of Birmingham. (For further information contact Dr Rutherford at Advisory Service on Teaching Methods, University of Birmingham, Birmingham B15 2TT.)

Villemur, A. (ed.) (1983). *Directory of Grant-Making Trusts.* Tonbridge, Kent: Charities Aid Foundation.

APPENDIX: SOME SOURCES OF RESEARCH FUNDING

Alzheimer's Disease Society,
Third Floor, Bank Buildings,
Fulham Broadway,
London SW6 IEP.   Tel: 01 381 3177

Association for Spina Bifida and
Hydrocephalus,
22 Woburn Place,
London WC1H OEP.   Tel: 01 388 1382

Association to Combat Huntington's Chorea,
34a Station Road,
Hinckley, Leicestershire LE10 1AP.   Tel: 0455 615558

Back Pain Association,
31–33 Park Road,
Teddington, Middlesex TW11 OAB.   Tel: 01 977 5474/5

British Diabetic Association,
10 Queen Anne Street,
London W1M OBD.   Tel: 01 323 1531

British Foundation for Age Research,
49 Queen Victoria Street,
London EC4N 4SA.   Tel: 01 236 4365

British Migraine Association,
178A High Street,
Byfleet,
Weybridge, Surrey KT14 7ED.   Tel: 09323 52468

Cancer Research Campaign,
2 Carlton House Terrace,
London SDW1Y 5AR.   Tel: 01 930 8972

The Chest Heart and Stroke Association,
Tavistock House North,
Tavistock Square,
London WC1E 9JE.   Tel: 01 387 3012

Children Nationwide Medical Research Fund,
Nicholas House, 181 Union Street,
London SE1 0LN.   Tel: 01 928 2425

Department of Health and Social Security,
Alexander Fleming House,
Elephant & Castle,
London.   Tel: 01 407 5522

Education and Social Research Council,
1 Temple Avenue,
London EC4Y OBD.   Tel: 01 353 5252

The Epilepsy Association of Scotland,
48 Govan Road,
Glasgow G51 1JL.   Tel: 041 427 4911

Foundation for the Study of Infant Deaths
5th Floor, 4 Grosvenor Place,
London SW1X 7HD.   Tel: 01 235 1721

Iris Fund for the Prevention of Blindness,
York House (ground floor),
199 Westminster Bridge Road,
London SE1 7UT.   Tel: 01 928 7743

Medical Research Council,
20 Park Cresent,
London W1N 4AL.   Tel: 01 636 5422

The Mental Health Foundation,
8 Hallam Street,
London W1N 6DH.   Tel: 01 580 0145

The Migraine Trust,
45 Great Ormond Street,
London WC1N 3HD.   Tel: 01 278 2676

The Multiple Sclerosis Society of Great
Britain and Northern Ireland,
25 Effie Road, Fulham,
London SW6 1EE.   Tel: 01 381 4022

The Muscular Dystrophy Group of Great
Britain and Northern Ireland,
Nattrass House,
35 Macaulay Road,
London SW4 0QP.   Tel: 01 720 8055

National Fund for Research into Crippling
Diseases,
Vincent House,
North Parade,
Horsham, West Sussex RH12 2DA.   Tel: 0403 64101

National Schizophrenia Fellowship,
78 Victoria Road,
Surbiton, Surrey KT6 4NS.   Tel: 01 390 3651

Parkinson's Disease Society of the
United Kingdon,
36 Portland Place,
London W1N 3DG.   Tel: 01 323 1174

Royal National Institute of the Blind,
224 Great Portland Street,
London W1N 6AA.   Tel: 01 388 1266

Schizophrenia Association of Great Britain,
International Schizophrenia Centre,
Bryn Hyfryd, The Crescent,
Bangor, Gwynedd, Wales.   Tel: 0248 354048

Scottish Home and Health Department,
Chief Scientist Office,
St. Andrew's House,
Edinburgh EH1 3DE.   Tel: 031 556 8501

Spastics Society,
12 Park Crescent, London W1N 4EQ.   Tel: 01 636 5020

The Wellcome Trust,
1 Park Square West,
London NW1 4LJ.   Tel: 01 486 4902

Part II: Methods

8 Experimental Abnormal Psychology

Fraser N. Watts
MRC Applied Psychology Unit, Cambridge CB2 2EF.

Experimental abnormal psychology is concerned with the investigation of the psychological dysfunctions of patients with mental health problems. Many such patients show impairment of a wide range of psychological functions, so it is relatively easy to select a psychological task and to demonstrate that a clinical group performs less well at it than a control group. This is especially true of people suffering from schizophrenia (Neale & Oltmanns, 1980) or depression (Watts, 1988) as these have a broad impact on psychological functioning. At this level, experimental psychology is easy, indeed *too* easy, to do.

The challenge is to carry out an experiment that does more than add to the catalogue of psychological dysfunctions shown in a particular group of patients. To meet this challenge, you need a good reason for choosing to study a particular dysfunction. The key difference between worthwhile and trivial studies in experimental abnormal psychology lies in the rationale for the experiment. No amount of technical competence in the execution of the experiment makes up for not having a good reason for doing it.

There can be various reasons for choosing to study a particular dysfunction. This chapter will be organised around three such reasons.

First, you may select a particular dysfunction for study because it is a prominent symptom of the condition that you wish to treat. The reason for investigating it lies in the hope that understanding it better will enable you to treat it. A variant of this strategy is to select for investigation a dysfunction that is a close analogue of the symptom of therapeutic interest, but this raises difficult issues about the choice of the right analogue.

A second possible reason for studying a particular dysfunction is more theoretical. To help in reaching a theoretical formulation of a particular condition, you may want to know what are the most striking impairments of the patients concerned. Identifying specific tasks which are affected particularly severely may guide you towards a theory of the disorder concerned. A key technical issue here, as we shall see, is demonstrating clearly that patients are significantly more impaired on the task of interest than on a related control task.

Thirdly, a researcher may focus on a particular dysfunction because he or she has a hypothesis that it plays an important part in the aetiology of the clinical condition in which it is found, or that it influences the risk of relapse after symptomatic improvement. Such 'vulnerability' factors are important both theoretically and practically. They make an important contribution to understanding the nature of the disorder; they also indicate where preventive clinical work should be targeted.

These three rationales for studying particular dysfunctions will be considered in turn. Space does not permit a more general discussion of the design of psychological experiments, though these are obviously relevant to abnormal psychology. Kerlinger (1973) may be useful on experimental design and Barber (1979) on common pitfalls.

RESEARCH ON CLINICALLY IMPORTANT DYSFUNCTIONS

If a dysfunction is selected for study because of its clinical importance, in the hope that better understanding will have implications for treatment, two alternative strategies are available. One is to do experimental research on the target dysfunction itself; the other is to select for initial investigation a close analogue of the target dysfunction. For example, if learned helplessness (Garber & Seligman, 1980) is a close analogue of depression, studying learned helplessness in detail may have important implications for clinical work with depressed people.

Analogues can be classified on various dimensions. Firstly there is the range of subjects in whom the analogue is found. Some analogues are laboratory phenomena found only in the group of patients concerned, not in the normal population. An intermediate situation is where the analogue phenomenon is found in a sub-group of non-patients with personality characteristics somewhat similar to those of the patients concerned. For example, people with obsessional personalities may provide phenomena which are a useful analogue of symptoms found in obsessional patients. Secondly, there is the dimension of the closeness of the analogue phenomenon to the clinical phenomenon. For example, intrusive, repetitive, adhesive, upsetting thoughts in non-patients may be considered a close analogue of obsessional ruminations, and have 'face validity' as such. Lack of confidence in performance on a reality monitoring task (in which subjects have to distinguish events that have been externally supplied from those that have been internally generated) is a less obvious but nevertheless interesting, analogue of the checking problems of obsessionals (Sher, Frost & Otto, 1983). A third distinction between analogues concerns whether they occur naturally, or whether, like learned helplessness, they are experimentally created.

The reasons for choosing to study experimental research on analogues of clinical phenomena rather than on the phenomena themselves are not difficult to discern. Firstly, laboratory analogues are more tractable. More reliable measures can be obtained, background conditions can be manipulated more readily, and so on, Secondly, by choosing the kind of measure that has been studied in general experimental psychology, a large body of knowledge and theory relating to those measures becomes immediately applicable. The application of experimental psychology to the study of the psychological functioning of clinical groups is thus facilitated.

However, there are also reasons to be cautious about this strategy of studying 'analogue' tasks (i.e. tasks that are interesting because they appear to be an analogue of clinical phenomena). In experimental research, minor changes to a task can make a decisive difference to whether or not a particular phenomenon is demonstrable. If the phenomenon does not generalise from one laboratory paradigm to another slightly different one, the chances of it generalising from the laboratory to the outside world are not good. Further, there are many clinical phenomena that are known to be powerfully affected by the social context. For example, compulsive checking is generally much worse when patients are on their own. For similar reasons, the artificial context of the laboratory will often be unlikely to produce a good analogue of some clinical phenomena. Similarly, some clinical phenomena, such as responses to threat, may only be manifest in the context of really significant threats that cannot be manufactured in the laboratory.

These concerns certainly do not provide grounds for the condemnation of all analogue research in experimental abnormal psychology. The situation is parallel to that which obtains for evaluations of treatments with 'analogue' populations. Borkovec and Rachman (1979) have argued that the generalisation of results from treatment research with 'analogue' subjects depends less on whether they have the administrative status of patients than on the nature and intensity of the problems they present. Similarly, a particular analogue dysfunction can be considered as a candidate for research on its merits. Some will repay study, others will not.

The issues can be illustrated in connections with Hemsley's (1977) instructive review of the possible relationships between the symptomatol-

TABLE 8.1

Possible relationships between clinical phenomena and adaptations to information overload (from Hemsley, 1977; reproduced by permission of the *British Journal of Psychiatry*)

Method of adaptation	Clinical phenomena
Errors intrusion of associated responses	Inappropriate responding Incoherence of speech
Omission lowered responsiveness Raised threshold for response	Under responsiveness* Poverty of speech* Flatness of affect*
Approximation simplified categorising system. Several stimuli elicit the same response rather than there being a differentiated response to each	Undifferentiated responding Delusions
Escape reduction of exploratory responses. Avoidance of situations of high information load	Social withdrawal* Catatonic symptoms
Queuing delayed responding	Retardation
Filtering increased attention of certain classes of sensory input	Narrowed attention*

*More prominent in chronic patients.

ogy of schizophrenics and types of responses to information overload (Table 8.1). The question is how close are the analogies between the two columns of this figure? How similar, for example, are the phenomena found in schizophrenics' performance in a laboratory card-sorting task to clinical symptoms of over-inclusive thinking? Such questions require more careful empirical investigation than has generally occurred. It would be relevant to know the magnitude of the correlation between the occurrence of the clinical symptoms and the laboratory phenomena; also how similar are the situational conditions that influence the occurrence of the two sets of phenomena.

Perhaps one of the analogue phenomena that has been studied most fruitfully in recent years is the relative accessibility of positive and negative memory in depression. It is a common clinical observation that depressed people are likely to dwell on negative things about themselves and neglect positive ones. This probably applies to various kinds of thought content, but it is often best to choose one example that you hope will prove paradigmatic and to study it in detail. Recent research has focused on the relative accessibility of positive and negative memories, and has provided abundant evidence that memories are biased towards those that are congruent with mood (e.g. Teasdale, 1983).

Such research needs to make assumptions about exactly how an experimental task parallels a clinical phenomenon. For example, it is assumed that what is found for autobiographical events will also be true of 'supplied' materials in laboratory experiments. It is also assumed that latency of recall when people *try* to recall material in the laboratory is an indication of the likelihood of their recalling such material spontaneously in real life. Unfortunately, such assumptions are often made only tacitly and it is simply assumed, without discussion or evidence, that the analogy between an experimental result and a phenomenon of direct clinical interest is close.

Analogue research should exploit its potential to clarify issues that are not clear from clinical observation. For example, if people are clinically depressed, both when negative events occur and when they remember them, it is not clear whether it is a mood at encoding or mood at retrieval which is responsible for the effect. By using mood induction procedures to create depressed mood at encoding but not at retrieval, it is possible to disentangle the processes that produce the mood congruency effect. Another issue concerns the size of the pool of memories on which people draw when remembering particular events. It might be argued that depressed people remember negative events relatively frequently simply because more such things have happened to them. To rule out this explanation, it is necessary to work with a pool of memories of known size. For this purpose, memory for a specially constructed list of hedonically biased words can be studied.

If the investigation of an analogue of a clinically important target variable is to be really worthwhile, it should be carried to the point where it does more than simply demonstrate in the laboratory what most clinicians thought they know already from direct observation. Rather, research should seek to advance our understanding of how and why the phenomenon arises, in a way that has treatment implications. Research on the effects of mood on the accessibility of personal memories is only just reaching this point—after 10 years. It is now clear that the difficulty that depressed patients have in recalling positive events arises at the stage of accessing a *specific* positive event (Williams & Broadbent, 1986). Depressed people are able to recall general classes of positive events, but these probably have less impact on mood than accessing specific events. We are close to the point of understanding enough about cues for autobiographical memories (Rubin, 1986), and where problems arise for depressives, to be able to suggest retrievial strategies they could use to recall more easily the positive things that have happened to them.

One class of clinical phenomena for which it is particularly difficult to find a good analogue are those that are qualitatively different from anything that occurs in the normal population, rather than being a quantitative extension of a problem that is continuously distributed through the normal population. Psychotic symptoms are the most obvious example of the former, and present a particular problem for the application of experimental psychology derived from the normal population. However, even where it *appears* that a clinical symptom is just an extension of a phenomenon that occurs in the normal population, the processes underlying it may be quite different. The avoidance of social situations by a paranoid patient might look like an extension of the social avoidance of a "normal" shy introvert, but this would probably be a misleading assumption. Superficial analogies between clinical symptoms and phenomena found in the normal population often break down on close examination. However, it is sometimes possible to find unusual conditions under which qualitatively distinct clinical symptoms begin to be demonstrable in normal subjects.

Shapiro (1960) has provided an instructive discussion, illustrating this latter point, of the effects on visual perception of parietal–occipital lobe damage demonstrated by Bender and Teuber (1949). There were four principle phenomena: (a) a decrease in the intensity of percepts, (b) systematic changes in space values, (c) a tendency to see objects as smaller than they really were, and (d) increased fluctuation in visual thresholds. Because these phenomena were produced in normals by prolonged stimulation, Bender and Teuber hypothesised that very brief stimulation might reduce or eliminate the perceptual abnormalities of their parietal–occipital patients. Their results confirmed this prediction, with the exception of the size distortion phenomenon. It thus seems that a quantitative change in exposure durations regulates the appearance of a qualitatively distinct perceptual phenomena. All that is needed is the assumption of a different threshold in the brain-damaged patients.

A similar approach has been taken to formulating a psychological model of hallucinations, another phenomenon that is apparently qualitatively distinct from anything that occurs in normals (Slade, 1976). In fact, there is evidence that hallucinations can be induced, at least in people with a history of hallucinations, by physiological manipulations such as hyperventilation. This argues for the role of physiological arousal in inducing hallucinations. Though such interventions are apparently not sufficient to induce hallucinations in all people, those who are prone to hallucinations may not be qualitatively distinct from the rest of the population. Mintz and Alpert (1972) have proposed that high scores on two dimensions with continuous distributions in the normal population, vivid mental imagery and poor reality testing, constitute this predisposition to hallucinations.

Another component in Slade's model comes from subsuming hallucinations under the more generally occurring category of task-irrelevant thoughts. These are increased in the normal population by psychological distress, and by situations where tasks being undertaken require relatively little processing resources, and this has been shown to be true of hallucinations too. Desensitisation to sources of psychological stress, and increasing the demands made by a concurrent task, both reduce the frequency of hallucinations. This multi-component theory of hallucinations provides a good example of how the study of psychological parameters in normal people can be applied to the explanation of a qualitatively distinct phenomenon. Both here and in the work of Bender and Teuber discussed above, theorising based on general psychology has led to direct experimental work on the psychological symptom concerned.

If the objective of experimental research on clinical symptoms (or their analogues) is to suggest treatment strategies, the central objective must be to bring the symptom under experimental control. Because general experimental psychology is largely devoted to investigating the conditions under which psychological phenomena occur, it is highly relevant to this enterprise. Understanding how to control a phenomenon in the laboratory can suggest how to 'treat' it in the clinic.

DIFFERENTIAL DEFICIT HYPOTHESES

Next, I shall consider investigation of dysfunctions which are interesting because they are particularly severe, and can be shown to be significantly greater than deficits among similar tasks. Demonstrations of differences between a clinical and a control group on a task are much more interesting theoretically if it is also shown that the groups do not differ (or differ less) on a control task. Thus the relevance of judgements of body size to anorexia are much clearer if it is known that it is *just* body judgements that are distorted. If all size judgements were equally distorted it would be much less clear how this was related to a clinical condition characterised specifically by reduced body weight. Similarly, an attentional disorder has been postulated as being fundamental to schizophrenia and it has been predicted that schizophrenics will be especially impaired on tasks where they are subject to distraction. However, for the relevance of this to be clear a control condition is needed so that it can be demonstrated that the deficit in performance is greater under conditions of distraction than without it. Without such controls, the demonstration of psychological deficit in a patient group is too poorly specified to be theoretically interesting. For example, it seems that some of the supposedly specific deficits that researchers claim to have demonstrated in schizophrenia might be due to nothing more than the fact that it takes schizophrenics longer than controls to learn to perform optimally on almost all psychological tasks. Familiarity with materials has quite a powerful effect on task performance (Baron & Treiman, 1980) and many of the chronic schizophrenics studied have probably under-performed on particular tasks solely for this reason. Interpretations of results that assume that a specific deficit has been demonstrated may thus miss the point.

We will now consider some of the technical problems of design and interpretation that arise in seeking to demonstrate specific (or 'differential') deficits.

First, if you wish to demonstrate that a deficit is specific to a particular clinical group, the choice of control groups is crucial. If a 'normal' control group is used, care must be taken to ensure that it does not differ in unintended ways from the clinical groups. For example, no good can come from comparing a depressed and a normal group on memory if the groups also differ on intelligence. However, an appropriate 'normal' control group is insufficient if you wish to claim that a specific deficit is unique to a particular clinical group. For example, if you want to claim that a particular deficit is unique to schizophrenia and may explain schizophrenic symptoms, it is necessary to show that it is not also found in depression (Chapman & Chapman, 1973a).

Suppose that we wish to test the hypothesis that depressed patients are more impaired, relative to controls, in memory for positive materials than for neutral materials. The experiment might be arranged so that each subject was tested on both kinds of material. This has two advantages over the alternative arrangement in which two different groups of depressed subjects (and two different control groups) are tested on the two memory measures. One is the practical advantage that fewer subjects need to be recruited; the other is that it eliminates at a stroke the problems of ensuring that the two depressed groups are comparable (e.g. equally depressed, etc.). The snag is that testing subjects on one measure may influence their performance on the next. There may be either practice effects or fatigue effects. Usually these can be dealt with by 'counterbalancing' the order of the tests, i.e. some subjects have one test first and some the other. However, this solution breaks down in the case where the practice effect is asymmetrical i.e. where test (a) leads to an improvement on test (b) when it is given subsequently, but test (b) has less effect on test (a). Such asymmetrical transfer effects certainly occur (Poulton, 1982) and they can only be dealt with by having a design in which each subject is given only one test. However, it is generally reasonable, at least in a preliminary experiment, to give both tests to the same subjects and to evaluate statistically whether transfer has occurred.

An experiment of this kind is likely to lead to statistical tests employing a two-way analysis of variance (see Chapter 5). Such an analysis yields three main statistical tests. First, there will be the 'main effect' of subjects. In the present example, this would indicate that depressed subjects performed worse *overall*. This may well be the case, but will be of little theoretical interest as depressed patients tend to be at least slightly impaired on so many functions. Next, there will be the 'main effect' of tests, which, unlike the previous one, will probably be a 'within-subjects' main effect that is computed differently from a 'between-subjects' one. In the present example, this would refer to whether all subjects taken together tend to do better at one memory test than the other. This would probably not be the case, but, even if it were, it would not be of direct relevance to abnormal psychology. The interesting test in the analysis would be the *interaction* between groups and tests. It is here then that the prediction that depressed patients are more impaired, relative to normals, in remembering positive than neutral material would be tested.

A great deal of contemporary experimental psychology is built on predictions relating to such interaction effects. In abnormal psychology, one of the tems in the interaction almost always concerns different groups of subjects (a clinical and a control group), though in general psychology other kinds of interaction are tested too. Hypotheses concerning interaction effects in abnormal psychology are sometimes termed 'differential deficit' hypotheses, i.e. that a clinical group is relatively more impaired on one task than on another. A closely related statistical approach to testing a differential deficit hypothesis is to examine the *difference* between each subject's scores on the two measures using a one-way analysis of variance (or a 't' test) to compare groups on this difference score. This is mathematically equivalent to the interaction term in a two-way analysis of variance but, because it provides fewer cell means, provides a less useful description of the results of the experiment. Because a significant interaction term can mean so many things, it is essential to report the means for the various conditions. *Post-hoc* tests to compare two means should also be used if it is to be claimed that they differ significantly. It is also often helpful for the researcher to plot out the interaction effect as a graph. The analysis of variance alone is not enough.

The research literature on differential deficits, as Chapman and Chapman (1978) concluded at the end of a review, is 'rather a mess'. Though studies testing such hypotheses have been extremely common, the majority have been methodologically unsound and have probably drawn incorrect conclusions. Too few research workers have yet grasped the problems and what needs to be done to remedy them. The issues are complex and technical, and it will not be possible here to provide more than a general introduction. Unfortunately, there is not yet complete agreement on the most appropriate solution. More detailed discussions of this issue have been published in relation to schizophrenia (Chapman & Chapman, 1973b, Chapter 4; Chapman & Chapman, 1978) mental handicap (Chapman & Chapman, 1974) children (Bogartz, 1976), and the elderly (Kausler, 1982, Chapter 5). More general discussions have been published by Chapman and Chapman (1973c), Loftus (1978) and Baron and Treiman (1980).

With all hypotheses relating to interaction effects, the success of the experiment depends on how well matched are the two measures. The basic principle here is the familiar one that in a controlled experiment two measures (just like two groups) should differ only on the variable of interest, but be alike in all other ways. There is one particular problem that arises so commonly here that it deserves special comment, which is where the two tasks differ in their general level of difficulty as well as on the dimension of theoretical interest. Suppose we hypothesize that what an amnesic group finds difficult is the active retrieval of material, but that their ability to recognize material is unimpaired. If we could demonstrate this, it would appear to be an important step in identifying the exact locus of the memory deficit in the amnesic group. However, the two tasks could easily differ, not only in whether or not they required active retrieval, but also in their overall level of difficulty. If the tasks differed in both respects the interpretation of an interaction involving them would be ambiguous. In experiments testing the differential deficit hypotheses, the most common situation has been to have one task of moderate difficulty (e.g. free recall) and one easy task (e.g. recognition). The finding is usually that groups differ on the former more than on the latter. The researcher then reaches for an explanation of this fact that ignores the implications of these differences in difficulty.

The difficulty of a task has important implications for how well it differentiates groups. In general a task on which 50% of people succeed on each of the component items will differentiate groups better than a very easy or very difficult task. Constructors of intelligence tests have long understood the value, for this reason, of including items that around 50% of the population will pass. Difficulty also has implications for the variance of the scores. With easy or difficult tasks, the variance tends to be restricted and the distribution skewed. Equating difficulty is valuable in part because it equates the variance of the two measures. It is less essential that the difficulty level should be 50%, though this will maximise the variance and hence the capacity of the tests to differentiate groups.

To press home the seriousness of this issue, it may be helpful to summarise some of the points made by Chapman and Chapman (1978) in applying it to the literature on differential deficit in schizophrenia. Two-thirds of the relevant studies have found that schizophrenics show more thought-disordered responses to affective than to neutral materials, but this may well be a product of greater discriminability of measures based on the former. In two studies where the tests were matched on psychometric properties, differences between schizophrenics and controls disappeared. Similarly, two-thirds of the relevant studies found that schizophrenics showed greater deficits in learning passages with high contextual constraint, but again this may have been an artefact of the different psychometric properties of measures based on the two kinds of passage. When a study was done in which these were matched, the difference between schizophrenics and normals disappeared.

Matching tasks on psychometric properties (difficulty of items, variance of scores, internal homogeneity of the scale) avoids generating interaction effects that are in reality just an artefact of differences in those properties. However, it may have costs. It is often necessary to introduce some other difference between the tasks to avoid differences in psychometric properties such as difficulty. For example, Raulin and Chapman (1976) equated the difficulty of high and low contextual constraint by making the low constraint word lists shorter. An interaction effect of these matched tasks is thus still ambiguous, but in a new way. Is it due to differences in list length or contextual constraint? In principle the implications of varying both textual constraint and list length could have been explored by introducing additional versions of the tasks. Most problems of design and interpretation can in principle be resolved by an escalation of the number of groups or tasks, but this is not always sensible. A judgement needs to be made about the scientific pay-off of this method of choosing between alternative interpretations. A course needs to be steered between designs that are watertight at the cost of being prohibitively cumbersome and designs that are so leaky they are effectively useless. It is often prudent to take a calculated risk, whilst keeping a clear head about how the problems might affect the interpretation of results.

Having discussed the value of matching pairs of tasks in their level of difficulty, we should note that there are often good theoretical reasons to compare tasks of *different* levels of difficulty. Suppose for example, that the gap between the performance of schizophrenic patients and controls is greater on digits backwards than on digits forwards. A common theoretical approach to such a situation is in terms of 'component processes' (Sternberg, 1977), that there is a common process that underlies performance on both tasks, and an additional process that is required for the more difficult one. The assumption is then made that this additional component is more sensitive to the effects of schizophrenia than the component process common to both tasks. Another common theoretical approach is in terms of limited resources. The basic assumption is that the clinical group has less capacity to allocate processing resources to a task than the control group as Ellis and Ashbrook (1987) have argued for depression. This will result in their being at a relatively severe disadvantage in performing a demanding task that requires resources greater than they generally have available, but which are within the scope of the control group.

Matching of tasks on psychometric properties such as difficulty is not the only approach to the problems of differences in discriminability, and three others involving supplementary analyses will now be discussed briefly.

None is foolproof, but they each make at least a limited contribution to guarding against claiming spurious support for a differential deficit hypothesis.

1. Tests designed to be sensitive to the properties of a clinical group often produce not only a different mean for the clinical group but also a different variance. The variance in the clinical group is often higher and the distribution skewed. Transforming the scales (e.g. applying a log transformation to the skewed scale) to eliminate such differences in variance does not deal with underlying differences in the discriminating power of tests, but it does deal with some statistical artefacts produced by having tests with different kinds of variances (Winer, 1971, pp. 449–452). If a particular interaction survives this treatment, the amount of confidence the experimenter can have in it is increased.

2. If one test differentiates between a clinical and a control better than another simply because of its psychometric properties, this pattern of results should also be found when two normal groups with different levels of performance are compared. To check on this, you might divide the control subjects into high-IQ and low-IQ subgroups, and examine whether they also differed on one test more than the other. If an interaction is found only when one of the groups is clinical, and not with two normal groups, you can be more confident that the interaction is due to the characteristics of the clinical group rather than the different psychometric properties of the test.

3. There are some interaction effects involving a 'cross-over' that are *not* subject to the problems of interpretation that have bedevilled so much abnormal psychology. For example, if a depressed group performs better than a control group in memory for negative materials, but worse in memory for positive materials, this cannot be an artefact of psychometric differences between tests. This suggests another post-hoc method of dealing with the problems of interpreting an interaction effect where the tasks are not matched on difficulty. Take, for example, an experiment in which the clinical group has performed worse than the control group on both tasks. You can select for a post-hoc analysis just the better clinical subjects and the poorer control subjects. This may change the relative positions on the graph of the lines representing the clinical group and the control group so that they now cross over (Fig. 8.1). If this happens, it is relatively unlikely that the interaction effect is an artefact of differences in the discriminating power of the tests.

However, obtaining convergent data from different kinds of experiment

FIG. 8.1. How a cross-over interaction may emerge in a sub-groups clinical and control subjects matched on overall performance.

probably provides the most powerful support for the theory from which a particular interaction effect is predicted. Where there is a clear theory underlying the prediction of an interaction, there are often two or more interaction effects that can be predicted from the same underlying assumptions. For example, it might be hypothesised that imaginal processes in memory are relatively unimpaired in elderly subjects. Imagery can be introduced into a memory experiment either through direct instructions to use imagery, or through materials that lend themselves to imagery (e.g. concrete *vs.* abstract nouns). It would be predicted that in both cases the gap between the performance of elderly and young subjects would be narrowed. Clearly it is advantageous to have such converging experiments relating to the same basic hypothesis.

Another approach to the specification of differential deficits which has been less widely employed, but which has considerable promise, is based on task decomposition (i.e. breaking it down into its components). Decomposition research is well established as a way of identifying the effective components in a treatment package. For example, imaginal desensitisation can be decomposed into (a) relaxation alone and (b) imagery without relaxation. However, decomposition of tasks on which performance is impaired is attempted less often.

When a researcher is faced with the phenomenon of a clinical group which performs a task conspicuously badly, it is often possible to decompose it into its constituent parts to discover where the difficulty comes in. Levy (1973) has provided an excellent exposition of the decomposition approach to the construct validity of psychological tests. One of the unpublished studies he cites is a decomposition of the Digit–Symbol subtest of the WAIS. Several simplified versions of the tasks were devised including a test of writing speed in which the same symbol has to be written repeatedly for 90 seconds, a version in which there were just two possible symbols rather than the usual nine. This study has a single 'normal' group and the study focused on correlations between these simplified tests and the normal versions (and consequently the variance in the normal versions accounted for by the simplified version). With a clinical and an abnormal group to compare, an analysis could be undertaken of where the deficit in the abnormal group arose. For example, there might be no difference between groups in writing speed, but the abnormal group might become slower than the control group as soon as a choice of symbols was introduced. (Issues about the effect of the relative difficulty of components, parallel to those already discussed in this section, arise again here.) It might also be found that writing speed correlated with the normal version less highly in the clinical than the control group. The work of Luria (1966, part III) represents another example of the study of intra-individual discrepancies in performance.

DYSFUNCTIONS OF AETIOLOGICAL IMPORTANCE

A third reason for being interested in a particular psychological dysfunction rests on it being hypothesised to have an important role in aetiology. It should be noted here that 'dysfunction' is being used in an extended sense and can include any dimension along which people differ in the normal population and which has consequences for the development of clinical conditions. Vulnerability factors are obviously of enormous importance, though unfortunately they are very difficult to study. We will consider some of the problems that arise and the solutions that can be attempted.

The first step is relatively simple. Clearly, people who manifest a particular abnormality would also be predicted to show high levels of the hypothesised vulnerability factors. Thus to return to an example used earlier in the chapter, hallucinators would be expected to have vivid imagery and poor reality testing. The main issue at this first stage (apart from constructing reliable measures of the hypothesised vulnerability factors) is the choice of the control group. As in studies of differential deficits, this should be similar to the target group in all respects except the presence of the particular abnormality in question. Thus Mintz and Alpert (1972) compared hallucinating schizophrenics, not with normal controls, but with non-hallucinating schizophrenics. When two such generally similar groups are shown to differ on the hypothesised vulnerability factors, the chances are much increased that they really are relevant to the target symptom. This is too often neglected, and when it is eventually done the results tend to be disappointing. For example, though conflict between the verbal and non-verbal components of communications may be characteristic of the families of schizophrenics, it is not specific to them. When Bugenthal, Love, Kaswan and April (1971) investigated the families of delinquents, they too proved to have a high level of double-bind communications.

A number of models of onset assume a 'diathesis-stress' process in which it is assumed that the vulnerability factor interacts with a triggering event to generate symptoms. Such models require a 2 × 2 factorial design including groups with/without the vulnerability factor and with/without the triggering event. The diathesis–stress model that is currently attracting most interest is the learned helplessness model of depression, though so far studies claiming to support it have often not produced the required evidence that the vulnerability factor predicts symptoms significantly better in those who have experienced the triggering event than those who have not (Williams, 1985).

The first step in any vulnerability model is to show that the vulnerability factor is characteristic of people with a particular abnormality. However, at best, this only establishes an association between the two variables and you cannot infer a causal relationship from a correlation. The alternative causal hypotheses, that the abnormality has caused the hypothesised vulnerability factor, or that they have both been caused by a third variable, cannot yet be ruled out.

The ideal solution to this problem is a prospective study in which you identify which people have the vulnerability feature, and predict on this basis which ones will develop the abnormality concerned. However, prospective studies tend to be cumbersome. The problem is partly that the rate of inception of a disorder is often so low that you have to use extremely large groups. Sometimes, if the hypothesis relates to a delayed effect, like the effect of early upbringing in increasing the risk of schizophrenia in adulthood, a very long-term study is also needed. The problem of low numbers can be alleviated somewhat by studying a high-risk group, like people in families with a history of the disorder concerned (e.g. Mednick & McNeill, 1968). Depression, being such a ubiquitous disorder, is probably the most feasible to study prospectively. For example, you might obtain a high-risk group by studying people about to undergo an event such as childbirth that is thought to increase the risk of depression.

It is important to notice that there can be considerable variation in how unusual each of the two factors are (Meehl, 1973, pp. 244–250). The extremes are (a) cases where the vulnerability factor is common, but the triggering stress is rare; and (b) cases where the vulnerability factor is rare, but the triggering stress is common. Which of these patterns is presumed to apply will affect exactly how you test a diathesis–stress model. There is a particular need for caution over hypothesising that a common variable is a vulnerability factor for a relatively rare disorder.

Even a prospective study has potential problems (see the sections on path analyses and cross-lagged correlations in Chapter 10). There is always a possiblity, even if a strong correlation is found between the vulnerability factor at time one and symptomatology at time two, that what is taken to be a vulnerability factor is in fact an early prodromal symptom. This is most likely when only one premorbid occasion is sampled, and it is quite close in time to the full onset of symptomatology. Also, there is the possibility that in those subjects who have had symptoms on a previous occasion, the presence of the hypothesised vulnerability factor at time one is really a residual symptom of a previous episode of depression. This last problem can be handled to some extent by selecting for a supplementary analysis subjects who have *never* been depressed.

Prospective studies are sufficiently problematic that it is reasonable to look for alternatives to them. Let us now consider some of those available. The available designs are summarised in Table 8.2. A general caution about retrospective studies is that a clinic-based sample may be unrepresentative in their aetiological processes, and that a general population study

TABLE 8.2
Methods of investigating vulnerability factors and their problems

1. Prospective studies:
    Often needs a very large sample (or a 'high-risk' sample).
    The supposed vulnerability factor may be just an 'early' symptom.
2. Concurrent assessment of stable vulnerability factors (e.g. sex):
    Few sufficiently stable vulnerability factors.
3. Retrospective assessment of vulnerability factors:
    Need to use objective measures so as to minimise retrospective distortion.
4. Use of 'recovered' groups as a guide to what pre-morbid groups would be like:
    Need to check that supposed vulnerability factors are not just residual symptoms.
5. Prediction of response to induction procedures:
    Susceptibility to the induction procedure may not accurately reflect vulnerability to the clinical condition.

is the best way of avoiding this potential problem (see the section on Hypothesis testing epidemiology in Chapter 14).

There are also problems in assessing vulnerability factors retrospectively, though this problem melts away like snow in the sun if the vulnerability factor you are concerned with is known to be stable. Sex is an unusually stable characteristic. Therefore, when you find that most agoraphobics are women, it is entirely reasonable to infer that being a woman increases vulnerability to agoraphobia, though of course it says nothing about how this vulnerability is mediated. Irritability, in contrast, is not stable. So, if you find that patients with angina tend to be irritable, you can make no causal inferences. (Much of the older research on personality factors that are assumed to increase vulnerability to psychosomatic illness is flawed in this way.) There are in-between cases of hypothesised vulnerability factors that are not necessarily stable (like sex) but are presumed to be so. Conditionability is an interesting example. If patients with neurotic problems show higher-than-average conditionability, this might be interpreted as a vulnerability factor. The assumption here is that conditionability is a stable characteristic, but the alternative hypothesis that the clinical condition has affected conditionability cannot be ruled out.

A variant of this strategy is to get self-report measures of stable (i.e. 'trait') aspects of personality. The state/trait measures of anxiety (Spielberger et al., 1983) are the most widely used example of this approach. Though the subject completes both scales at the same time, it has often been shown that they have different patterns of correlates that are consistent with their different intentions.

Another approach is to try to get retrospective measures of vulnerability characteristics. The problem with these is that they are likely to be unreliable. However, there are important exceptions. Sometimes a pre-morbid feature can be found that is a sufficiently good marker of the hypothesised vulnerability factor to be of interest and also sufficiently objective that there is no reliability problem. For example, school records have been used as a source of objective information about the pre-morbid sociability of people who subsequently became schizophrenic. Obviously the availability of such indices is severely limited, but researchers have so far been less ingenious than they might have been in generating them. Rawls' (1971) report on the capacity of variables drawn from pre-morbid life to predict readmission to mental hospital is a good model of ingenuity.

Thirdly, there are 'recovered' groups. The current spate of studies of whether recovered depressives show the cognitive vulnerability factors hypothesised by Beck and others is a good example of this approach. But how far are you justified in assuming that 'recovered' people have reverted to their pre-morbid state? One problem is that recovery is often only partial. If you take an administrative criterion of recovery (e.g. discharged from treatment) you will probably have many people who still have mild symptoms. On the other hand, if all people with mild symptoms are excluded, it will be difficult to find an adequate sample and they may be so highly selected as to be unrepresentative in other ways. Statistical techniques are sometimes helpful in disentangling the effects of (a) current mood state from (b) whether or not people have had a depressive illness. Monitoring the relapse process carefully may also provide rich time-course data that are helpful in disentangling alternative hypotheses. However, even people whose symptoms have fully remitted may show residual effects of a depressive episode that render them different from people who are vulnerable to depression but who have not yet actually become depressed.

There is no statistical solution to this problem. When recovered depressives are shown to have particular characteristics, we can never be sure whether they are pre-morbid vulnerability features or the permanent residue of a depressive episode. Finally, there is the problem of finding a *comparable* 'never-ill' group with whom to compare the recovered group. The group may differ in various incidental ways from the clinical group, producing differences on the measure of the hypothesised vulnerability factor that will be misinterpreted. Researchers can and should match groups on some of the more obviously relevant variables, but other unnoticed differences between groups may remain.

Related to hypotheses about pre-morbid vulnerability factors are hypotheses that a particular symptom of a clinical condition is 'primary'. Many psychological disorders have features that span multiple domains. Depression, for example, affects physiological, cognitive and behavioural systems. In such cases there is a tendency to claim primacy for one or other domain of dysfunction, for example, that negative cognitions are the primary symptoms of depression. In fact, primacy seems to be rather rare in abnormal psychology. It is probably much more common for there to be mutual interactions between the different systems of a complex condition such as depression. Thus cognitive and physiological aspects often affect each other. A 'primacy' theory would be refuted by such a state of affairs; the thesis that negative cognitions are the primary aspect of depression predicts not only that cognitions generate other features of depression including dysphoria, but also that dysphoria does *not* similarly generate negative cognitions. The latter claim is clearly incorrect, as evidence for the effects of mood on negative memories indicates (Teasdale, 1983). In its strongest form, a primacy theory would also claim that all cases of the primary symptom should lead to the other symptoms of the condition, and would be refuted by cases in which the primary symptom occurs alone, except as a temporary phase of the aetiological processes. Primacy theories also make predictions about the course of onset. The symptoms should always develop first and the secondary symptoms later. The converse pattern of development would refute a strong primacy theory.

Strong primacy theories are perhaps something of a 'will o' the wisp', and perhaps scarcely worth chasing. However, within the framework of the more plausible assumption of mutual interaction between symptoms, it can be important to know whether one aspect of disorder can induce its other aspects. This requires an experimental manipulation such as psychological or physiological induction procedures. Studies of the effects of mood induction procedures (currently the best known example of a psychological induction procedure) have made a substantial contribution to research on depression (Goodwin & Williams, 1982). Studies of the effects of alcohol (see Huesmann, 1982, p. 238) are an example of a physiological induction procedure that has contributed to the understanding of alcoholism. Two cautions are required in such studies. One is that care should be taken not to over-extrapolate from rather loose similarities between clinical symptoms and the state induced by the experimental procedure. The other is to ensure that the effects of the procedure do not merely reflect the effects of demand characteristics. This is more problematic with psychological than with physiological procedures because they are less easily disguised. However, it is possible to include a condition in which counter-demands are given, in which for example an elation induction procedure is used but subjects are told it will make them feel unhappy (e.g. Polivy & Doyle, 1980). One of the uses of such induction studies is to allow theories about vulnerability factors to be tested directly, but this assumes that susceptibility to the induction procedure is determined by the same variables as vulnerability to the clinical condition. Hypotheses about the antecedent events that lead to particular conditions can also in principle be tested by the use of procedures designed to induce the disorder concerned. The use of insoluble problems in the 'learned helplessness' paradigm is a widely used example. The application of conditioning procedures to produce a sexual fetish (Rachman, 1966) is another. Clearly, there can be ethical problems with such procedures. There is a research dilemma here that applies to all induction procedures in abnormal psychology. If the state induced is *too* close to a clinical disorder there will probably be ethical problems in inducing it. Alternatively, if it produces only a weak simulation of the disorder, its relevance to the explanation of the clinical disorder is doubtful. But even if the simulation of the clinical disorder is perfect, all that is established is that the clinical disorder *can* be induced in this way, not that this is the normal genesis. There may be different paths to the same disorder, and the route represented by the experimental procedure may be an atypical one.

An alternative approach to studying the genesis of a clinical condition is to look at the course it follows after inception. Knowing how to predict, or even control, changes in the severity of a condition is clearly of practical value. Of course, nothing can be inferred about the original genesis of the disorder, but it is always a plausible hypothesis that factors known to affect the course of a disorder might also contribute to its genesis. Ideas about possible vulnerability factors can be translated into hypotheses about factors which will predict the course of the disorder, and in this new form are much more tractable. Thus research on the prediction of the course of schizophrenia from patterns of communication involving high levels of expressed emotion in the family (e.g. Leff & Vaughn, 1985) has been more fruitful than research on the role of family processes in the genesis of schizophrenia. Research on prognostic factors is always difficult to interpret causally, though sometimes careful analysis can at least be suggestive. For example, current marital status predicts outcome in schizophrenia but it seems that both are predictable from pre-morbid sociability (see Watts, 1983, pp. 300–301), suggesting that current marital status does not have a direct casual impact.

Sometimes social variables known to be associated with the course or severity of a disorder can be manipulated experimentally, such as in the work of Purcell and Weiss (1970) showing the beneficial effects of separating a small group of asthmatic children (those who were less steroid dependent) from their parents. Of course, when children leave home too many aspects of the environment are changed simultaneously for unambiguous conclusions to be drawn. The key manipulation was one in which children were cared for in their own homes by a substitute mother while the rest of the family were away. It was shown that this led to improvements in the children's asthmatic symptoms. Where manipulations are used to test hypotheses about causal factors the key requirement is for a 'clean' intervention whose effects are known. Because a substantial component of the effectiveness of so many interventions can be attributed to non-specific factors, the fact of their effectiveness doesn't necessarily confirm the principles on which they are based. For example the clinical success of an intervention designed to reduce the level of expressed emotion in the family of a schizophrenic doesn't necessarily confirm the specific relevance of expressed emotion. The intervention may have achieved its clinical results in other more non-specific ways.

CONCLUSIONS

Inevitably, this chapter has focused on some of the difficulties of doing research in abnormal psychology. The intention has not been to discourage the reader, but to lay bare the scientific process. Researchers are naturally always ambitious in the sense of wanting to draw bold conclusions from their work, but it is an essential characteristic of the scientific process that this must be balanced by caution. Because it is so easy to draw incorrect conclusions from research, scientists need to be constantly on their guard. The methodological cautions of experimental research should not be seen as off-puttting, arcane or elitist. They are just the distillations, from much research experience, of how scientists can avoid fooling themselves into thinking they have proved something when they haven't. Only in this way can we decide whether our bold conjectures about clinical conditions are actually true.

REFERENCES

Barber, T. X. (1979). *Pitfalls in Human Research: Ten Pivotal Points*. Oxford: Pergamon Press.

Baron, J. & Treiman, R. (1980). Some problems in the study of differences in cognitive processes. *Memory and Cognition*, **8**, 313–321.

Bender, M. B. & Teuber, H. L. (1949). Disturbances in visual perception following cerebral lesion. *Journal of Psychology*, **28**, 233–234.

Bogartz, R. S. (1976). On the meaning of statistical interactions. *Journal of Experimental Child Psychology*, **22**, 178–183.

Borkovec, T. & Rachman, S. (1979). The utility of analogue research. *Behaviour Research and Therapy*, **17**, 253–261.

Bugenthal, D. E., Love, L. R., Kaswan, J. W. & April, C. (1971). Verbal–non-verbal conflict in parental messages to normal and disturbed children. *Journal of Abnormal Psychology*, **77**, 6–10.

Chapman, L. J. & Chapman, J. P. (1973a). Selection of subjects in studies of schizophrenic cognition. *Journal of Abnormal Psychology*, **86**, 10–15.

Chapman, L. J. & Chapman, J. P. (1973b). *Disordered Thought in Schizophrenia*. New York: Appleton-Century-Crofts.

Chapman, L. J. & Chapman, J. P. (1973c). Problems in the measurement of cognitive deficit. *Psychological Bulletin*, **79**, 380–385.

Chapman, L. J. & Chapman, J. P. (1974). Alternative to the design of manipulating a variable to compare retarded and normal subjects. *American Journal of Mental Deficiency*, **79**, 404–411.

Chapman, L. J. & Chapman, J. P. (1978). The measurement of differential deficit. *Journal of Psychiatric Research*, **14**, 303–311.

Ellis, H. & Ashbrook, P. W. (1987). Resource allocation model of the effects of depressed mood states on memory. In K. Fiedler and J. Forgas (eds) *Affect, Cognition and Social Behaviour*. Toronto: Hogrefe.

Garber, J. & Seligman, M. E. P. (1980.) *Human Helplessness: Therapy and Applications*. London: Academic Press.

Goodwin, A. & Williams, J. M. G. (1982). Mood induction research: its implications for clinical depression. *Behaviour Research and Therapy*, **20**, 373–382.

Hemsley, D. R. (1977). What have cognitive deficits to do with schizophrenic symptoms? *British Journal of Psychiatry*, **130**, 167–173.

Huesmann, L. R. (1982). Experimental methods in research in psychopathology. In P. C. Kendall and J. N. Butcher (eds) *Handbook of Research Methods in Clinical Psychology*. New York: John Wiley.

Kausler, D. H. (1982). *Experimental Psychology of Human Aging*. New York: John Wiley.

Kerlinger, F. N. (1973). *Foundations of Behavioural Research: Educational, Psychological and Sociological Enquiry*. New York: Holt, Rinehart & Winston.

Leff, J. & Vaughn, C. (1985). *Experienced Emotion in Families: Its Significance for Mental Illness*. New York: Guildford Press.

Levy, P. (1973). On the relation between test theory and psychology. In P. Kline (ed.) *New Approaches in Psychological Measurement*. London: John Wiley.

Loftus, G. R. (1978). On the interpretation of interactions. *Memory and Cognition*, **6**, 312–319.

Luria, A. R. (1966). *Higher Cortical Functions in Man*. New York: Plenum.

Mednick, S. A. & McNeil, T. F. (1968). Current methodology in research on the etiology of schizophrenia. *Psychological Bulletin*, **70**, 681–693.

Meehl, P. E. (1973). Why I do not attend case conferences. In P. E. Meehl (ed.) *Psychochognous: Selected Papers*. Minnesota: University of Minnesota Press.

Mintz, S. & Alpert, M. (1972). Imagery vividness, reality testing and schizophrenic hallucinations. *Journal of Abnormal Psychology*, **79**, 310–316.

Neale, J. M. & Oltmanns, T. F. (1980). *Schizophrenia*. Chichester: Wiley.

Polivy, J. & Doyle, C. (1980). Laboratory induction of mood states through the reading self-referent mood statements: affective changes or demand characteristics. *Journal of Abnormal Psychology*, **89**, 286–290.

Poulton, E. C. (1982). Influential comparisons: effects of one strategy on another in within-subjects designs of cognitive psychology. *Psychological Bulletin*, **91**, 673–690.

Purcell, K. & Weiss, J. H. (1970). Asthma. In C. G. Costello (ed.) *Symptoms of Psychopathology: A Handbook*. New York: John Wiley.

Rachman, S. (1966). Sexual fetishism: an experimental analogue. *Psychological Record*, **16**, 293–296.

Raulin, M. L. & Chapman, L. J. (1976). Schizophrenic recall and contextual constraint. *Journal of Abnormal Psychology*, **85**, 151–155.

Rawls, J. R. (1971). Toward the identification of readmissions and non-admissions to mental hospitals. *Social Psychiatry*, **6**, 58–61.

Rubin, D. (1986). *Autobiographical Memory*. Cambridge University Press.

Shapiro, M. B. (1960). Introductory notes to the work of Bender and Teuber on disorders of perception. Unpublished observations. Institute of Psychiatry, University of London.

Sher, K., Frost, R. O. & Otto, R. (1983). Cognitive deficits in compulsive checkers: an exploratory study. *Behaviour Research and Therapy*, **21**, 357–363.

Slade, P. D. (1976). Towards a theory of auditory hallucinations: outline of an hypothetical poor-factor model. *British Journal of Clinical Psychology*, **15**, 415–423.

Spielberger, C. D., Gorsuch, R. L., Lushene, R., Vagg, P. R. & Jacobs, G. A. (1983). *Manual for the State–Trait Anxiety Inventory (Form Y)*. Palo Alto: Consulting Psychologists Press.

Sternberg, R. J. (1977). *Intelligence, Information Processing and Analogical Reasoning.* Hillsdale, N. J.: Lawrence Erlbaum.

Teasdale, J. D. (1983). Affect and accessibility. In D. E. Broadbent (ed.) *Functional Aspects of Human Memory*. London: The Royal Society.

Watts, F. N. (1983). Socialization and Social Integration. In F. N. Watts and D. H. Bennett (eds) *Theory and Practice of Psychiatric Rehabilitation*. Chichester: John Wiley.

Watts, F. N. (1988). Cognitive impairments. In J. M. G. Williams, F. N. Watts, C. M. MacLeod and A. Mathews (eds). *Cognitive Psychology and Emotional Disorders*. Brighton: Lawrence Erlbaum.

Williams, J. M. G. (1985). Attributional formulation of depression as a diathesis–stress model: Metalshy *et al.* reconsidered. *Journal of Personality and Social Psychology*, **48**, 1572–1575.

Williams, J. M. G. & Broadbent, K. (1986). Autobiographical memory in suicide attempters. *Journal of Abnormal Psychology*, **95**, 144–149.

Winer, B. J. (1971). *Statistical Principles in Experimental Design*, 2nd edn. New York: McGraw Hill.

9 Outcome Research

David A. Shapiro
*MRC/ESRC Social and Applied Psychology Unit, Department of
Psychology, University of Sheffield, S10 2TN.*

Mental health practice is composed of a large variety of interventions. These range from admission to a psychiatric ward to participation in a self-help group or taking a course of psychotropic medication. In relation to any of these, it seems reasonable and indeed socially important to ask, 'Does it work?', or 'Does intervention X work better than intervention Y?' This chapter sets forth the basic principles of outcome research, which lies at the heart of efforts by clinical psychologists and others to build a scientific foundation for mental health practice. The aim is to provide a guide both to the design of outcome studies and to the critical reading of published outcome research. Examples will be taken from research on psychological treatments, because this is the field I know best. However, most of the principles discussed are common to all mental health interventions. Indeed, the basic research approach or paradigm of outcome research was originally developed for the evaluation of drug treatments.

CHOICE, COMPROMISE AND INFORMATIVENESS

The investigator seeking to establish the effectiveness of one or more interventions is faced with a large number of decisions about how to proceed. Research design is the discipline governing such decisions. It incorporates a number of key principles which must be attended to in framing an outcome study. Given the practical and resource constraints limiting any one study, however, the demands of these principles have an unfortunate tendency to conflict with one another; beginners should take heart from the fact that it is therefore impossible to design the 'perfect' study. The art of outcome research design thus becomes one of creative compromise based upon explicit understanding of the implications of the choices made.

A good way to go about research design is to imagine that we have already completed the study we envisage, and that the results are available (Horowitz, 1982). This imaginative exercise should be repeated assuming all the patterns of results that we can envisage. Such an exercise will enable us to fulfil the central purpose of research design, which is to maximise the informativeness of the results by minimising the number of plausible explanations for them.

CHOOSING A DESIGN

The simplest approach to evaluating a treatment is to measure the symptoms or well-being of a series of patients before they undertake the treatment, and to repeat this measurement when treatment is complete. However, many competing explanations will reduce the informativeness of data obtained using this 'pre-post' design. In the technical terminology of outcome research, this method lacks 'controls' to exclude these alternative explanations (Table 9.1). Thus if patients are found to be, on average, no better off at the end of treatment than before, then this appears to suggest that the treatment, as practised, is ineffective. However, one of several plausible alternative explanations is that the patients were on a deteriorating course which was effectively stemmed, albeit not reversed, by the treatment.

TABLE 9.1
Outcome designs

Design	Features	Controls for:
Pre-post	One group, compare post-treatment with pre-treatment scores	
No-treatment control	Patients assigned to treatment or to no-treatment control group	(1) 'Spontaneous remission' or passage of time
Placebo control	Patients assigned to treatment or placebo-treatment control group	(1) As above (2) Expectations of benefit
Comparative outcome study	Patients assigned to one of several active treatments	(1) As above (2) As above but more convincing and ethical

If, on the other hand, patients are on average much better off at the end than at the beginning of treatment, different explanations suggest themselves. There is of course the optimistic interpretation that the treatment is effective. However, alternatives include the possibility that the patients would have got better anyway. In psychotherapy research, this is known as 'spontaneous remission' (Lambert, 1976). Even if patients do not invariably improve without treatment, their mental health will undoubtedly vary over time and with changing circumstances, and they tend to seek help when they are at their worst.

Considerations such as these have led to the use of no-treatment control groups in the basic design for outcome research (Table 9.1). Rather than simply following a single group of treated patients, changes in those undertaking a treatment are compared with changes in others, the control group, not receiving that treatment. The logic of this comparison is that any changes in the control group give us an estimate of what would have happened to the treated group if they had not undertaken the treatment. This logic requires, of course, the assumption that the groups are composed of individuals whose personal characteristics and circumstances are comparable or interchangeable. Formally speaking, this assumption is expressed as follows: the treatment and control groups are comprised of individuals drawn and assigned to one or other treatment at random from the same parent population, every member of which enjoyed an equal probability of being assigned to either of the two groups.

So far, we have considered alternative explanations arising from changes in the treated individuals not attributable to treatment. Other alternative explanations arise from the possibility that the mere fact of receiving a treatment that participants believe to be effective may predispose them to experience or report benefits, irrespective of the efficacy or otherwise of the treatment procedures themselves. In the evaluation of drugs, this consideration gave rise to the use of placebo controls—the administration of inert tablets. In drug research, this preferably takes the form of a double-blind placebo trial, in which patients receiving an active drug are compared with others receiving an apparently identical but pharmacologically inert placebo, with both the patient and the administering personnel ignorant of (i.e., 'blind' to) the nature of the tablets taken by any one person. This contrasts with the simpler, single blind, method in which only the patient is unaware of the nature of the treatment.

Unfortunately, however, this method has limitations. First, there may be side-effects or other features that distinguish the active and placebo treatments and thus enable participants to 'break the blind'. In psychological treatments, participants (patient and therapist alike) cannot be ignorant of the procedures they are following, and cannot be prevented from formulating their own hypotheses and expectations as to the effectiveness or otherwise of the activities in which they are engaged. Personnel employed to interview patients to assess their progress are seldom able to avoid exposure to information (especially within patients' accounts of their experiences) that gives away the nature of the treatment they have undergone.

In addition, the conceptual distinction between 'active' and 'placebo' treatments that is so clear with pharmacological treatments is blurred when we consider psychological treatments (Wilkins, 1984). With physical treatments, the efforts of physicians to encourage the belief that the treatment is helpful are clearly separable, in terms of both operations and impact, from the biochemical pathways differentiating active from placebo treatments. In contrast, the encouragement of positive expectations is a psychological process much closer to those mediating the effectiveness of psychological treatments. Indeed the engendering of such positive expectations is probably a part of every psychological treatment, although different psychological treatments achieve this via differing means.

These considerations have led many outcome researches to elaborate their designs one step further. Instead of—or sometimes as well as—comparing an active treatment with a placebo, they very often compare two or more active treatments in the same study (Basham, 1986). To the extent that all active treatments share the non-specific benefits arising from participants' belief in their value, this design reduces the need for a placebo condition. Dispensing with the placebo condition has the ethical advantage that no one is denied treatment, and that all patients are receiving something that has at least a good chance of being helpful. This design has the practical advantage of mirroring the actual choices available in clinical practice, which are more often between alternate courses of action than between 'doing something' and 'doing nothing'. Such comparative studies provide a concurrent opportunity to compare the contents or processes of the two treatments, which may help us identify the active ingredients within each treatment, and to find out just how different or similar these may be in the methods under comparison (Stiles, Shapiro & Elliott, 1986).

Important practical and ethical problems arise from any study in which the decision about which treatment a patient receives is influenced by research considerations as well as by the likely benefit to that patient. Practically, the researcher must consider the likely impact on the patient of becoming aware that alternatives to the treatment actually received are available within the same facility. Thus, for example, in-patients, or out-patients living or working in the same setting as one another, can encounter other patients receiving different treatments. If one treatment is apparently superior (e.g. involves more patient-therapist contact), knowledge of this may well influence the reactions of patients assigned to the different treatments. Ethically, many would consider that the principle of informed consent requires that the patient be told that there are alternative treatments under comparison.

The investigator designing an outcome study should begin with a careful specification of the research question or questions to be answered in the study. This should define the nature of the two or more conditions to be compared. Next, the possible outcomes and their implications should be evaluated to ascertain to what extent each would provide unambiguous answers (i.e. answers not susceptible to alternative explanations) to the research questions. Several attempts at this may be necessary to yield a worthwhile design. The next step is to consider the details of its implementation. The methodological problems that must be overcome in carrying out an outcome study are considered next.

FOUR TYPES OF INVALIDITY

Many of the methodological problems faced in outcome research (Kazdin, 1978, 1986; Mahoney, 1978) may be subsumed within Cook and Campbell's (1979) discussion of validity and invalidity (Shapiro & Shapiro, 1983).

Cook and Campbell (1979) distinguish four types of validity, shown in Table 9.2. *Statistical conclusion validity* refers to the validity with which a study permits conclusions about covariation between the assumed independent and dependent variables. Threats to statistical conclusion validity typically arise from unsystematic error rather than systematic bias. *Internal validity* refers to the validity with which statements can be made about whether there is a causal relationship from independent to dependent variables, in the form in which they were manipulated or measured. Threats to internal validity typically involve systematic bias. *Construct validity* of putative causes and effects refers to the validity with which we can make generalisations about higher order constructs from research operations. Finally, *external validity* refers to the validity with which conclusions can be drawn about the generalisability of a causal relationship to and across populations of persons, settings, and times. Frequently encountered threats to each of the four types of validity will now be considered in detail.

Statistical Conclusion Validity

A central issue in statistical conclusion validity concerns statistical power, the probability of rejecting the null hypothesis when it is false. This depends primarily upon the size of the effect an experimenter is seeking to detect, and the numbers of subjects in the groups being compared (Cohen, 1962, 1977). Comparing a psychological treatment with no treatment, it is

TABLE 9.2
Aspects of validity

Validity type	Focus	Major issues
Statistical conclusion	Covariation between independent and dependent variables	1. Statistical power 2. Treatment delivery 3. Heterogeneity of patients
Internal	Causal relationship between independent and dependent variables	1. Bias from pre-treatment differences 2. Bias from attrition
Construct	Theoretical constructs	1. Representativeness of treatments 2. Concomitant variation in non-specifics 3. Investigator bias 4. Reactivity of measures 5. Specificity and relevance of measures 6. Timing of assessment
External	Generalisability over persons, settings and times	Representativeness of: 1. Patients 2. Therapists 3. Settings

reasonable to expect a large effect of around one standard deviation unit (i.e. mean of treated group one standard deviation better than mean of untreated group). To detect such an effect, sample sizes of no more than 10 in each group are necessary (Kraemer, 1981). However, if the experiment is seeking to detect a weaker effect, as may be the case when different treatments are compared rather than treatment versus no treatment, then much larger groups are necessary (Kazdin, 1986). For example, if the effect size is around one-third of a standard deviation unit, samples of around 150 per group are required for the secure detection of the effect. Power problems are exacerbated by attrition (missing data), which reduces the available sample size (in addition to introducing possible bias).

Uncontrolled variation in the way a treatment is delivered or implemented presents a second major threat to statistical conclusion validity. Shapiro and Shapiro (1983) found that the majority of the outcome studies they reviewed were deficient in this respect. However, this problem is increasingly being overcome by the preparation of manuals defining the treatment procedures to be followed (Beck, Rush, Shaw & Emery, 1979; Klerman et al., 1984; Luborsky, 1984). Project therapists are then trained to implement the techniques as specified in the manual, and their adherence to the manual is empirically assessed via process analysis of recorded sessions (De Rubeis, Hollon, Evans & Bemis, 1982; Evans et al., 1983; Hardy & Shapiro, 1985). The importance of this methodological advance is heightened by recent concern with variations in the skillfulness with which therapists are found to deliver a treatment procedure (Schaffer, 1982). Just how far it is feasible or appropriate to go in the direction of specifying an intervention in writing will, of course, vary with the nature of that intervention. In principle, however, this should be done as much as possible (Luborsky & DeRubeis, 1984).

A third threat to statistical conclusion validity arises from excessive heterogeneity amongst the patients treated in an outcome study. It is often argued that patients differing in presenting problems, personality or life circumstances must be expected to differ in their response to a given treatment. On this argument, investigators admitting varied individuals to their treatment groups are subscribing to a 'uniformity myth' that invalidates their research. The increasingly common solution to this problem is to select patients on the basis of specified inclusion criteria, such as minimum scores on questionnaries such as the Beck Depression Inventory (Beck et al., 1961) or psychiatric diagnoses based on such systems as DSM-III (American Psychiatric Association, 1980) or the PSE-ID-CATEGO system (Wing, Cooper & Sartorius, 1974).

Despite the obvious logical attractions of this approach, it has drawbacks. At a purely practical level, the more restrictive the inclusion criteria the longer it will take to locate suitable patients and the less willingly will other professionals refer to the research programme. Notoriously, patients meeting given criteria suddenly become much rarer when a researcher launches a trial requiring such patients! Furthermore, the more restricted the population from which the patients are drawn, the narrower the range is the range of patients to whom the results may be generalised. In addition, making the patient population homogeneous may prevent the investigator from finding out which patient characteristics are prognostic of good versus poor outcome in the treatments being studied.

Another problem is that the measures used to select patients may not tap the most important and treatment-relevant similarities and differences between individuals—for example, similarities in terms of symptoms could conceal large differences in terms of underlying personality or be overshadowed by differences in social integration. Finally, it must be acknowledged that the available selection criteria often fail to meet the rigorous scientific standards of precision that inspired their introduction into an outcome design. For example, DSM-III criteria for affective disorders are based upon an interviewer's judgement as to the presence of a certain number of symptoms drawn from a menu-like list. Thus although homogenous patient groups are in principle desirable in outcome research, the gains may sometimes be more apparent than real, and, like most design advances, carry some drawbacks too.

A different perspective on statistical conclusion validity derives from the growing concern with *clinical* as opposed to statistical significance of results. From a practitioner's perspective, statistical power may be counterproductive if it enables researchers to report statistically reliable results based upon trivially small differences between groups assigned to alternative treatments. Although there is no agreed standard procedure to ascertain the clinical significance of change, several proposals have been made, such as measurement of the extent to which treatment returns clients to normative levels of functioning, the magnitude of change, and the degree to which change is perceptible to significant others in clients' everyday lives (Hugdahl & Ost, 1981; Jacobson, Follette & Revenstorf, 1984; Kazdin & Wilson, 1978; Yeaton & Sechrest, 1981).

Internal Validity

Threats to internal validity chiefly concern sources of possible bias in the comparison between experimental conditions. A primary requirement is to ensure that the groups of individuals assigned to different experimental conditions are comparable at the outset.

The most common solution to this problem is random assignment (Shapiro & Shapiro, 1983). However, randomisation can often result in nonequivalent groups, especially if the samples are small, with consequent opportunities for the groups to differ by chance. When this happens, investigators can only attempt to 'correct' for the initial differences in some way. One solution is the use of 'residual gain scores' from which the effects of initial differences are statistically partialled out. The principles underlying this are illustrated in Figs 9.1 and 9.2.

In Fig. 9.1, every individual is represented by either a circle or by a cross, depending on which of two treatments they received. The individual's position in the figure is determined by that person's scores before treatment (along the horizontal axis) and after treatment (along the vertical axis). The relationship between pre- and post-treatment scores for the sample as a whole is represented by the *regression line* shown. This line provides the 'best fit' to the complete set of data. This fit is determined by the criterion that the sum of the squares of all the vertical distances from individual points to the line be as small as possible. Note that, in the example shown, the circles tend to be above the regression line, and the crosses below it. These vertical distances are known as residuals. Figure 9.2 shows these rescaled, as residual gain scores. Here, the regression line is now the horizontal axis, so that points on the line have a score of zero.

FIG. 9.1. Regression of post-treatment on pre-treatment scores.

Thus this method substitutes for each raw post-treatment score the difference between that score and the score that would have been expected,
given the pre-treatment score obtained for that individual and the relationship for the sample as a whole between pre- and post-treatment scores.
This method is only useful if the correlation between pre- and post-
treatment scores is large enough for sufficient correction to be obtained
(Mintz, Luborsky & Christolph, 1979).

Another solution is to analyse arithmetic differences between post- and
pre-treatment scores. However, these difference scores compound the
error components in the two scores from which they are derived, with a
consequent loss in statistical power. A third solution is known as 'blocking'. This comprises dividing the participants into two or more groups,
according to the level of their pretreatment scores, and then using two-way
analysis of variance to establish whether the post-treatment difference
between treatments is similar or different for people at different levels on
the pretreatment variable. However, no merely statistical manipulation

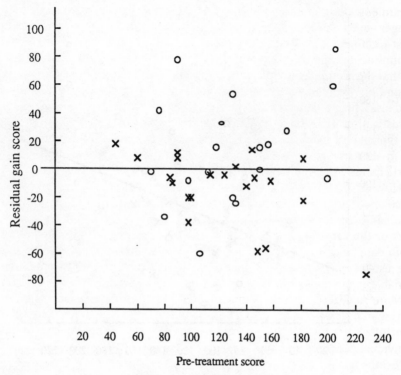

FIG. 9.2.   Residual gain scores.

can guarantee that the initial difference between the groups under comparison was not responsible for the post-treatment differences observed; such corrections do not address the question of whether the two samples were drawn from the same population and would have changed similarly if given similar treatments. In order to avoid these problems, some investigators have abandoned randomisation in favour of prematched groups, but this raises tricky statistical issues.

A second, related source of bias derives from attrition or loss of subjects from the study (Howard, Krause & Orlinsky, 1986). Howard *et al.* point out that this begins before inclusion in the study, as there is a natural filtering process whereby some members of the population deemed to be appropriate for inclusion in a study become unavailable, either through choice or through intervening circumstance; whereas other members have a disproportionately greater chance of inclusion.

After inclusion in a study, subjects may be lost for a variety of reasons, most of which threaten to bias the study because they cannot be dissociated from the treatment and subjects' reactions to it. People may discontinue treatment, opting to seek alternative treatment or believing that they no longer need help. They may continue treatment, but fail or refuse to supply post-treatment data. When the rates of post-inclusion attrition differ across groups being compared, the causes of that attrition are likely to differ also, so that the groups are no longer comparable. It is difficult to place an upper bound on acceptable attrition rates, as these will vary with the treatment and assessment demands of the study and with the population under investigation. In the light of data presented by Shapiro and Shapiro (1983) on typical post-inclusion attrition rates, however, it is reasonable to expect of investigators the loss of no more than the reported mean 10% of participants from any treatment group.

Howard *et al.* (1986) review several methods that have been developed to compensate for the effects of attrition, but note that these all rest on the untenable assumption that 'attritors' and 'completers' are equivalent samples of the same population. These authors recommend the elimination from data analyses of all cases missing any independent variable data and the use of only those cases that are not missing data on a dependent variable in any analysis involving that particular dependent variable.

More radically, however, Howard *et al.* (1986) propose a reorientation of research strategy away from the pretence of control for what cannot be controlled, towards a new perspective in which the basic unit of study is the individual case, described with as much dependent and independent variable information as is required at the present state of development of psychotherapy research. In this new strategy, it is the knowledge of which points in the independent variable space are associated with the best average outcomes that is ultimately of clinical importance. Thus if dependent variable data are missing from a point in the independent variable space represented by the combination of two independent variable values each of which is associated with better than average outcomes, it becomes important to design a study that will capture data at this point.

Construct Validity

Representativeness of Treatments.   Cook and Campbell (1979) consider the adequacy with which the independent variable is represented within a study as an important aspect of construct validity. It is important that the treatments incorporated within a study be designed to represent the techniques of interest, both with respect to such obvious structural features as the number and duration of sessions, and more subtle aspects such as the specific interventions or general interpersonal style of the therapist. Kazdin (1986) presents a careful discussion of 'treatment integrity', noting that in some comparative studies it may be appropriate to allow some features of the treatments to vary to represent the treatments more faithfully, even though the variations may also be looked upon as confounds. This arises, for example, when different treatments are expected to require differing numbers of sessions to attain their optimal effectiveness.

Control for Non-specific Effects. A major issue in psychotherapy research has been the exent to which treatment effects are attributable to the specific techniques under investigation, rather than to so-called 'non-specific' factors such as the arousal of expectations on the part of clients that the treatment will be beneficial. If such factors are present to different degrees in different treatments, this concomitant variation threatens the construct validity of the research by suggesting that the mechanism whereby one treatment is more effective than another may be quite different from the more specific one envisaged by the theory underlying that treatment. In the 1960s and 1970s, increasingly sophisticated controls for such effects were incorporated into research designs, on the basis of an explicit analogy with the use of pharmacologically inert placebos in drug research (Shapiro & Morris, 1978). An early example of this was Paul's (1966) incorporation into his comparative outcome study of an 'attention placebo' condition.

Subsequently, however, the adequacy of such controls was questioned (Borkovec & Nau, 1972; Kazdin & Wilcoxon, 1976; Shapiro, 1981). Specifically, it was suggested that optimal control for non-specific effects required empirical demonstration that the control condition was as credible as the active treatments with which it was to be compared. Failing that, Kazdin and Wilcoxon (1976) advocated a *treatment–element control* strategy, in which the control procedure resembles the active treatment as closely as possible. For example, Holroyd *et al.* (1984) found that tension headache sufferers improved as much with electromyographic (EMG) feedback increasing muscle activity as with feedback reducing it. Shapiro and Shapiro (1983) report that only a small minority of comparative outcome studies incorporated such controls.

More recently, however, it has been argued that the predominant conceptualisation of non-specific effects in psychotherapy as analogous with the placebo effect in drug therapy (Shapiro & Morris, 1978) is misguided (Wilkins, 1984; Parloff, 1986).

For example, Parloff (1986) argues that under the necessarily nonblind experimental conditions of psychotherapy research, it is well-nigh impossible to ensure that therapists and their patients will view the experimental and placebo treatments as equally credible. The neat medical distinction between core somatic pathology and symptoms cannot be sustained with respect to psychological disorder. The effectiveness of all psychological treatments is likely to be based in part upon common factors arousing hope and expectation of benefit. Thus it is misguided to seek a true placebo, controlling for the actual active ingredients of a treatment, whether such ingredients are characteristic or incidental, unique or common. These considerations lead Parloff (1986) to recommend research designs comparing known alternate treatment forms and modalities, which can serve as natural placebo controls for each other (Rosenthal & Frank, 1956).

Investigator Bias. Closely linked with the question of non-specific effects is the likely impact of experimenter bias upon psychotherapy studies. Reasons for suspecting the influence of subtle, unwitting demands by investigators upon the responses made by subjects include the substantial evidence for experimenter effects in psychological research (Rosenthal & Rubin, 1978). These effects are the social influences at work in a situation defined as one in which one person is professionally engaged in the task of helping another, the strong and enthusiastic allegiances of psychotherapists to their preferred orientations and treatment methods, and the above-noted impossibility of double-blind conditions in psychotherapy research.

Smith, Glass and Miller (1980) found a substantial correlation between the allegiance of investigators (inferred from analysis of their published reports) and the results they obtained for a given treatment. There is a tendency for new psychotherapeutic methods to show outstandingly good results in early studies published by their originators, followed by more modest findings characteristic of the field as a whole when studied by less committed workers. For example, Berman, Miller and Massman (1985) attribute the failure of recent studies to confirm earlier reports of the superiority of cognitive therapy over other methods (Shapiro & Shapiro, 1982a) to the greater allegiance of earlier investigators to cognitive therapy. Independent replication in several institutions is required for the true importance of any mental health treatment to be established.

Reactivity of Outcome Measures. A further, related construct validity issue concerns the vulnerability of outcome measures to the biasing effects discussed above. For example, measures administered 'blind' by individuals unaware of the treatment condition to which subjects have been assigned tend to yield smaller treatment effects (Shapiro & Shapiro, 1983). This is despite the fact that the impact of the blind is in reality reduced by unavoidable disclosures to experimenters of the subject's treatment assignment. For example, during interviews subjects often refer, directly or indirectly, to their treatment experiences; if the interviewer knows which treatments are under comparison, it is often impossible to avoid matching these incidental remarks to the treatment conditions.

Different outcome measures vary in the extent to which they are vulnerable to bias. Thus therapist ratings or self-report measures of the severity of the problem for which the person is seeking help are highly reactive to demand characteristics, whereas a physiological index is much less so. There is evidence that more reactive measures yield more favourable results (Shapiro & Shapiro, 1983; Smith *et al.*, 1980). Whilst therapist ratings and self-reports have their place, this implies that every study should include at least one non-reactive measure of change.

Specificity and Relevance of Measures. The construct validity of a study is threated if the outcome measures used are not sufficiently specific to the problem under treatment, or not relevant to the goals of treatment. Some investigators (e.g. Rachman & Wilson, 1980) attribute the equivocal findings of much outcome research to excessively general, crude outcome measures based upon simplistic models of such constructs as anxiety. Shapiro and Shapiro (1983) found more powerful effects with measures that were more specific to the goals of treatment.

It is a commonplace observation in psychotherapy research that different outcome measures applied to the same clients in the same treatments may yield quite different results. For this and other reasons, there is general agreement (Lambert, Christensen & DeJulio, 1983; Kazdin, 1986; Lambert *et al.*, 1986) that outcome assessment needs to be multifaceted, involving different perspectives (the treated individual, significant others, professional observers), different aspects of the individual (e.g. behaviour, affect, and cognition) and different modalities of assessment (e.g. self-report, direct observation, and clinician ratings). However, Shapiro and Shapiro (1983) found that most investigators confined themselves to only one or two out of five assessment modalities.

Another measurement issue is that it may be important to distinguish the effects of a mental health treatment from the value attached to such effects. Some investigators have argued that different psychotherapies may have different and potent effects that are valued differently by different people (Stiles, 1983; Strupp & Hadley, 1977). Projecting multiple dimensions onto a single dimension of 'improvement' or 'change' by using averaged scales makes therapies comparable but at a cost of masking their diversity and potency of effect (Stiles *et al.*, 1986).

A final aspect of measurement that bears on construct validity relates to the timing of outcome assessment. In principle, outcome research should demonstrate the maintenance of treatment effects over time. Although Nicholson and Berman (1983) have provided persuasive evidence that follow-up data are typically very similar to data obtained immediately after the completion of treatment, there are striking exceptions to this generalisation for particular problems and treatments (Kazdin, 1986). For example, Kingsley and Wilson (1977) found that individual behaviour therapy was more effective in achieving weight reduction at post-treatment when compared with a group treatment based on social pressure; 1 year later, however, weight loss data favoured the social pressure treatment. In the review by Shapiro and Shapiro (1983), 77% of outcome data were obtained immediately after treatment, and only 6% were obtained 4 or more months after the end of treatment. Investigators' reluctance to present long-term follow-up data is readily explicable: such data are costly to obtain, and are often compromised by attrition or by participation in additional treatment.

External Validity

External validity is defined by Cook and Campbell (1979) in relation to problems of generalising to particular target persons, settings, and times; and of generalising across types of persons, settings, and times. For psychotherapy research, the central problem is the extent to which the persons and settings studied in the literature represent those of clinical practice.

Much psychotherapy research has taken the form of 'analogue' studies in which undergraduate students are solicited to participate in brief treatments designed to help them overcome circumscribed and relatively minor problems such as public speaking anxiety or specific phobias (Kazdin, 1978; Mathews, 1978; Borkovec & Rachman, 1979), conducted in laboratory or academic rather than in clinical settings. There is some evidence that such studies may show larger gains in treatment than are found in settings and with populations more representative of clinical practice (Smith *et al.*, 1980; Shapiro & Shapiro, 1983). On the other hand, therapists in such research tend to be trainees, unrepresentative of qualified and experienced therapists, and likely, if anything, to yield less favourable outcomes. Krupnick, Shea and Elkin (1986) reviewed 14 studies presenting direct comparisons between solicited and non-solicited patients receiving treatment in clinically representative settings. These authors concluded that results of studies using solicited patients alone must be interpreted with caution. Not only may such studies over- or under-estimate response to treatment, but they may also yield conclusions concerning the relative efficacy of different treatments that do not hold up when tested with non-solicited patients.

Of course, there are often good reasons to choose solicited populations. Within the resource limitations and practical constraints under which mental health researchers operate, the demands of external validity are often in conflict with those of internal or construct validity. For example, random allocation to different treatments may not be feasible in an established clinical service, with referral patterns based on the reputations and preferred treatment methods of individual practitioners. A comparative design that allowed individuals to be assigned to treatments in such a biased way would confound the treatment variable under test with features of the therapists, the patients and their circumstances which influenced the referral decisions. These same features would also probably contribute substantially to the outcome obtained in each case. This would present a fatal threat to the internal validity of the study as a comparison between treatments. In these circumstances, the preferred compromise would almost certainly be to sacrifice external to internal validity and solicit patients via new channels outside the established referral system, to enable random assignment to treatments.

MAKING SENSE OF EXISTING OUTCOME RESEARCH

A vast number of controlled and comparative outcome studies of mental health treatments have been published over the past 35 years. This large amount of information is difficult to integrate in such a way as to provide clear guidelines for future practice, training and research. Indeed, reviewers attempting such integrations of outcome research on mental health treatments, particularly psychotherapy, have reached disparate conclusions. In relation to 'verbal', non-behavioural therapies, for example, the negative conclusions drawn by Eysenck (1952) and by Rachman and Wilson (1980) conflict sharply with the more optimistic evaluations of Bergin (1971; Bergin & Lambert, 1978), Meltzoff and Kornreich (1970), and Luborsky, Singer, and Luborsky (1975).

Such debates may in part reflect subjective and unsystematic elements of the traditional approach to reviewing scientific literature. The term *meta-analysis* denotes a family of approaches and techniques based upon the application to the literature review process of the methodological principles of empirical social science (Glass, McGaw & Smith, 1981; Shapiro & Shapiro, 1982a; Shapiro, 1985). Meta-analysis entered clinical psychology with the appearance of Smith and Glass's (1977; Smith, Glass & Miller, 1980) review of psychotherapy outcome studies. This work has been widely praised (Fiske, 1983; Rosenthal, 1978), criticised (Eysenck, 1978; Wilson & Rachman, 1983) and built upon (Andrews & Harvey, 1981; Landman & Dawes, 1982; Prioleau, Murdock, & Brody, 1983; Shapiro & Shapiro, 1982b) by other reviewers.

Table 9.3 summarises the differences between traditional and meta-analytic reviews. A traditional, narrative review is qualitative in orientation, with rational and interpretive considerations governing its scope, procedures and conclusions. It is common to exclude studies from consideration which the reviewer considers severely deficient from a methodological point of view. Studies may be grouped according to characteristics shared in common, and results of such grouped studies may be presented in tabular form.

TABLE 9.3
Traditional versus meta-analytic reviews

	Traditional	*Meta-analytic*
Orientation	Qualitative	Quantitative
Coverage	Selective	Representative or exhaustive
Quality control	By exclusion	Empirical evaluation
Organisation	Study by study	By features
Representation of findings	Narrative statements	Quantitative and/or probabalistic
Description of study features	Qualitative	Systematic coding schemes
Linking study features to outcomes	Narrative statements	Disaggregation and statistical analysis

In contrast, a meta-analysis is primarily quantitative in orientation. Selection of studies is governed by sampling principles; a sample of studies is drawn, following replicable procedures, from the population of studies addressing the issue at hand. Exclusion of individual studies on the basis of evaluative judgements of their quality, made in full knowledge of the findings of the study, is typically avoided. Rather, studies are scored for their methodological attributes, using defined coding schemes of proven reliability, and these methodological attributes are subsequently correlated with the findings of each study, to determine empirically the impact of study quality on the results obtained. Meta-analysis thus takes account of study quality, but in a quantitative fashion rather than by selection of 'good' studies. This process does not eliminate the need for human judgement in evaluating research, but, rather, attempts to systematise the exercise of such judgement in accordance with the canons of social science.

Other attributes of each study are similarly coded, so that the study-by-study narrative of the traditional review can be replaced by generalisations across studies, organised according to features common to or differing between groups of studies. In mental health treatment research, for example, the literature can be described in terms of such parameters as the types of patients treated, the treatment methods used, the length and format of treatment, and the instruments used to assess client change.

Meta-analysis differs from traditional reviews in how the findings of each study are represented. The outcome of each study, or of each treatment comparison contained withing each study, is expressed quantitatively. Most commonly, a difference between group means is expressed in standard deviation units. Such a standardised difference score is known as an

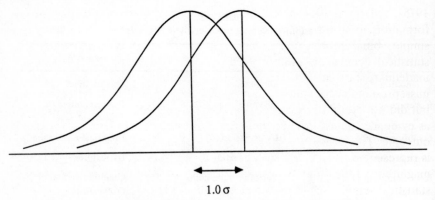

FIG. 9.3.   Effect size of one standard deviation.

effect size. The meaning of this statistic can be illustrated with reference to a hypothetical example shown in Fig. 9.3. This diagram represents a study in which the difference between treated and untreated control subjects is equal to an effect size of 1.0.

If we assume that the scores on the outcome measure follow the familiar, bell-shaped normal distribution, an effect size of 1.0 implies that 84.1% of the members of the treated group are better off in terms of the outcome measure than the average member of the control group. Another way to think of an effect size is in terms of the percentage of variance it accounts for. Considering the variation in outcome between all the individuals in both groups, for an effect size of 1.0 it turns out that 20% of this variation amongst individuals can be attributed to their membership of one or other of the two groups, with the remaining 80% of the variation being due to other factors probably unrelated to treatment. Yet a third way of understanding an effect size is based upon the idea of dividing the combined sample into 'successes' and 'failures' according to a dichotomous criterion appropriate to the particular sample and circumstances. In the case of an effect size of 1.0 as between treated and untreated groups, we find that treatment enhances subjects' success rate by 45% (Rosenthal, 1983).

Another approach involves cumulative testing of the null hypothesis of no treatment differences across studies by combining the probabilities obtained in each study (Rosenthal, 1978). Yet another method is to divide mean pre-post difference scores by mean pre-treatment scores in each group (Blanchard, Andrasik, Ahler, Teders & O'Keefe, 1980). This method takes no account of within-group variation.

Reviewers summarising data from a series of studies have traditionally tallied the number of positive (i.e. statistically significant) and null (i.e. not statistically significant) findings in a 'box score' total (e.g. Luborsky *et al.*,

1975). All the meta-analytic methods described here preserve more information about the magnitude of effects obtained in each study than this simple, binary, box score. The box score procedure compounds the statistical conclusion validity problems which ensue if each study has inadequate statistical power when considered alone. The box score method misrepresents every study whose results were in the predicted direction, but did not attain significance on account of inadequate statistical power, as evidence against the hypothesised relationship between treatment and outcome. This difficulty is overcome in meta-analysis, because each finding is represented as an effect size, expressing in standard deviation units the magnitude of the difference between treatment groups, irrespective of the statistical significance of each result considered alone.

Finally, meta-analysis involves statistical analysis of the correlates of study outcomes. Effect sizes or other indices of outcome are considered as dependent measures to be predicted from substantive and/or methodological features of each study. The relations of single parameters such as treatment method or sample size to outcome can be examined via simple statistics such at t tests or zero-order correlations. More complex questions (such as the identification of independent predictors of outcome from amongst sets of predictors, or the search for interactions between client and treatment parameters in the determination of outcome) can be addressed with correspondingly complex statistical procedures such as multiple regression. Large and varied data sets (such as are found in mental health treatment outcome research) are particularly suited to this type of analysis, which offers the potential for a much richer account of the relationships between study parameters and outcome than the traditional narrative review.

Meta-analysis has an established place in the integration of research data on the outcomes of mental health treatments (Garfield, 1983; Michelson, 1985), and meta-analytic findings were drawn upon to illuminate several of the methodological issues discussed earlier in this chapter. Indeed, the contrast between meta-analytic and traditional reviews is becoming less pronounced than implied by the presentation in Table 9.3, as increasing numbers of reviewers use and adapt meta-analytic techniques as appropriate. However, meta-analysis must be used carefully and with due regard for the impact of the assumptions made in carrying out the meta-analysis upon the conclusions drawn. Furthermore, there may be insufficient studies looking at new or unusual treatments to permit a meaningful meta-analysis. The advent of meta-analysis has thrown into new relief some recurrent weaknesses of outcome studies, together with avoidable limitations in the precision with which their methods and data are reported. Investigators planning outcome research should anticipate the inclusion of their published work within future meta-analytic reviews. This has implications both for the conduct of the research itself and for how it is reported. For example, the informativeness of meta-analyses is enhanced if investigators use closely comparable outcome measures and patient inclusion criteria in different studies, and if they ensure that all necessary information is included in their reports (Shapiro & Shapiro, 1983).

COSTS, BENEFITS AND EFFECTIVENESS

In health service practice, it is painfully obvious that the availability of mental health treatments is limited by resource constraints. Treatment decisions for individual patients are influenced by the availability of therapists, office space and other resources. For example, the waiting list for the best available treatment may be so long that immediate access to a less oversubscribed intervention may be preferable for the patient. Underlying such individual dilemmas are the strategic choices made by health districts in deciding how much of which kinds of service to make available, which would in an ideally rational world be governed by evidence showing how to gain the maximum benefit to the patient population from available resources. If outcome research is to facilitate such rational policy formulation, therefore, it must measure the costs as well as the effects of interventions (Yates & Newman, 1980; Newman & Howard, 1986).

Following Newman and Howard (1986), we may define the costs of an episode of treatment in terms of the cost of each 'unit of service activity' (such as an individual psychotherapy session). Each unit cost consists of the salary and fringe benefit cost for the professional(s) involved for that proportion of their working time, plus the costs of material resources used and of allocated overheads (such as accommodation, support staff, heating, etc., also expressed as a proportion of annual figures). The total cost of an episode of treatment is obtained by summing the costs of the units of service it comprises. As noted by Newman and Howard (1986), however, such cost measures are no more than an estimation procedure for describing the human efforts and material ingredients invested in an intervention. In addition, these authors have extended the cost concept to that of 'therapeutic effort', also encompassing the degree to which an intervention imposes restrictions upon the freedom of the patient.

Costs can be related to effects in two ways. First, *cost–effectiveness* analysis expresses the yield of an intervention in terms of units of effectiveness per unit of cost, without attempting to scale effectiveness in monetary terms. Thus we might compare treatments in terms of the costs in £s per symptom point reduction on a standard measure such as the Present State Examination. In a study by Piper, Debbane, Bienvenu, and Garant (1984) comparing four forms of psychotherapy (long-term versus short-term variants of both individual and group therapy), cost considerations altered the relative merits of the four conditions as compared with their ordering with respect to effectiveness alone. In contrast, *cost–benefit* analysis takes the further step of assigning financial value to the effects of treatment. For example, the financial benefits to the state of a successful psychotherapy might include the reduced benefits liabilities and increased taxation income consequent upon the patient's return to employment. Cost–benefit analysis entails several complex and debatable economic assumptions and value judgments, and is thus too ambitious and fraught an enterprise for many outcome researchers. Cost–effectiveness analysis, on the other hand, can be recommended as a helpful addition to most comparative outcome studies. In summary:

1. Treatment decisions depend on costs as well as effectiveness of treatment.
2. Therapeutic effort reflects costs of treatment episode plus restrictions on patient's freedom.
3. Cost-effectiveness analysis expresses yield in terms of units of effectiveness per unit of cost.
4. Cost-benefit analysis expresses yield in terms of financial benefit per financial unit of cost.

CONCLUSION

This chapter has reviewed the most common designs for outcome research studies, discussed methodological issues bearing upon the validity of such studies, outlined the recently developed meta-analytic approach to summarising existing research findings, and introduced the appraisal of costs as an important element in the evaluation of mental health treatments. As noted at the outset, the art of outcome research design is one of creative compromise, since practical constraints and the countervailing demands of different methodological criteria preclude the 'perfect' study. In practice, the definitive evaluation of a given method requires complementary and convergent evidence from a body of methodologically diverse studies ranging from laboratory analogues with good internal and statistical conclusion validity to field trials with good external validity.

Under-resourced and possibly inexperienced investigators working in service settings should take heart from this state of affairs. Careful attention to the principles discussed here will enable them to make worthwhile contributions to outcome research. The goal in planning such studies, of course, is to maximise the yield from the design strengths available whilst minimising the weaknesses stemming from unavoidable deficiencies. Given the benefits of methodological diversity in outcome research, there is a countinuing need for soundly designed, albeit modestly resourced, studies in service settings.

ACKNOWLEDGEMENTS

I thank Bill Stiles for comments on a draft of this chapter.

REFERENCES

American Psychiatric Association (1980). *Diagnostic and Statistical Manual of Mental Disorders*, 3rd edn. Washington, DC: American Psychiatric Association.

Andrews, G. & Harvey, R. (1981). Does psychotherapy benefit neurotic patients? A reanalysis of the Smith, Glass and Miller data. *Archives of General Psychiatry*, **38**, 1203–1208.

Basham, R. B. (1986). Scientific and practical advantages of comparative design in psychotherapy research. *Journal of Consulting and Clinical Psychology*, **54**, 88–94.

Beck, A. T., Ward, C. H., Mendelson, M., Mock, J. & Earbaugh, J. (1961). An inventory for measuring depression. *Archives of General Psychiatry*, **4**, 561–571.

Beck, A. T., Rush, A. J., Shaw, B. F. & Emery, G. (1979). *Cognitive Therapy of Depression*. New York: Guilford Press.

Bergin, A. E. (1971). The evaluation of therapeutic ourcomes. In A. E. Bergin and S. L. Garfield (eds.), *Handbook of Psychotherapy and Behaviour Change: An Empirical Analysis*. New York: John Wiley.

Bergin, A. E. & Lambert, M. J. (1978). The evaluation of therapeutic outcomes. In S. L. Garfield and A. E. Bergin (eds.), *Handbook of Psychotherapy and Behavior Change: An Empirical Analysis*, 2nd edn. New York: John Wiley, pp. 139–189.

Berman, J. S., Miller, R. C. & Massman, P. J. (1985). Cognitive therapy versus systematic desensitization: Is one treatment superior? *Psychological Bulletin*, **97**, 451–461.

Blanchard, E. B., Andrasik, F., Ahler, T. A., Teders, S. J. & O'Keefe, D. O. (1980). Migraine and tension headache: A meta-analytic review. *Behavior Therapy*, **11**, 613–631.

Borkovec, T. D. & Nau, S. D. (1972). Credibility of analogue therapy rationales. *Journal of Behavior Therapy and Experimental Psychiatry*, **3**, 257–260.

Borkovec, T. D. & Rachman, S. (1979). The utility of analogue research. *Behaviour Research and Therapy*, **17**, 253–261.

Cohen, J. (1962). The statistical power of abnormal-social psychological research: A review. *Journal of Abnormal and Social Psychology*, **65**, 145–153.

Cohen, J. (1977). *Statistical Power Analysis for the Behavioral Sciences*, 2nd edn. New York: Academic Press.

Cook, T. D. & Campbell, D. T. (1979). *Quasi-experimentation: Design and Analysis for Field Settings*. Chicago: Rand McNally.

DeRubeis, R., Hollon, S., Evans, M. & Bemis, K. (1982). Can psychotherapies for depression be discriminated? A systematic investigation of cognitive therapy and interpersonal therapy. *Journal of Consulting and Clinical Psychology*, **50**, 744–756.

Evans, M., Hollon, S., DeRubeis, R., Tuason, V. B., Wiemer, M. & Auerbach, A. (1983). Development of a system for rating psychotherapies for depression. Paper presented at *The 14th Annual Meeting of the Society for Psychotherapy Research, Sheffield, England*.

Eysenck, H. J. (1952). The effects of psychotherapy: An evaluation. *Journal of Consulting Psychology*, **16**, 319–324.

Eysenck, H. J. (1978). An exercise in mega-silliness. *American Psychologist*, **33**, 517.

Fiske, D. W. (1983). The meta-analytic revolution in outcome research. *Journal of Consulting and Clinical Psychology*, **51**, 65–70.

Garfield, S. L. (1983). Introduction to special section. *Journal of Consulting and Clinical Psychology*, **51**, 3.

Glass, G. V., McGaw, B. & Smith, M. L. (1981). *Meta-analysis in Social Research*. Beverly Hills, CA: Sage.

Hardy, G. E. & Shapiro, D. A. (1985). Therapist verbal response modes in prescriptive vs. exploratory psychotherapy. *British Journal of Clinical Psychology*, **24**, 235–245.

Holroyd, K. A., Penzien, D. B., Hursey, K. G., Tobin, D. L., Rogers, L., Holm, J. E., Marcille, P. J., Hall, J. R. & Chila, A. G. (1984). Change mechanisms in EMG biofeedback training: Cognitive changes underlying improvements in tension headache. *Journal of Consulting and Clinical Psychology*, **52**, 1039–1053.

Horowitz, M. J. (1982). Strategic dilemmas and the socialization of psychotherapy researchers. *British Journal of Clinical Psychology*, **21**, 119–127.

Howard, K. I., Krause, M. S. & Orlinsky, D. E. (1986). The attrition dilemma: Toward a new strategy for psychotherapy research. *Journal of Consulting and Clinical Psychology*, **54**, 106–110.

Hugdahl, K. & Ost, L. (1981). On the difference between statistical and clinical significance. *Behavioral Assessment*, **3**, 289–295.

Jacobson, N. S., Follette, W. C. & Revenstorf, D. (1984). Psychotherapy outcome research: Methods for reporting variability and evaluating clinical significance. *Behavior Therapy*, **15**, 336–352.

Kazdin, A. E. (1978). Evaluating the generality of findings in analogue therapy research. *Journal of Consulting and Clinical Psychology*, **46**, 673–686.

Kazdin, A. E. (1986). Comparative outcome studies of psychotherapy: Methodological issues and strategies. *Journal of Consulting and Clinical Psychology*, **54**, 95–105.

Kazdin, A. E. & Wilcoxon, L. A. (1976). Systematic desensitization and non-specific treatment effects: A methodological evaluation. *Psychological Bulletin*, **83**, 729–758.

Kazdin, A. E. & Wilson, G. T. (1978). *Evaluation of Behavior Therapy: Issues, Evidence, and Research Strategies*. Cambridge Mass.: Ballinger.

Kingsley, R. G. & Wilson, G. T. (1977). Behavior therapy for obesity: A comparative investigation of long-term efficacy. *Journal of Consulting and Clinical Psychology*, **45**, 288–298.

Klerman, G., Rounsaville, B., Chevron, E., Neu, C. & Weissman, M. (1984). *Manual for Short-term Interpersonal Therapy for Depression*. New York: Basic Books.

Kraemer, H. C. (1981). Coping strategies in psychiatric clinical research. *Journal of Consulting and Clinical Psychology*, **49**, 309–319.

Krupnick, J., Shea, T. & Elkin, I. (1986). Generalizability of treatment studies using solicited patients. *Journal of Consulting and Clinical Psychology*, **54**, 68–78.

Lambert, M. J. (1976). Spontaneous remission in adult neurotic disorders. A revision and summary, *Psychological Bulletin*, **83**, 107–119.

Lambert, M. J., Christensen, E. R. & DeJulio, S. S. (eds) (1983). *The Assessment of Psychotherapy Outcome*. New York: Wiley.

Lambert, M. J., Shapiro, D. A. & Bergin, A. E. (1986). The effectiveness of psychotherapy. In S. L. Garfield & A. E. Bergin (eds). *Handbook of Psychotherapy and Behavior Change*, 3rd edn. New York: Wiley.

Landman, J. T. & Dawes, R. M. (1982). Psychotherapy outcome: Smith and Glass's conclusions stand up under scrutiny. *American Psychologist*, **37**, 505–516.

Luborsky, L. (1984). *Principles of psychoanalytic psychotherapy: A manual for supportive-expressive treatment*. New York: Basic Books.

Luborsky, L. & DeRubeis, R. J. (1984). The use of psychotherapy treatment manuals: A small revolution in psychotherapy research style. *Clinical Psychology Review*, **4**, 5–14.

Luborsky, L., Singer, B. & Luborsky, L. (1975). Comparative studies of psychotherapies: Is it true that 'Everyone has won and all must have prizes'? *Archives of General Psychiatry*, **32**, 995–1008.

Mahoney, M. J. (1978). Experimental methods and outcome evaluation. *Journal of Consulting and Clinical Psychology*, **46**, 660–672.

Mathews, A. M. (1978). Fear reduction research and clinical phobias. *Psychological Bulletin*, **85**, 390–404.

Meltzoff, J. & Kornreich, M. (1970). *Research in Psychotherapy*. New York: Atherton Press.

Michelson, L. (1985). Editorial: Meta-analysis and clinical psychology. *Clinical Psychology Review*, **5**, 1–2.

Mintz, J., Luborsky, L. & Christolph, P. (1979). Measuring the outcomes of psychotherapy: Findings of the Penn Psychotherapy Project. *Journal of Consulting and Clinical Psychology*, **47**, 319–334.

Newman, F. L. & Howard, K. I. (1986). Therapeutic effort, treatment outcome, and national health policy. *American Psychologist*, **41**, 181–187.

Nicholson, R. A. & Berman, J. S. (1983). Is follow-up necessary in evaluting psychotherapy? *Psychological Bulletin*, **93**, 261–278.

Parloff, M. B. (1986). Placebo controls in psychotherapy research: a sine qua non or a placebo for research problems? *Journal of Consulting and Clinical Psychology*, **54**, 79–87.

Paul, G. L. (1966). *Insight vs. Desensitization in Psychotherapy*. Palo Alto: Stanford University Press.

Piper, W. E., Debbane, E. G., Bienvenu, J. P. & Garant, J. (1984). A comparative study of four forms of psychotherapy, *Journal of Consulting and Clinical Psychology*, **52**, 268–279.

Prioleau, L., Murdock, M. & Brody, N. (1983). An analysis of psychotherapy versus placebo studies. *Behavioral and Brain Sciences*, **6**, 275–310.

Rachman, S. & Wilson, G. T. (1980). *The effects of psychological therapy*, 2nd edn. New York: Pergamon Press.

Rosenthal, R. (1978). Combining results of independent studies. *Psychological Bulletin*, **85**, 185–193.

Rosenthal, R. (1983). Assessing the statistical and social importance of the effects of psychotherapy. *Journal of Consulting and Clinical Psychology*, **51**, 4–13.

Rosenthal, R. & Frank, J. D. (1956). Psychotherapy and the placebo effect. *Psychological Bulletin*, **53**, 294–302.

Rosenthal, R. & Rubin, D. B. (1978). Interpersonal expectancy effects: The first 345 Studies. *Behavioural and Brain Sciences*, **3**, 377–415.

Schaffer, N. D. (1982). Multidimensional measures of therapist behavior as predictors of outcome. *Psychological Bulletin*, **92**, 670–681.

Shapiro, A. K. & Morris, L. A. (1978). Placebo effects in medical and psychological therapies. In S. L. Garfield & A. E. Bergin (eds.) *Handbook of Psychotherapy and Behavior Change*, 2nd edn. New York: Wiley.

Shapiro, D. A. (1981). Comparative credibility of treatment rationales: Three tests of expectancy theory. *British Journal of Clinical Psychology*, **20**, 111–122.

Shapiro, D. A. (1985). Recent applications of meta-analysis in clinical research. *Clinical Psychology Review*, **5**, 13–34.

Shapiro, D. A. & Shapiro, D. (1982a). Meta-analysis of comparative therapy outcome studies: A replication and refinement. *Psychological Bulletin*, **92**, 581–604.

Shapiro, D. A. & Shapiro, D (1982b). Meta-analysis of comparative therapy outcome research: A critical appraisal. *Behavioural Psychotherapy*, **10**, 4–25.

Shapiro, D. A. & Shapiro, D. (1983). Comparative therapy outcome research: Methodological implications of meta-analysis. *Journal of Consulting and Clinical Psychology*, **51**, 42–53.

Smith, M. L. & Glass, G. V. (1977). Meta-analysis of psychotherapy outcome studies. *American Psychologist*, **32**, 752–760.

Smith, M. L., Glass G. V. & Miller, T. I. (1980). *The Benefits of Psychotherapy*. Baltimore: Johns Hopkins University Press.

Stiles, W. B. (1983). Normality, diversity and psychotherapy. *Psychotherapy: Theory, Research and Practice*, **20**, 183–189.

Stiles, W. B., Shapiro, D. A. & Elliot, R. K. (1986). "Are all psychotherapies equivalent?" *American Psychologist*, **41**, 165–180.

Strupp, H. H. & Hadley, S. W. (1977). A tripartite model of mental health and therapeutic outcomes: With special reference to negative effects in psychotherapy. *American Psychologist*, **32**, 196–197.

Wilkins, W. (1984). Psychotherapy: The powerful placebo. *Journal of Consulting and Clinical Psychology*, **52**, 570–573.

Wilson, G. T. & Rachman, S. (1983). Meta-analysis and evaluation of psychotherapy outcome: Limitations and liabilities. *Journal of Consulting and Clinical Psychology*, **51**, 54–64.

Wing, J. K., Cooper, J. E. & Sartorius, N. (1974). *The Measurement and Classification of Psychiatric Symptoms*. Cambridge University Press.

Yates, B. T. & Newman, F. L. (1980). Approaches to cost-effectiveness analysis and cost-benefit analysis of psychotherapy. In G. R. VandenBos (ed.) *Psychotherapy: Practice, Research, Policy*. Beverly Hills, Cali.: Sage.

Yeaton, W. H. & Sechrest, L. (1981). Critical dimensions in the choice and maintenance of successful treatments: Strength, integrity, and effectiveness. *Journal of Consulting and Clinical Psychology*, **49**, 156–167.

10

Patient Series and Quasi-Experimental Designs

R. Glynn Owens
University of Liverpool.

P. D. Slade
University of Liverpool.

D. M. Fielding
St. James Hospital, Leeds.

Experimental procedures have become widely accepted as an appropriate means of conducting research in the mental health field. Such experimentation may range from the small-N ABAB and similar designs beloved of applied behaviour analysts to large-scale statistical studies of experimental and control groups. Common to all such procedures, however, is the general principle of holding constant all factors except the independent variable under study; where these cannot be controlled directly, some form of statistical control, involving the 'balancing' of these factors between conditions, is adopted. Most frequently such balancing of factors is achieved by some form of randomisation; either baseline and experimental conditions are randomly varied, or subjects in large-N designs are randomly allocated to one or other group.

Such an approach has a clear strength in permitting any differences between conditions to be attributed to the only factor which has been permitted to vary systematically, and designs following such principles are now commonplace in mental health research. Often, however, there are reasons that render a tight experimental design undesirable or impractical. As a result researchers have developed a number of alternative approaches to the study of various types of problem, permitting topics to be studied that lie outside the scope of traditional experimental methods. Two

189

methods that have had particular impact in psychological settings are the patient series and quasi-experimental designs, approaches which, whilst not without their own problems, side-step certain difficulties encountered by straightforward experimentation.

PATIENT SERIES DESIGNS

Even the slightest acquaintance with clinical problems brings an awareness that patients are very much individuals (Kiesler, 1966). A corollary of this is that a researcher's behaviour is likely to vary considerably from patient to patient. Such variation may present problems to a traditional experimental design, producing considerable heterogeneity within comparison groups and also considerable overlap between them. Thus a therapist who attempted to compare, say, directive and non-directive psychotherapy would probably find it difficult to be entirely directive to one group and entirely non-directive to another group (the difficulty of being non-directive has been demonstrated by Truax (1966)). In consequence, groups that were meant to be distinct may in fact turn out to be not at all dissimilar. Where a therapist would normally, in practice, use elements of both of the methods being compared, an attempt to use only one for the purposes of an experiment might result in a totally artificial experiment whose results would have little or no relevance to actual clinical practice.

The problem is compounded when it is recognised that in many cases such groups as 'no treatment' control groups may be unacceptable on ethical grounds. In such cases it may be appropriate to provide treatment to all individuals involved, reporting the results of such interventions as they stand without direct comparison with similar untreated individuals. Finally, it is notable that the similarities between individuals often become apparent only at a relatively abstract level; that is, while similar processes may operate, the specific factors may none the less be quite disparate (Shapiro, 1966). For example, two people may show aggressive behaviour in response to some disturbing or irritating event, yet the specific events may be peculiar to each. In such cases it may be important to study in detail each individual, rather than to summarise the subjects in terms of means and variances. Indeed a number of writers have pointed out how similarities of process may be masked by such activities as averaging. Sidman (1960) for example illustrates how subjects showing basically similar (but parametrically different) performances may give rise to a totally different average performance.

Because of problems such as these a number of important works have presented their results not as experimental findings but rather as a description of a series of patients. Such a 'Patient Series' design may be traced back to the case history reports of workers like Freud. Modern patient series designs, however, show considerably more sophistication than these early reports. Two well-known and much-quoted examples are Masters and Johnsons' studies of psychological methods of treatment for sexual dysfunction patients (Masters & Johnson, 1970) and Becks' studies of cognitive processes and therapy in patients presenting with depressive and anxiety problems (Beck, 1976). The basic underpinning of patient series research designs was formulated by Cronbach (1975) in his principle of 'intensive local observation', as follows:

> An observer collecting data in one particular situation is in a position to appraise a practice or proposition in that setting, observing effects in context. In trying to describe and account for what happened, he will give attention to whatever variables were controlled. But he will give equally careful attention to uncontrolled conditions, to personal characteristics, and to events that occurred during treatment and measurement. As he goes from situation to situation, his first task is to describe and interpret the effect anew in each locale, perhaps taking into account factors unique to that locale. . . . As results accumulate, a person who seeks understanding will do his best to trace how the uncontrolled factors could have caused local departures from the modal effect. That is, generalization comes late and the exception is taken as seriously as the rule.

It can be seen from the above that the basic principle underlying the 'patient series approach' involves a combination of systematic observation and manipulation of relevant variables, where possible, while maintaining a clear focus on the individual rather than the average group member. As such this research lends itself to many clinical problems and situations. We shall now consider some of the methods and possibilities associated with such an approach.

Prediction of Outcome

When a more or less standard psychological treatment is given to a group of patients who apparently share a similar problem (for example, an exposure treatment for agoraphobic patients or a controlled drinking programme for problem drinkers) the outcome of treatment is likely to vary. Some patients are likely to show a good response, others a poor response, while the outcome for still others will be intermediate between the two extremes. This is a common clinical observation and one that lends itself to analysis by the clinician-researcher.

There are good reasons why the clinician may wish to investigate the issue of which patients respond well and which poorly to the treatment. If the patients who are likely to respond poorly can be predicted in advance from pretreatment variables, such patients can be offered a different type of treatment by the clinician or referred on to someone else who offers a different kind of treatment. Similarly, if the likelihood of a poor eventual outcome can be predicted from variables relating to initial treatment response, the clinician may change the treatment approach at an early stage. Thus the investigation of prediction of treatment response has much to commend it for practical reasons.

The common approach to this issue is to collect data on the nature and severity of the target problems in a sizeable and unselected sample of patients, both before and after exposure to a standard treatment regime. Such measures are likely to be quantitative in nature, such as how close a snake-phobic patient can approach to a live snake or an agoraphobic patient's rating of their anxiety at various distances from home. A quantitative index of improvement can be obtained by subtracting the post-treatment from the pre-treatment values. (For a discussion of the complex statistical issues in the measurement of change, see Harris, 1963.) These 'change' scores can be treated *either* as continuous treatment–outcome measures *or* used to establish discrete outcome categories such as 'good', 'intermediate' or 'poor response'. In either case, they can be used as dependent measures in the analysis of treatment prediction. As previously indicated, the predictors of interest will either be *pretreatment* variables or *treatment* variables. The former may well include demographic variables (e.g. age, sex, occupation, marital status, etc.), severity of problem variables (e.g. duration of drink problem, severity, etc.), assessments of personal, social and marital satisfaction, general measures of anxiety, depression and other problems, expectancies for treatment success, etc. Treatment variables may include number of attendances, number of homework assignments completed, rapport achieved by therapist, etc. Initial response to treatment is a particularly useful treatment variable as research with a variety of different treatment approaches and clinical problems has shown that response to the first one of two sessions of treatment is a good predictor of eventual clinical improvement.

The type of statistical analysis which can be performed with the data will depend largely on the nature of the outcome criterion variable used (Table 10.1). If it is *continuous*, correlational measures will probably be the most appropriate: if *discrete*, then analyses of variance and discriminant function analysis will be required. However, whether the dependent variable is continuous or discrete the clinician will no doubt wish to know which of the predictor variables has the strongest influence on outcome. For this the clinician–researcher will need to carry out 'multiple regression analyses'.

One cautionary point needs to be raised when carrying out statistical analyses of outcome prediction data. Often the relationship between the 'dependent or criterion' variable and a 'predictor' variable is not linear (i.e. a straight line). For example, the relation between severity of agoraphobic

TABLE 10.1
Summary of methods for investigating response to treatment

| | Predictor variables | | Methods of statistical analysis |
Outcome criteria	Pretreatment	Treatment	
Continuous, i.e Degree of change	Age, sex, severity of problem, etc.	No. of attendances No. of homework assignments completed, etc.	Correlations, multiple regression analyses, etc.
Discrete, i.e. Good vs. intermediate Very poor response	Same	Same	ANOVAS, discriminant function analyses, multiple regression analyses

symptoms and treatment response may be curvilinear one, with 'mild' and 'very severe' patients showing much less of a response than 'moderately severe' patients. There may also be an asymmetrical relationship between the predictor and the criterion, an example that patients with good motivation may show varied responses to treatment though patients with poor motivation never respond well. Where such non-linear relationships obtain, the statistical methods outlined in Table 10.1 are probably inappropriate. Bivariate plots or scattergrams taking two variables (one dependent one predictor) at a time will usually serve to sort out this complication. Non-linear relationships should not be regarded merely as a statistical nuisance; they can be of theoretical interest and practical importance.

Model-Building

As well as lending itself to investigations of prediction of treatment outcome, or indeed any kind of prognostic outcome such as for example recovery of function following post-traumatic amnesia, the 'patient series' approach is useful for model-building. In such an exercise the clinician–researcher is concerned with extracting general principles or processes from consideration of a sample of individual patients presenting with apparently similar problems. One method of model-building which is becoming increasingly popular is that of *functional analysis*. The interested reader is referred to the paper by Owens and Ashcroft (1982) for a succinct, general exposition of this methodology.

In essence the functional analysis approach involves analysis of behaviour in terms of *A*ntecedents, *B*ehaviour and *C*onsequences—the

FIG. 10.1.   Outline of a functional analysis of aggression. (Reproduced from Owens & Bagshaw, 1985, by permission of Plenum Publishing.)

A-B-C paradigm. Examples of each of these may be seen in the functional model of aggressive behaviour of Owens and Bagshaw (1985). This model is summarised in the form of a flow diagram in Fig. 10.1. Basically *antecedents* include such factors as aversive stimulation (reactive aggression paradigm), personality factors, physiological factors, drugs (including alcohol), etc. whereas the *consequences* include the various pay-offs or reinforcers to the individual.

Clearly, whilst the model points to the types of factor that may be involved in aggressive behaviour, it does so only in a very general way, with reference to 'aversive stimuli', 'reinforcers', etc. In any given episode of violent behaviour the actual variables may be specific to the individual concerned. Thus for one individual the aversive stimulus may take the form of being mocked by a friend; for another it may be a physical blow. Stimuli that are aversive to one individual may not be so to another, as has been demonstrated elegantly by Vernon and Ulrich (1966), who showed how particular learning experiences could result in previously neutral stimuli acquiring aversive properties and giving rise to reactive aggression. This individuality is a common aspect of models derived from a patient series design, particular features of each case being grouped according to their functional, rather than their physical similarities. Thus rather than listing each different type of aversive stimulus encountered in the patient series it is recognised that the various stimuli play similar roles and may therefore be grouped together. In the same way other functionally similar but physically different events (e.g. reinforcers) may be subsumed under a single heading.

The model presented in Fig. 10.1 illustrates several aspects of patient series designs. First, it should be recognised that different processes may operate in the development and the maintenance of a problem; in extreme cases these two aspects may reflect almost totally different formulations. Secondly, it is clear that not all of the variables potentially used in the problem may be present in any given episode or example. Thirdly, and perhaps most importantly, the variables involved are usefully classified in terms of their functional status within the system rather than in terms of their physical property.

Practical Aspects

Developing a model of a clinical problem or phenomenon from a patient series study comprises several practical aspects if such development is to proceed effectively. The data on which such a model is based must of course cover the whole range of possible phenomena if the model is to be comprehensive; it is important, therefore, that observation of an adequate range of patients be combined with a thorough understanding of the relevant literature. Typically the series will develop from analyses of individual cases, the common features of such cases being extracted to form a general model. Producing an analysis of an individual case com-

FIG. 10.2.   The cyclical nature of functional analysis.

prises firstly gathering and categorising relevant data, secondly drawing together the interrelationships between the various aspects of such data, and thirdly testing out hypotheses generated by the model. The process is thus a cyclical one of assessment, formulation and intervention leading to further assessment, reformulation and so on (Fig. 10.2). For example, the clinician may on the basis of data gathered from interviews and other forms of assessment produce a model according to which the behaviour or the problem 'makes sense'. Armed with this understanding of the problem it is possible to devise an intervention which, in principle, will alleviate the problem. By further assessing the results of such an intervention the adequacy of the original model may be tested and on the basis of such testing the model refined further as necessary.

Patient series studies thus provide a framework for the derivation of general models of specific psychological phenomena. Such designs have permitted the construction of functional analyses of a number of psychological problems including anorexia nervosa and bulimia nervosa (Slade, 1982), childhood enuresis (Fielding, 1982), alcohol abuse (Sobell & Sobell, 1981), etc.

Strengths and Weaknesses of Patient Series Designs

As with any approach to research, patient series designs have both advantages and disadvantages. Perhaps the most obvious strength of a patient series design is its clear ecological validity. That is to say, since the use of such a design requires little if any alteration to a clinician's normal practice, results obtained are easy to link with the 'real world'; the artificiality of the experimental laboratory may be completely avoided. A second clear advantage is the avoidance of many of the ethical problems which constrain more traditional designs, particularly in the use of 'no-treatment' or placebo control groups. Failure to use any form of control procedure, however, may also constitute one of the major disadvantages of such a design, making it difficult to determine exactly how much of any result obtained is due to the procedures adopted. It may be argued, for example, that individuals treated in patient series designs may have improved irrespective of the treatment used. Whilst this may be evaluated to some extent by using a waiting list or similar control, the problem of interpretation will remain. Even if the rate of improvement by patients in treatment is greater than the rate in the waiting list, the possibility remains that the improvement is due to some non-specific aspect of the treatment. In most cases, therefore, investigation of a topic by means of a patient series design will need to be supplemented by consideration of experimental material. Such experimental material may reflect existing literature on the topic (as in the functional analysis of aggression) or may suggest its own experimental research (as in the functional analyses of anorexia and bulimia nervosa).

A second difficulty with the patient series design stems from its dependence on the specific individuals included. In most cases the individuals taking part in such studies will be, at least to some extent, unrepresentative. Rarely will their participation reflect random sampling from a suitable population. To some extent such a problem may be overcome by careful selection of participants in the series so as to permit a degree of systematic replication (as in single case research). That is to say, individuals are selected so as to produce a systematic variation of factors suspected to be of relevance. For example, a young male patient may be followed by an older female patient; if the results are similar, doubt is cast on the possible involvement of age and gender in the process. Whilst it will not usually be possible for patient series to adopt such systematic variation, careful monitoring of the status of individuals with respect to such variables may permit *post-hoc* consideration of their role.

For many researchers, however, there is little to compare with direct experimental manipulation of relevant variables. Such direct manipulation permits a degree of assessment of the role of such variables widely surpassing that provided by simple observation. The desirability of investigating problems of real clinical significance experimentally in a naturalistic setting has thus led to the development of procedures capable of direct application in a number of contexts; these include the procedures that have come to be known as quasi-experimental designs (Campbell & Stanley, 1963; Cook & Campbell, 1979).

QUASI-EXPERIMENTAL DESIGNS

Often a topic will be suitable in principle for experimental investigation but a truly experimental treatment will be inappropriate for practical, political, ethical or other reasons. In such cases it may be appropriate to approximate as far as possible an experimental procedure within the constraints that are operating. Thus, in a traditional experimental design, subjects may be randomly allocated to experimental or control groups. In some circumstances such random allocation may be impossible. Amongst the factors that may restrict the use of such random elements we may include the following.

Practical Issues. The investigation of such questions as the effects of natural disasters obviously rules out the production of a truly random design. Comparing psychological morbidity in survivors of the Hiroshima and Nagasaki atrocities with that in other similar cities provides some information as to the effects of such events, but a number of confounding variables inevitably remain. Each city is, for example, to some extent individual; the factors that led to the choice of Hiroshima and Nagasaki as targets may in principle also be the factors that produce any subsequent findings in research studies.

Political Issues.   Often it is desired to investigate the effects of some event whose occurrence depends largely on political circumstances. Perhaps one of the best known of such questions concerns the investigation of the effect of introduction or withdrawal of capital punishment on the incidence of violent crime. Experimentally, it is desirable that the introduction and withdrawal of the death penalty take place at random points in time. By observing the effect of such introduction and withdrawal on the incidence of violent crime a link to the penalty could be established, since the latter is the only factor varying systematically. However, such random introduction and withdrawal is usually politically (and arguably morally) unacceptable. Rather, changes in judicial policy tend to be associated with other political and social changes, and it can always be argued that it is these, rather than the change of punishment, that are responsible for any changes observed.

Ethical Issues.   Often the evidence that a measure will be of benefit is associated with such a high initial plausibility that to withold it from certain individuals would be questionable on ethical grounds. Thus evaluation of the compulsory wearing of seat belts in motor cars, or crash helmets on motor cycles might ideally be done by imposing such a requirement on a randomly selected subgroup of such individuals. Yet not only would such a procedure be politically impractical, it would also be tantamount to deliberately increasing the risk of death or injury amongst those on whom no such obligation was placed. In the same way, the evaluation of the benefit of introducing pedestrian crossings or subways near schools would not normally be considered an appropriate subject for a truly randomised design.

Methodological Issues.   In many cases the appropriate use of randomisation design may itself produce a degree of confounding in the experiment. A study by Dean, Chetty & Forest (1983), for example, looked at the psychological benefits of breast reconstruction in mastectomy patients by providing reconstruction to a randomly determined subgroup and comparing psychological morbidity in the two groups thus obtained. Unfortunately, such a design immediately encounters its own problems as a direct consequence of the randomisation. Firstly, since the experiment required informed consent on the part of the patients, it is perhaps unsurprising to find that a substantial proportion (almost half) of the patients refused to participate. Not surprisingly, many women were unwilling to have the decision of being given breast reconstruction determined by a toss of a coin in the operating theatre. Generalisation of the results is therefore limited as a result of the patients participating being an atypical subgroup. Secondly, there is the possibility that the randomisation may have its own psychological effects. In this example, some women who awake from the operation to find that they *had* been given reconstruction may have seen this as evidence that they were 'lucky', and a good omen for their future prognosis; others who were not given reconstruction may have interpreted this as evidence of being unlucky and an omen for poor prognosis. Comparison of the data obtained with other studies on the psychological outcome of mastectomy lend some support to such an argument (Owens, Ashcroft, Leinster & Slade, 1986).

As a result of problems such as these much research has adopted what have come to be known as 'quasi-experimental' designs, defined as those in which, for some reason, random allocation of subjects to groups is not possible (Campbell & Stanley, 1963). Quasi-experimental designs in which a cause is studied after it has exerted its effect (as in the Nagaski/Hiroshima example) are sometimes decribed as 'ex post facto' or 'causal comparative' designs; for the purpose of the present chapter the term 'quasi-experimental' will be used throughout. In a quasi-expermental design, the basic structure is that of a traditional experiment, but it is acknowledged that certain factors in addition to the one under study will vary between experimental and control conditions. Thus in dealing with the problems described above, a study of the effects of nuclear bombing might include a comparison between the survivors of Hiroshima and Nagasaki and other inhabitants of similar, unbombed cities. Studies of the effects of road safety measures, or of capital punishment, have typically used either before and after measures (acknowledging that other changes in society may be concurrent with those under study) or comparison of settings which are broadly similar except with respect to the dimension of interest (e.g. the comparison of adjacent American states that differ in policy on capital punishment). Examples of such studies may be found in Campbell, 1969 (road safety) or Walker, 1968 (capital punishment). Ethical problems of withholding treatment may be circumvented by making comparisons between all current patients who are given a treatment and others seen before the treatment became available (e.g. Owens, Ashcroft, Leinster & Slade, 1986). A similar strategy may be employed to circumvent methodological problems associated with randomisation.

Example: The Effect of Choice of Treatment on Well-being of Breast Patients

In a study reported in detail elsewhere (Ashcroft, Leinster & Slade, 1986) a quasi-experimental design was used to investigate the psychological consequences of allowing women with early breast cancer to make their own choice of treatment. The study arose from recognition by a number of surgeons that for certain patients there was no medical basis for selecting one of two different treatments, lumpectomy with radiotherapy or mastectomy. In effect the surgeon could provide no better way of choosing treatment than tossing a coin. Whilst such random selection of treatment would provide a classic experimental method for investigating the effects of various treatments, it is perhaps unsurprising to note that few women were willing to have their treatment selected in this way. In consequence, since there was no basis according to which the surgeon could determine the treatment for these women, it was decided to allow the women themselves to make the choice. Such a procedure immediately renders a true experimental design impossible. Consideration of the psychological outcome of the different treatments, for example, is confounded by the fact that other systematic differences would exist between those choosing mastectomy and those choosing the lumpectomy/radiotherapy combination (e.g. differences in degree of concern about body image). Whilst it could be argued that the effect of choice itself could be investigated by making choice available to only a random subgroup of women, ethical considerations argued against this; those women not given choice would be having their choice made (by no better method than the toss of a coin) by the surgeon, and as has already been noted few women were willing to allow this. Nevertheless, the issue was of obvious importance and investigation of the effects of choice desirable.

As a consequence of these considerations a decision was made to allow all suitable patients (i.e. all those for whom no medical grounds for preferring a particular treatment could be determined) to make, if they wish, their own choice of treatment. A battery of psychological tests was administered and scores along these dimensions compared with similar measures used in studies of breast patients where choice had not been permitted. The results are too complex to go into detail here, but perhaps the most remarkable finding was that these patients, unlike similar patients in the literature, showed good psychosocial adaptation to their disease and treatment. Such good adaptation could not be attributed to the particular treatment chosen, with no differences being found between those opting for each of the two treatments. However, a significant difference was found between those patients who were allowed to chooose their own treatment and those who were not. The results were thus consistent with the notion that allowing patients to choose their own treatment, where this is feasible, is associated with improved psychological outcome. Such a conclusion is implied from the observations that (a) women in this study given a choice showed a better outcome than those who were not given such a choice, and (b) women in this study given a choice showed a better outcome than comparable patients in other studies who were not given a choice.

Although the findings were *consistent* with the conclusion that choice is associated with improved psychological outcome, such a conclusion is not *necessarily* implied. Patients in the present study given a choice differed in ways additional to their choosing their own treatment, most notably in the staging of the disease (only those patients at a suitably early stage were permitted to choose). Similarly, the choice patients in the present study differed from patients of similar staging in the literature in a number of ways, most obviously in terms of the individuals concerned with their treatment (a surgeon sufficiently progressive to consider allowing patients their own choice of treatment and a clinical psychologist available to help women make their decision). In principle, these or other differences may have accounted for the results obtained. Nevertheless, the study provides support for the provision of choice of treatment where practical; the notion that choice is beneficial may thus be considered to have passed at least minimal testing. Although the study does not permit the definite conclusion that choice is of benefit, to have obtained the opposite results would have dealt a severe blow to such a notion.

To summarise, then, in the above example the use of a quasi-experimental design permitted investigation in an area where practical and ethical constraints would have precluded a conventional experiment. The information gathered, whilst not permitting definite conclusions, provided a reasonable preliminary test of the hypothesis that choice is a significant variable and encourages further work in the area. According to the notion that a concept is scientific to the extent that it is falsifiable, the use of such a design permits at least one route to possible falsifiability, in that, for example, the patients concerned may have turned out to have shown no psychological benefit relative to others reported in the literature or to others in the same study not given a choice.

Practical Aspects of Quasi-Experimental Designs

Implicit in the definition of a quasi-experimental procedure is that any results obtained will be open to more than one possible interpretation. It is the responsibility of the researcher, therefore, to take whatever steps are possible to minimise the number of such alternative explanations. In general such steps enhance as much as possible the comparability of comparison conditions, and then taking whatever steps are possible to assess the potential significance of any remaining differences.

Enhancing the comparability of the comparison conditions requires, first and foremost, a good understanding of the subject matter under investigation. The researcher should know what factors are likely to have an effect on the dependent variables and take whatever steps are possible to match these between the two groups. In the case of the breast cancer project, for example, it would obviously have been more difficult to interpret the results if the patients given a choice of treatment for breast cancer had been compared with women suffering from some totally different disease. The researcher establishing a quasi-experimental design needs to identify as many as possible of the factors that may affect the dependent variables and attempt to equalise these across the comparison conditions. Thus in examining the effects of the death penalty on rates of offending, it is more sensible to compare American states which are similar in terms of population density, urban/rural distribution etc., as well as in rates of other offences for which penalties differ only slightly or not at all (Sutherland & Cressey, 1970). The identification of a good comparison group requires considerable skill and knowledge on the part of the quasi-experimental researcher.

Another obvious method for minimising alternative interpretations of data obtained from quasi-experimental studies is to include relevant and robust pre-intervention/post-intervention measures. Even more powerful still is a design in which change during an experimental phase is compared with change during a control phase, with measures taken before and after each phase. The strongest form of this design is probably that in which a treatment is introduced, withdrawn and then reintroduced, with measures being taken between each phase of the design. Even when the inclusion of a carefully matched no-treatment control group is impossible, the results obtained with satisfactory pre/post-measures may still prove convincing and difficult to set aside.

Supplementary Analyses

No matter how much effort the experimenter puts into increasing comparability of comparison groups and ensuring the inclusion and relevant pre/ post-measures, it is likely that some variables will still be confounded. Supplementary analyses may therefore be useful. The first stage is to test whether there were any unintended differences between the experimental condition and the comparison condition (or comparison phase). If it can be shown that there were not, the case for a causal interpretation of the data is enhanced. However, if unintended differences between conditions are discovered, further analyses may focus on either reducing the total amount of data variance or eliminating the confounding influence of uncontrolled variables. For example, if the experimental and comparison samples were found to differ in terms of average age, several methods might be used to rule out the hypothesis that the age factor was responsible for the important group differences in the dependent variable.

One method (the age-matched subgroup analysis) would involve selecting subsamples from the experimental and comparison groups who were comparable in age and then determining whether or not they differed in terms of the crucial dependent variables. An alternative method would be to use an analysis of covariance statistical approach in which group differences on crucial dependent variables would be adjusted in terms of group differences in age and then tested for significance.

Finally, when carrying out analyses of a clinical data set, it may be helpful to test out clinical formulations of the cause-effect relationships between hypothesised variables. A number of statistical methods are available for doing this, including 'path-analysis' and 'cross-lagged correlation analysis'.

Path Analysis.   Path analysis can contribute to causal theory building in two different ways: first in terms of general theoretical clarification and secondly in the estimation of specific causal impacts. For a general introduction to the area the reader is referred to the book by Cook and Campbell (1979).

We will illustrate the theoretical contribution that 'path analysis' can make to the understanding of one clinical problem, namely anorexia nervosa. Several years ago, Slade (1982) developed a functional–analytic account of this disorder involving two major setting conditions (general dissatisfaction and perfectionism) which, it was argued, could lead to anorexia nervosa if the individual went on a serious diet. It was suggested that general dissatisfaction in turn developed from three further factors (adolescent problems, interpersonal problems, and stress and failure experiences). The two major setting conditions were hypothesised to lead to a 'need for total control' which might then lead on to pathological dieting. The important point is that the theoretical model of anorexia nervosa was spelt out in a form suitable for path-analysis.

We will consider the application of this statistical method by reference to a restricted part of the above model. Namely, that adolescent problems (A) and interpersonal problems (B) contribute independently to general dissatisfaction (C) and that the latter contributes directly to dieting behaviour (D). The path diagram based on this model is outlined in the upper, left-hand quadrant of Fig. 10.3. The corresponding correlation coefficients are shown in the upper, right-hand quadrant.

The less-specific model against which the latter could be tested is shown in the lower quadrants of Fig. 10.3. This model suggests that not only do (A) and (B) contribute to (C), which in turn affects (D) but that (A) and (B) have an independent effect on (D). Thus the models outlined in the upper and lower quadrants of Fig. 10.3 give rise to testable differences in terms of correlations.

Cross-lagged Correlations.   The cross-lagged correlation technique may be useful for investigating the cause–effect relation between two variables

FIG. 10.3.   Hypothetical path diagrams and the corresponding correlation coefficients.

assessed concomitantly at two points in time (Fig. 10.4) (Cook & Campbell, 1979). As an example, of where it might be used, we may be interested in the causal relationship between 'negative self-statements' (NSS) and 'depressed mood' (DM) where either direction of causality is possible. Another example is the investigation of Golin, Sweeney and Shaeffer (1981) of the role of attributions in the onset of depression. Although the statistical technique is subject to major deviations and problems (Rogosa, 1980), well-balanced and normally distributed data such as those presented in Fig. 10.4 are open to clear interpretation. Basically, a causal influence is suggested where the correlation between one variable at time one (NSS 1) and the other variable at time two (DM 2)

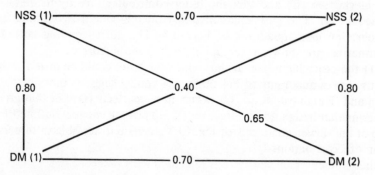

FIG. 10.4.   Hypothetical cross-lagged correlation pattern between negative self-statements (NSS) and depressed mood (DM).

exceeds the correlation observed between the second variable at time one (DM 1) and the first variable at time two (NSS 2).

Strengths and Weaknesses of Quasi-experimental Designs

Clearly quasi-experimental designs may share with the patient series designs the benefits of ecological validity and the circumvention of numerous ethical problems. Thus in the example of the breast cancer and choice of treatment study it was possible to investigate a variable of significance without the ethical problem of withholding choice from a subsample of patients. In such circumstances it may be the case that the use of a quasi-experimental design provides methodological as well as ethical advantages. Comparison of the studies of breast reconstruction reported by Dean *et al.* (1983) and Owens *et al.* (1986) reveals that the former, although a true randomised trial, is at least as difficult to interpret as the latter quasi-experimental procedure. Firstly, the percentage of patients willing to participate in the former is low, leaving open the question of generalisability to other patients similar to those who refused. Secondly it is apparent that those randomly allocated the the 'no treatment' control group showed a poorer outcome than might have been expected, suggesting that the relatively good results of the experimental group may be confounded. It is thus possible then that the use of a traditional random trial may create at least as many problems as a quasi-experimental procedure.

Besides the advantages of ethical simplicity and ecological validity a quasi-experimental design has the advantage of permitting the direct assessment of the role of variables under investigation by their systematic manipulation. To the extent that an outcome variable fluctuates systematically with changes in an experimental variable, the hypothesis that the two are indeed related is supported. Whilst such a test of a relationship is obviously not as strong as in a true experimental design (because of the presence of confounding variables), it may nevertheless prove highly informative.

On the other hand, the use of a quasi-experimental design will always, by its very nature, permit alternative interpretations as a result of confounding variables. It is thus an inherent weakness of the quasi-experimental design that positive results do not unequivocally indicate the role of the variables under study. However, it will often be possible, in the light of data obtained from quasi-experimental procedures, to initiate further studies which clarify remaining doubts. Consider, for example, the investigation of the effects of introducing a speed limit on a road where the accident rate has been high. It can be argued that any reduction following introduction of the limit reflects nothing more than the effect of confounding factors; accidents may, for example, have been random, but the limit prompted by a particular peak. Since such a peak would (on a random model) occur only infrequently, research may indicate a spurious reduction. If, however, such a quasi-experimental study *does* indicate a reduction, it may then be possible to introduce further limits on other roads without requiring an accident 'peak' to prompt such introduction. Reduction of the accident rate on these additional roads following reduction in the speed limit would not be explicable in terms of the random model and would thereby strengthen the case for reduction. Thus although a quasi-experimental study may not in itself give strong evidence for a relationship, a series of such studies may permit greater and greater confidence in the results obtained. Often the use of a quasi-experimental procedure on an exploratory basis will lead to the removal of objections on political or ethical grounds and permit the introduction of a full-scale experimental design.

SUMMARY AND CONCLUSIONS

Whilst the experimental tradition is of considerable value in the conduct of psychological research, it is not without its problems. Statistical large group designs may have difficulty with participation rates, drop out rates, and other sampling problems; even with single subject designs there may be problems in isolating the experimental variable of interest. Attempts at statistically balancing variability by averaging may give rise to results which can be generalised only to groups, not to individuals, or may require such distortion of procedure to prevent overlap between groups that the techniques under investigation bear only a slight resemblance to real clinical practice. Difficulties such as these are exacerbated when political, ethical or similar issues constrain the extent to which an experimental design can be initiated.

In the light of difficulties such as these it may often be appropriate to withhold traditional experimental procedures and look instead to patient series or quasi-experimental designs. Figure 10.5 indicates a possible basis for choosing between patient series, quasi-experimental or more traditional experimental designs. In the patient series design, careful investigation of individual patients, coupled with a thorough analysis of the features of each case, may permit considerable clarification of important issues to do with treatment (e.g. Masters & Johnston, 1970) or indeed the whole theoretical analysis of a topic (e.g. Slade, 1982). In the case of a quasi-experimental designs, the presence of confounding variables may limit the confidence which may be placed in the results, but the information provided may none the less be of considerable value; indeed such a design

FIG. 10.5.   A possible strategy for choosing research procedures.

may often turn out to be at least as useful as a traditional randomisation once consideration is given to issues such as participation rate, and the status of control groups. In many instances, the minimal interference with normal clinical procedures required by patient series and quasi-experimental designs may permit a study that is much less artificial than one following more traditional approaches. Reasons such as these suggest that they will continue to complement more conventional research designs.

REFERENCES

Ashcroft, J. J., Leinster, S. & Slade, P. D. (1985). Breast cancer; patient choice of treatment. *Journal of the Royal Society of Medicine*, **78**, 43–46.

Beck, A. T. (1976). *Cognitive Therapy and the Emotional Disorders*. Meridan.

Campbell, D. T. (1969). Reforms as experiments. *American Psychologist*, **24**, 409–429.

Campbell, D. T. & Stanley, J. C. (1963). Experimental and quasi-experimental designs for research. In N. L. Gage (ed.) *Handbook of Research on Teaching*. Chicago: Rand McNally.

Cook, T. D. & Cambell, D. T. (1979). *Quasi-experimentation; Design and Analysis for Field Settings*. Chicago: Rand McNally.

Cronbach, L. J. (1975). Beyond the two disciplines of scientific psychology. *American Psychologist*, **30**, 116–127.

Dean, C., Chetty, U. & Forest, A. P. M. (1983). Effects of immediate breast reconstruction on psychosocial morbidity after mastectomy. *Lancet*, **i**, 459–462.

Fielding, D. M. (1982). An analysis of the behaviour of day and night wetting children; towards a model of micturition control. *Behaviour Research and Therapy*, **20**, 49–60.

Golin, S., Sweeney, P. D. & Shaeffer, D. E. (1981). The causality of causal attributions in depression: a cross-lagged panel correlational analysis. *Journal of Abnormal Psychology*, **90**, 14–22.

Harris, C. W. (ed.) (1963). *Problems in Measuring Change*. Madison: University of Wisconsin Press.

Kiesler, D. J. (1966). Some myths of psychotherapy research and the search for a pradigm. *Psychological Bulletin*, **65**, 110–136.

Masters, W. H. & Johnson, V. (1970). *Human Sexual Inadequacy*. Boston: Little Brown.

Owens, R. G. & Ashcroft, J. B. (1982). Functional analysis in applied psychology. *British Journal of Clinical Psychology*, **21**, 181–189.

Owens, R. G. & Ashcroft, J. B. (1985). *Violence; A Guide for the Caring Professions*. Beckenham: Croom Helm.

Owens, R. G., Ashcroft, J. J., Leinster, S. & Slade, P. D. (1986). Psychological effects of the offer of breast reconstruction in mastectomy patients. In M. Watson and S. Greer (eds.) *Psychosocial Issues in Malignant Disease*, Vol. 2, Oxford: Pergamon.

Owens, R. G. & Bagshaw, M. (1985). First steps in the functional analysis of aggression. In E. Karas (ed.) *Current Issues in Clinical Psychology*, Vol. 2. New York: Plenum.

Rogosa, D. (1980). A critique of cross-lagged correlation. *Psychological Bulletin*, **88**, 245–258.

Sidman, M. (1964). *Tactics of Scientific Research*. New York: Basic Books.

Shapiro, M. B. (1966). Generality of psychological processes and specificity of outcomes. *Perceptual and Motor Skills*, **23**, 16.

Slade, P. D. (1982). Towards a functional analysis of anorexia nervosa and bulimia nervosa. *British Journal of Clinical Psychology*, **21**, 167–179.

Sobell, M. and Sobell, L. (1981). Functional analysis of alcohol problems. In C. K. Prokop and L. A. Bradley (eds.) *Medical Psychology; Contributions to Behavioural Medicine.* New York: Academic Press.

Sutherland, E. H. & Cressey, D. R. (1970). *Criminology.* Philadelphia: J. P. Lippincott.

Truax, C. B. (1966). Reinforcement and non-reinforcement in Rogerian psychotherapy, *Journal of Abnormal Social Psychology*, **71**, 1–9.

Vernon, W. & Ulrich, R. (1966). Classical conditioning of pain-elicited aggression. *Science*, **152**, 668–669.

Walker, N. D. (1968). *Crime and Punishment in Britain.* Edinburgh University Press.

11 Qualitative Research

David A. Good
Department of Social & Political Sciences, University of Cambridge, Cambridge CB2 3RQ.

Fraser N. Watts
MRC Applied Psychology Unit, Cambridge CB2 2EF.

The expression 'qualitative research' is a loose description for a varied set of techniques. An examination of relevant books yields a long list of qualitative methods, ranging from the familiar to the exotic, and including participant observation (e.g. Festinger, Riecken & Schacter, 1956; King, 1978); case studies (e.g. Yin, 1984; Bromley, 1986); discourse analysis (e.g. Labov and Fanshel, 1977); protocol analysis (e.g. Ericsson and Simon, 1984); conversation analysis (e.g. Schegloff, Jefferson & Sacks, 1977); photographic analysis (e.g. Becker, 1981); diary studies (e.g. Pollock, 1983); document analysis (e.g. Bogdan, 1974); computational modelling (e.g. Colby, Weber & Hilf, 1971; Hand, 1985) and many others. All these methods are concerned with both data collection and analysis. Some are purely qualitative, though many can also generate quantitative data. Most are relatively new to psychology, and have their origins in the related disciplines of anthropology, linguistics, and sociology. This is not to say, though, that the assumptions at the heart of good qualitative work are alien to the psychologist. Clinical psychologists, in particular, are well acquainted with making judgements of a qualitative character and one of the attractions of qualitative research is the possibility it offers for developing such judgements into a formal research strategy capable of yielding substantive and reliable contributions to knowledge.

Though recent years have seen growing sophistication in qualitative research, its foundations within mental health research are still not as secure as the more traditional methods. We shall therefore give particular attention to the problems that any qualitative method needs to solve, and examine how they have been addressed in particular pieces of qualitative research of clinical relevance. First, however, we will consider some common misapprehensions about qualitative research.

In the minds of many researchers, any move towards non-numerical forms of analysis is associated with a retreat from clarity and rigour into a conceptual and methodological quagmire. Quantitative and qualitative approaches are seen as representing fundamentally different perspectives on how research should proceed. It is often assumed that there is little, if any, constraint on what is done in qualitative research, and that at best it can only be used at the exploratory, hypothesis-generation stage of research. While it is true that qualitative methods face difficulties that are avoided by quantification, there is a growing recognition that good qualitative research is both necessary and possible. As Miles and Huberman (1984) note, a number of leading methodological specialists have increasingly turned to the collection and analysis of qualitative data, and for good reason.

The first point to make is that quantification is by no means the only way to rigour. In fact, quantification is often necessary in psychology because of the imperfection of its theories and measurement procedures. With greater precision, the statistical analysis of quantitative data can become redundant. Conversation analysis, perhaps the most rigorous qualitative technique, depends on the search for counter-examples to fully specified claims (see Wootton, 1987, for a discussion of this point, and Schegloff, 1968, for a classic case). Such work also emphasises the point that qualitative research need not be associated only with exploratory and descriptive studies, even though it is likely that it will have its greatest attractions for many at those stages of empirical research. Qualitative research may be a relatively open-ended endeavour, but it is not the case that 'anything goes'. Different methods have different requirements. For example, an anthropologist attempting 'thick descriptions' of the type recommended by Geertz (Geertz, 1983), will admit quite different materials than will the conversation analyst examining 'adjacency pairs' (Schegloff & Sacks, 1973). Each qualitative method has its own rules and constraints.

A related point is that far from being an alternative to quantification, good qualitative analysis is necessary for good quantitative analysis. It is easy to lose sight of the fact that the process of quantification both forces and enables the researcher to solve a number of problems that are always present, but harder to identify and solve in qualitative research. Some procedure is always necessary to turn observed performances into a numerical index. That index can only be as good as the procedure on which it is based, and this in turn is derived from a piece of qualitative work.

In orthodox quantitative research, there necessarily exist procedures that can provide the appropriate numerical values for the statistical model which is the basis of the study. These procedures are effectively a function (F) which takes as input the information-rich set of raw observations, and gives as output a value or set of values (V) as a representation of that initial set. Both F and V may be more or less complex, and aspects of F may be built into the very design of the study. For example, reaction time data are the product of a contrived situation which usually require little or nothing of significance in F to produce V. The contrivance has pre-empted the task F might have accomplished. At the other extreme, the raw data might be a video of a group of children playing. F could than be a complex coding scheme for categorising the behaviours, and V might be a set of frequencies, co-occurrence relationships, or the like.

In producing V, F clearly provides a representation of the subject matter of the study which permits the making of comparisons, and the drawing of inferences. The provision of access to this inferential machinery is clearly the major benefit of quantification, but it produces two others that are of great value to the researcher. It reduces the complexity of the data to a small number of indices, and it provides a simple concise way of displaying the data. These are essential to any research, and they are harder to achieve in qualitative work. Researchers using qualitative methods can quickly find themselves overwhelmed by a mass of data which cannot be easily inspected in the search for patterns and relationships, or corralled into a useful format for reporting and presenting.

We will give relatively little attention to the purported philosophical bases of qualitative methods, partly because we want this chapter to have a practical focus, but also because we suspect that the link between qualitative methods and philosophical assumptions is much weaker than some advocates claim. Of course, some advocates of qualitative methods regard any attempt at quantification as misguided. However, as Stalin once remarked, bourgeois trains can easily accommodate socialist passengers pursuing socialist goals, and so too can qualitative methods be turned to other ends, no matter what their origin.

Because qualitative clinical research is relatively unfamiliar, we will present good illustrative examples. In doing so, we will consider three key questions: How were the data collected? How were they transformed into a manageable and meaningful representation for both analysis and report? What kinds of inferences were drawn, and how were they validated?

Despite the heterogeneity of qualitative methods, three key issues will recur. These will be discussed in detail in specific contexts later in the chapter, but we want to draw attention to them in relatively abstract form at this stage:

1. It is seldom sufficient to use a single source of data. Usually, conclusions will be much more secure if supported by both direct and

indirect measures, both objective records and personal accounts, material with both participants and observers, etc. Exactly which combination of data sources is best will vary from one piece of research to another. Investigators should consider what will give them maximum assurance of validity within the constraints of time and feasibility. Campbell and Fiske (1959) coined the term 'triangulation' to refer to the use of multiple data sources to confirm an interpretation in a situation in which any single source would lack sufficient credibility. It is a common and important principle of qualitative research.

2. The researcher should be clear whether he or she is doing exploratory reconnaissance or hypothesis testing. There is a place for both, but their methodological requirements are very different, and attempts to switch into hypothesis-testing mode in mid-stream are not likely to be fruitful. In hypothesis testing it is always essential for the hypotheses to be sufficiently clear to ensure that they are actually testable. With qualitative research, it is especially important that the categories on which the research is based should be clearly specified. The question for the researcher to ask himself or herself before beginning is 'what would be a counter-example to this hypothesis?'

3. Because the qualitative researcher is not using the 'short-cuts' to apparent objectivity provided by quantification, he must take special care to consider his personal connection to what he is studying. The ideal is to be sufficiently in tune with the culture under study to understand the nuances of psychological transactions, but for impartiality and commitment to scientific validity to remain unclouded. This is often a counsel of perfection, but then researchers must realise where they fall short, what risks this brings, and how they can compensate. Clinicians will have no difficulty in principle with grasping the importance of their personal involvement with what they are trying to understand.

THERAPEUTIC DISCOURSE—AN ECLECTIC APPROACH TO CONVERSATION

Qualitative analyses of conversation are one of the best developed techniques currently available, and we will take as an example the study of a psychotherapeutic interview by Labov and Fanshel (1977). It is the most rigorous of a number of qualitative studies of psychotherapeutic discourse, though there are others (e.g. Havens, 1986; Russell, 1987). It is not representative of any particular school of thought on how conversation research should proceed, but draws on an eclectic background which includes the work of linguistic philosophers, e.g. Austin (1962), ethnomethodologists (e.g. Schegloff & Sacks, 1973), and linguistic micro-analyses (e.g. Pittenger, Hockett & Danehy, 1960). It is an interesting and informative example in that it attempts to move beyond the confines of simple exploration and description; it also illustrates the wealth of detail that is available in a single case. However, because of the great commitment of time and resources it required, it is not one that many would be able to imitate.

Labov and Fanshel sought to address not only the description and explanation of the particulars of psychotherapeutic exchange, but also the more general conversational rules and procedures upon which it was built. Clearly, most research has a less ambitious intent. The study was based on just 15 minutes of the twenty-fifth psychotherapy session between a 19-year-old anorexic woman and her therapist. The data collected were an audio recording of this exchange, and the observations of the therapist after listening to the tape and being interrogated by the authors. They offer two justifications for this empirical base. First, by this stage in the series, the therapist and client will have established a routine way of dealing with one another that will be repeatedly exemplified, so it would not matter exactly which session was sampled. Second, the detailed study of individual cases has often proved to be a powerful tactic in science (see Davidson and Costello, 1969; and Chapter 12); the conclusion they yield can be validated against further cases.

In their presentation of each part of the conversation, they detail the background knowledge relevant to the structure and character of the interchange, which they present in the form of an expansion of the observed utterances. This permits the representation of the conversation as a set of actions. An example of an analysis of a brief interchange is given in Table 11.1.

From such analysis of individual utterances, Labov and Fanshel were able to build a picture of the various significant characters and issues in the patient's life. The major criterion for the evaluation of this process was the internal consistency of the resulting representation of the dialogue, which is assessed by three sorts of questions.:

1. Do the rules for the designation of various speech actions group together utterances which are ostensibly similar in the eyes of the therapist and the authors?

2. Are the expansions of the utterances legitimised by the participants' subsequent reactions?

3. Did the final characterisation of the dialogue avoid implications which conflicted reconcilably with the therapist's knowledge of the client?

Two points are of specific interest. First, in looking for counter-intuitive characterisations that their procedures might produce, they are seeking disproof by single counter-example, which makes the claims more vulner-

TABLE 11.1
Example of Labov and Fanshell's analysis of a brief episode

Text	Cues
[a] Rhoda: And *then-n*, with everything,	Tension: *with everything* (ellipsis),
[b] my sister wanted to go to *work* again.	exasperation
[c] So sh- stayed *Tuesday*.	

Expansion

[a] Rhoda: And then, in spite of everything that happened and all the trouble that had been caused at her house and ours,

[b] my sister wanted to go to work and call on my mother to help some more which was an unreasonable thing to do,

[c] so my mother stayed at my sister's house one more day, Tuesday, but my sister didn't go to work after all so she wasn't being unreasonable because she had no good reason to have asked my mother to stay.

Interaction

Rhoda: continues the narrative, giving information to show that her mother did not have any obligation to fulfil in Household 2, and asserts indirectly that the circumstances for her problem were caused by her sister's unreasonable behaviour.

able and thus more interesting if they survive. Second, their use of different sources of information, such as therapists' intuitions, their own experience of other therapy sessions, the client's own subsequent behaviour, illustrates the use of 'triangulation' in qualitative research.

The way in which Labov and Fanshel achieve their extended description is similar to Kreckel's (1981) work on the Wilkins family, who were the subject of a 'fly-on-the-wall' documentary series. This reflects an approach to the study of social life as quasi-linguistic and open to the same research methods as language (Harré, 1979). Kreckel's findings emphasise the importance of studying the relevant social microcosm if we are to interpret properly the significance of the personal actions observed. This in turn depends on understanding the meanings that the participants ascribe to their actions. Labov and Fanshel see the correct characterisation of such interpretations as the key problem to be solved, as writers in the hermeneutic tradition have also realised (Bauman, 1978).

A different tradition of conversation analysis has examined the structural regularities which may be found in coversation. It is a (less adventurous) style of work than that of Labov and Fanshel in that it relies less heavily on interpretation, but is capable of producing more solid, if more limited, findings. Researchers in this field move inductively from corpora of recorded conversations to a claim about how some facet of a conversational sequence is organised, and then test it by seeking counter-examples in a wider range of cases. If one is found, the claim is reformulated and tested in the same way. For example, using this method Schegloff *et al.* (1977) have studied how the 'repair' of a conversational error or infelicity may be initiated and accomplished by each participant.

This approach has not often been applied to clinical materials, but is potentially of clinical relevance. For example, the ability to initiate and accomplish a 'repair' depends upon the ability to monitor one's own and someone else's speech at various levels, and to produce a suitable reformulation. The selective losses found in the aftermath of head injury will be reflected in which kinds of error (for example, phonological lexical or syntactic) are noticed and redressed in spontaneous speech, and so an analysis of an aphasic's repair strategies could provide a guide to the precise nature of the impairment. See, for example, Schlenck, Huber and Willmes (1987).

Another example is that of Rochester and Martin (1979) on schizophrenic discourse. Using Halliday and Hasan's (1976) analysis of discourse coherence they constructed a coding scheme which was then applied to schizophrenic productions. This resulted in both further qualitative and quantitative analyses, which revealed important differences between thought-disordered, non thought-disordered schizophrenics and normals in the cohesiveness of the texts produced.

PARTICIPANT OBSERVATION

Participant observation (PO) is a research method that has seen greatest use in sociology and anthropology. In contrast to the micro-analytic approach to conversation, PO ostensibly requires much greater effort in the data collection process, but given that the researcher is basing the primary data on his or her own interpretation of the events being witnessed, the division between data collection and data analysis is not so clear. In essence, it refers to a method that places the researcher in the community of interest as the recording apparatus, and thus its success depends greatly on the researcher's personal skills. It can provide data of great authenticity and validity, although it is fraught with many problems, and is probably of greatest use in the descriptive and exploratory stages of research when the researcher needs to develop greater insight into those in whom he or she is interested.

The aspect of PO to which most attention has been given is data collection. The main issues that need to be considered here are (a) gaining access, (b) sampling, and (c) investigation effects.

The normal problems of gaining access to subjects are heightened in qualitative research by the level of involvement required. Considerable preliminary work may well be needed before satisfactory access is gained. In fact, the form of participation that researchers achieve is often beyond their control, and they may be forced by the circumstances to be more or less active and overt than they intended. Also, the personal characteristics of the researcher will dictate the role taken. For example, it would be impossible for a middle-aged white researcher to be accepted as a participant in a black juvenile gang in the South Bronx.

It might be thought that clinical researchers could never be covert in their own institution, but it should be rememberd that the overt clinical status can provide a cover for research activity. Furthermore, the researcher's own background will radically affect their understanding of what they observe. As Alaszewski (1986) has pointed out, there is a sharp difference between operating in familiar and alien cultures. In the latter case the researchers can suffer from not knowing enough to make sense of what is observed. In the former, it can be difficult for the researcher to recognise the full significance of highly familiar actions.

The sampling problems in qualitative research are more familiar than might be imagined. If one is to make claims about some class of condition or person, it is necessary to ensure that the correct beast has been trapped. In qualitative research this sometimes results in a *post-hoc* appraisal of the class of entity which has been studied, rather than an attempt to identify the class precisely before the data collection is conducted.

In any research on humans, the investigator and the investigation can inevitably exert an influence. In experimental work, there is the problem of demand characteristics; in survey research, there is the concern with the exact wording of the question and the interviewer's style, and so on. Given the extent of the researcher's role in PO, these effects can be of such magnitude that they form the basis of the subsequent theorising. However, it is always the hope that the investigator will provoke more activities of the type that would have occurred anyway rather than changing the character of what is observed.

The PO researcher who is not completely covert always faces problems in concealing his or her purpose, and avoiding disingenuous presentations by the subjects. These take many forms, ranging from subtle evasions to blatant lies, and are conveniently summarised by Douglas (1976, Ch. 4). The separation of the investigator and observer roles, though unusual in PO work, can be highly beneficial, and was recommended long ago by Katz (1953). It forces the researcher to have a more explicit observational agenda, permits the use of a greater number of observers, and spreads the burden of responsibility for the conduct of the study, thus making it easier for competing views about the quality of the observations and their significance to surface.

Being covert, however, causes problems too. The report by Festinger *et al.* (1956) of their well-known study of the infiltration of an apocalyptic group is instructive here, because it gives more explicit attention than is usual to methods and observations. They noted that it was impossible for their observers to maintain a completely passive role because often they were directly requested to act; not to have done so may have lead to their expulsion from the group. Thus, inevitably, some of the events that were recorded would have had a different character, and perhaps would not have occurred at all, if the observers had not been there. Secondly, they could not enlist native informants in the same way that overt observers would have done, but this did not inhibit all the lines of questioning with informants. As new and keen members of this type of group the observers had every reason to ask many questions. Finally, covert observers face peculiar difficulties in recording their observations. The observers needed to find time alone when they could jot down their observations where such time is hard to find; the quality of observations will vary as a function of the memory load that the observers faced at different times.

The strategy of having several observers was a good feature of Festinger's study because it offers the possibility of 'triangulation' from different data sets. As Friedrichs and Ludtke (1975, p. 20) and Pelto and Pelto (1978) point out, this increases the probability of eccentric observations being rooted out when there are conflicting reports, and also enhances the prospects of building a richer account of specific events of which individual observers might only be able to offer a partial report. Pelto and Pelto also point out the necessity of estimating the knowledge base on which reports are made. For some simple concrete matters (such as the number of people present at a small meeting) the observer is well placed to provide reliable data; for some other issues (such as the projected internal states of other participants) observations will obviously be on a less sound footing.

This point brings us to the most difficult part of the observations of Festinger *et al.* They were interested in how individuals' reactions to events varied as a function of their previous commitment to the belief system. They attempted to validate observations of individual commitment, first by seeking confirmation of the level of commitment from a variety of different actions, second by always considering alternatives. They considered this to be like detective work (see Festinger *et al.*, 1956, p. 249). Bromley in another context has referred to it as the quasi-judicial method; we return to this later.

Festinger's work provides a good methodological model of PO, and is much more satisfactory from this point of view than the work of Goffman (e.g. Goffman, 1961) which, in terms of content, is of more direct relevance to the clinician. Goffman's work does not provide an instructive exemplar because so little of his method and direct observations are revealed in the final reports. This is regrettable as particular issues arise relating to PO in hospitals, which is where clinicians are most likely to carry out research. However, there is an instructive discussion of the problems in setting up clinical PO in Alaszewski's (1986) report of his study of a mental handicap hospital.

A particularly good and recent example of the psychological use of participation observation in *Ecological Studies of Family Life* by Vetere and Gale (1987). Though the families studied were not explicitly 'clinical', the relevance to clinical research of this approach to the study of family processes is clear. Vetere and Gale also provide a good discussion of the benefits and problems of participant observation.

ACCOUNT ANALYSIS

The observation of behaviour can be supplemented by analyses of people's accounts of their behaviour. Nisbett and Wilson (1977) argued that such protocols are of little use because people do not usually have access to the relevant cognitive processes, but their argument is flawed in several ways (Kraut & Lewis, 1982; Wright & Rip, 1981). Nevertheless, their general point that such reports must not be taken always at face value must be remembered.

The area where accounts have been studied most rigorously is in the analyses of people's accounts of performance on psychological tasks, such as how they solve problems. Ericsson and Simon (1984) have presented a full exposition of the case for studying protocols obtained from subjects as a supplement to the experimental study of task performance. Normally, 'think-aloud' reports are obtained during actual performance, and more likely to be accurate than those obtained subsequently. Ericsson and Simon make an important distinction between (a) verbalising covert encodings or articulating material that is in focal attention at least in a compressed internal format, and (b) explaining other task-related thoughts or hypotheses that are not in focal attention. They make out a good case that the former can normally be reported with a high degree of accuracy, and that doing so affects neither the speed nor quality of performance.

Think-aloud protocols have a potential, so far largely unrealised, to contribute to the analysis of performance deficits in clinical groups, and they can supplement the experimental methods described in Chapter 8. However, caution is needed about requiring subjects to verbalise material that would not normally be in awareness. For example, requiring subjects to articulate hypotheses in a problem-solving task is an example of a 'think-aloud' requirement that goes beyond what is already in focal attention, and is likely to change performance.

The first step in the analysis of a protocol is to transform it into segments, formed in a consistent vocabulary so that linkages can be identified, and to check the reliability of this transformation. Reliability can be maximised by fine segmentation of the protocol, though it may also be necessary to sacrifice a degree of detailed specification of each segment to achieve good reliability. There then follows an analysis of the implicit grammar represented by the protocol. The methods for doing this are similar to those already described in this chapter for analysing discourse. Ericsson and Simon (1984) also give many examples of the analysis of decision-making and problem-solving protocols. Another example of protocol analysis of clinical interest is Foulkes' (1978) analysis of the grammar implicit in protocols of dreams.

An extension of account analysis to a limited segment of social interaction is the technique of Interpersonal Process Recall, which is now well developed and researched (Kagan, 1984; Barker, 1985). As soon as possible after an interaction, a videotape of it is played to each of the participants separately. The researcher stops the tape frequently and asks for a detailed analysis of moment-to-moment thoughts and feelings. This technique yields a wealth of data, and has important professional uses, both in the training of novice therapists and in the 'unblocking' of cases which have become stuck. It has the potential to yield interesting research data (such as data showing that the perspectives of client and therapist on a single event can be very different; Caskey, Barker & Elliott, 1984), though as yet it has led to few well-substantiated general findings.

A different kind of account analysis, so far less rigorously developed but with wide potential application, is based on people's accounts of their social actions. This kind of account analysis makes the assumption that social behaviour is rule-based and that participants are capable of supplying the implicit rules. Such accounts can be an important constraint on social behaviour in two ways. First, knowledge of the alternative accounts which could be offered of an action will force consideration of possible consequences, and these will matter to the actor. Second, an account that has been publicly offered will crystallise the definition of an event, and this can either permit or prohibit other subsequent acts (see Semin & Manstead, 1983).

An interesting example is a study of the accounts of football violence given by fans who participated in it (Marsh, Rosser & Harre, 1978). However, this example also reveals a problem with account analysis. Marsh's protocols revealed two different kinds of account that were often closely intertwined. One emphasised the violent intentions of the behaviour of the fans, the other that is was constrained by conventions that limited the actual violence that occurred. Marsh accepted the latter as being the correct account, apparently on the grounds that it coincided with his observations of violent behaviour. However, it is not clear that the accounts alone revealed any basis for deciding which strand to accept as the correct one. The moral seems to be the value of seeking convergent data from different sources. This is, once again, the principle of 'triangulation'. Accounts of social action can provide valuable insights that can be checked against observations made in other ways. However, it cannot at present be regarded as a secure basis on its own for drawing conclusions.

There are, of course, incidents that are driven, stage by stage, by people's *perceptions* of what is happening. In such cases, accounts are of central explanatory relevance, regardless of whether the participant's accounts are veridical by some external criterion. An excellent example is Hans Toch's (1969) study of participants' accounts of how violent incidents arose. He obtained detailed participants' accounts of 344 incidents of assault on police officers. An interesting feature of the study was the use of 'peer' interviewers, albeit equipped with an interview schedule, to obtain these accounts. Thus a prison inmate would be interviewed by another prison inmate. As is normal in such qualitative research, the interviews were first transcribed. Each stage of the incident was then coded, so that the material was reduced to standard form (e.g. C2 = violence in an effort to prevent being transported or moved after being arrested). The analysis then focused on common sequences. Thus, the researcher would start with the 164 incidents that began with 'officers' orders or instructions'. A branching tree would then be constructed showing the possible routes from this starting point to violence against the police officer. The most frequent sequence that was discovered by this method of analysis is shown in Fig. 11.1. The presentation of results in this form is an elegant solution to

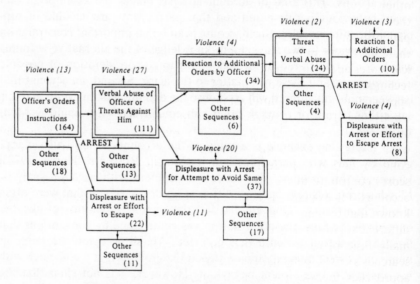

FIG. 11.1.   Sequences leading to police arrests (N = 344).

something that is often a problem in qualitative research. Clearly, this is a form of research that is of potential relevance to a wide range of clinical behaviour disorders.

CATEGORISATION STUDIES

Probably the form of qualitative research that has so far been most fruitful in the clinical field is that which seeks to establish a categorisation of a series of cases of 'instances'. The cases concerned are often individual patients (see the discussion of case series in Chapter 10), but there are of course other categorisations that are of potential clinical interest. At the other extreme, it would be possible to do a taxonomic study of recurrent events within a single case, such as a categorisation of meetings between a patient and a critical relative, of episodes of violent behaviour, or amnesic episodes. For such a categorisation study to be fruitful, it is of course necessary that there should be sufficient *variety* in the instances under study, and that this variety should be *lawful* in the sense that each of the categories of the taxonomy has a cluster of features spanning different domains that come together to define it. Again, categorisation studies normally draw on a variety of different data sources; both accounts and observations are often used.

A rigorous qualitative approach to clinical categorisation provides a clear example of the path between 'off-the-top-of-the-head' clinical methods on the one hand and quantitative approaches to taxonomy on the other. Both are in common use. Numerous clinicians have reflected on their clinical experience and derived an intuitive classification of the patients that they have seen, such as different types of depression. Equally, there have been numerous quantitative studies that have recorded numerical scores on features in a patient series, and subjected these to a statistical technique such as factor analysis that yields a categorisation. These approaches suffer from different problems. The purely clinical approach is wholly unconstrained, subject to no kind of empirical checking, and of unknown (and doubtful) reliability. The quantitative approach is in some ways too constrained, for example in the range of data that can be considered; only those features that can readily be captured in numerical scores contribute to the results of the analysis. Information from patient accounts, for example, is nearly always excluded. Also, though it is well known that techniques such as factor analysis can lead to a wide range of different solutions depending on the exact technique used, there is normally little place for the taxonomic process to be steered by the researcher's rich personal familiarity with the material. Qualitative approaches to categorisation seek to introduce greater rigour into the process than occurs with purely clinical approaches, but without the impoverishment both of data and the researcher's personal contribution, that often occurs with quantitative approaches.

There are three important methodological guidelines about qualitative approaches to categorisation.

1. The categories must be defined sufficiently explicitly for the allocation of instances to categories to be a reliable process, and the reliability should be checked empirically.

2. The set of categories used should be exhaustive, so that every instance can be allocated to one or other category.

3. Every category should be internally coherent; exhaustiveness should not be achieved by having a waste-basket category.

In practice it is often helpful to develop categories sequentially, beginning by grouping together instances that are very closely related. This produces an initial sorting into a large number of categories that have few instances each, but are at least coherent. These initial categories can then be combined as far as is compatible with the requirement that each resulting category should be internally coherent.

We shall illustrate qualitative approaches to categorisation with two main examples, one from cognitive performance, the other from social action research.

Our cognitive example is Baddeley and Wilson's (1986) study of autobiographical memory in amnesic patients. A standard technique of eliciting the data was used, in which subjects were presented with a series of cue words and asked to produce a memory suggested by each. The test was repeated after a week, and the interviews transcribed. Baddeley and Wilson then sought dimensions on which their amnesics' autobiographical memories varied, and on which a categorisation could be based. Some of the patients studied had normal autobiographical memory. Those in whom it was abnormal fell into three main groups:

1. 'Clouding' of autobiographical memory in which memories that were available on one occasion were largely unavailable on the next.

2. Those in whom fluency of memory was poor but there was little confabulation.

3. Those who were fluent but showed extensive confabulation.

The distinction between the latter two groups is of considerable theoretical interest in pointing to a distinction between the generation and checking of autobiographical memories. Indeed, the significance of this categorisation of pathologies of autobiographical memory comes largely from the integration of observation and theory that it represents. There is no need for qualitative research to be atheoretical.

Other important recent examples of qualitative categorisation studies in related fields are the studies of approaches to learning in higher education initiated by Ference Marton at Gothenburg (Marton, Hounsell & Entwistle, 1984). Analyses, both of students' *accounts* of how they approached the learning process, and of their *performance* when they recalled a passage they had studied, led to a distinction between deep and surface approaches to studying that had wide empirical ramifications. Recent work categorising slips of action (Reason & Mycielska, 1982) is also interesting both methodologically and substantively. In the field of social action, Toch's (1969) study of violent men is a good example of a categorisation study. He worked with detailed accounts of violent incidents from 69 people who had been engaged in them. Each case was then reduced to a summary pattern description or personality sketch. The cases were then subjected to a process of content analysis and grouping. The result was a list of 10 types of violence, six were classified as being self-preserving strategies, in which violence is used to bolster and enhance the person's ego in the eyes of himself and of others, the other four occurred in people who see themselves and their needs as being the only fact of social relevance.

One good methodological feature of this study is that is was subjected to a reliability check. It should be possible for any other investigator who spends the time to work through the protocols and correctly allocate each to one of the categories provided. A categorisation should ideally always be checked for reliability, and this should be included when the study is published. However, the presentation of results remains problematic, and it is usually necessary to fall back on the presentation of examples. It may be helpful to present delimiting as well as typical instances.

CASE STUDIES

Finally, we will consider qualitative case studies, which can be distinguished from both the experimental and intensive studies of individual cases discussed in Chapters 12 and 13 respectively. Qualitative case study research can also be distinguished from routine clinical case work both by its theoretical purpose, and its methodological rigour.

Case study research aims to make a general contribution to knowledge, which is not normally true of clinical case reports. The aims and objectives of the study should be clearly formulated, and determine both the selection of the case and the way in which it is studied. No case study can be fully comprehensive, but its limitations should flow from clearly specified objectives. A successful study from this point of view is Garfinkel's (1967) well-known study of 'Agnes', a patient who presented for a sex-change operation. This arose as part of his interest in how institutional realities are maintained; this unusual case permitted a rich study of the institution of gender. Similarly, Strauss and Glaser (1970) studied the dying trajectory of 'Mrs Abel' as part of a broader study of the dying process, examining how aware patients are of it and how they cope. Case studies are also frequently undertaken to illuminate the process of treatment; Dewald's (1972) study of a patient in psychoanalytic treatment is an exceptionally thorough study of this type.

Case studies can also draw explicitly on a particular theoretical background, such as the social-phenomenological position which influenced Garfinkel's study of Agnes. This is allied to the hermeneutic tradition of research which Packer (1985) has distinguished both from rationalistic research that seeks to discover an abstract system of relations in which social context and individual differences are minimised, and from empiricist research that sees behaviour as resulting from the interaction of causal forces. Hermeneutic research, in contrast, is said to investigate 'the semantic or textual structure of everyday practical activity' (p. 1086). In particular, hermeneutic analysis is concerned with how the significance of an action can be understood by reference to its setting, the personal and cultural practices within which it arises. However, as we have already observed, links between theoretical assumptions and practical methodology are often weak. Garfinkel's 'Agnes' is very different from the hermeneutic work on the laboratory game of 'Prisoner's Dilemma' that Packer presents; on the other hand 'Agnes' is very similar to other case studies that don't explicitly use Garfinkel's theoretical orientation.

Case study research aspires to a degree of methodological rigour beyond what is normally required in clinical reports. Like most other qualitative research they cannot afford to make do with a single source of data. Again, it is necessary to 'triangulate' from a variety of different vantage points. The principal sources are the subject's own account, the accounts of informants, relevant documentary evidence, and the researcher's direct observations. These can be checked against each other. As far as possible, any factual claims that are crucial to the case study should be corroborated from more than one source. Bromley (1977, 1986) has made the helpful suggestion that the evaluation of evidence in the case study is 'quasi-judicial'. Hearsay is not enough. Neither can researchers be content with simply stating how things appear to them. Evidence must be evaluated, and the conclusions reached must be ones that a reasonable and fair-minded group of people would accept if the evidence for them was set out. Moreover, evidence should be distinguished from conclusions in the way the case study is presented; the arguments and evidence for preferring one conclusion to another should be explicitly laid out. Unfortunately, many published case studies are unsatisfactory from this point of view, and present evidence and interpretations indistinguishably in a homogeneous narrative format.

Spence (1982) has argued that the truth criteria appropriate to ideographic material are those of 'narrative truth' rather than 'historical truth'. Narrative truth depends essentially on 'coherence' rather than 'correspondence' truth criteria. There can be legitimate debate over this point; what is essential is that if a case study is to be presented as having historical truth it must have satisfied the appropriate criteria. Clearly, meeting criteria for narrative truth does not mean that historical truth has been achieved.

Bromley is not the first to have made recommendations about how study research should be presented. A series of other rather similar recommendations have been made over the last 50 years (see Runyan, 1982, Chapter 8). However, Bromley's are perhaps the clearest and most comprehensive guidelines to have been set out so far. His suggestions regarding the content and organisation of a case report are set out in Table 11.2.

Concurrently, de Waele has developed methods for producing assisted autobiographies, in which the subject effectively writes his own case study with the assistance of an expert team (de Waele & Harré, 1979). Of course, this can also be seen as an application of account analysis, but we have included it here because of its similarity to case studies. The subject writes an initial autobiography in his or her own terms, but this is then subjected to negotiation with a team of experts. For this purpose, it is dismembered into a series of topics (e.g. living conditions; family and groups, etc.). An

TABLE 11.2
The contents and organisation of a case-report (adapted from Bromley, 1977)

1. The problem under investigation and the authorship of the report, including a statement of its purpose and terms of reference.
2. The identity of the individual, his physical appearance, location and other routine information.
3. The life-history and present circumstances of the individual and related issues.
4. The psychological attributes of the individual.
5. The social positions and social relationships of the individual.
6. The relationship of the individual to the investigator (or informants).
7. An evaluation of the individual in terms of accepted and explicit ethical standards.
8. A review of the evidence and arguments in relation to the purposes and terms of reference of the investigation.
9. A summary of the methods used in, and the conditions governing, the investigation, together with any associated reservations or implications.
10. Conclusions: findings, recommendations and forecasts.

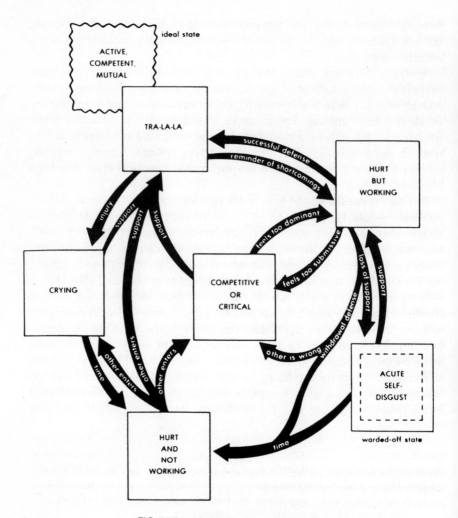

FIG. 11.2.   Model for the cycle of states.

extensive inventory has been developed covering nine such topics, which is used in the process of 'negotiating' the autobiography. The Focused Account Eliciting Interview is itself recognised as a social episode in which the material produced will be determined by how the interview is perceived; each interview therefore begins and ends with reflexive questions about the interview process. Finally, key longitudinal themes are identified, and the autobiography is often organised around how the subject has coped with conflicts or crises. It is a statement of how the subject interprets his own life, but because of the procedure of negotiation and authentication, everything included in the final version has been considered and evaluated by an expert team. Initially, de Waele has concentrated his research using this method on developing assisted autobiographies of murderers, but substantive conclusions have apparently not yet been published.

A variety of ideographic methods are available which do not aspire to the comprehensiveness of a case study, but which analyse in detail part of the material on which a case study would be based (see Runyan, 1982, Chapter 9). One example is Horowitz' study of Janice, a college student in psychotherapy, by his technique of 'configurational analysis' (Horowitz, 1979). One aspect of this technique is concerned with identifying key recurrent states and the patterns of change between them.

Analysis of the material from Janice's sessions led to the identification of several recurrent states. These were described, partly using her own terms, as 'tra-la-la', 'hurt and not working', 'hurt but working', 'acute self-disgust', etc. The second stage of the investigation focused on the circumstances that effected a transition from one state to another. For example, difficult material in therapy such as a reminder of shortcomings, often produced a change from 'tra-la-la' to 'hurt but working'. However, if this was followed by further difficulty, such as a loss of support, 'hurt but working' could give way in turn to 'acute self-disgust'. Such analyses led to the model of transitions between states given in Fig. 11.2. A further stage of the analysis focused on the recurrent images of self and others associated with each state. For example, when in the 'hurt but working' state, she perceived herself as an impaired but learning student, and the other person as a teacher.

Though Horowitz' initial 'configurational analysis' of Janice was a qualitative exercise, this can (and has been) supplemented by using intensive quantitative methods. Allport's analysis of over 100 letters written by the subject Jenny is another example of a partly qualitative, partly quantitative analysis of a corpus of material from a single subject (Allport, 1965).

CONCLUSIONS

Qualitative research techniques have enormous scope and adaptability. It can hardly be doubted that they are good at the research task of generating hypotheses. However, we have argued that some qualitative techniques are also sufficiently rigorous to yield conclusions in which researchers can have confidence. Recent years have seen growing enthusiasm for qualitative research, and as a result of this, it is now possible to be more precise than previously about *how to do it*. There remains a need for the refinement and specification of qualitative research methodologies, and this will happen as more researchers use these methods. At present, the greatest need is for good examples of projects that have produced significant findings. This is, in the end, the test by which qualitative research will properly be judged.

There are a growing number of books on qualitative methodology that researchers may find it useful to consult, including Patton (1980), Reason and Rowan (1981), Maanen (1983), Miles and Huberman (1984), Silverman (1985) and Walker (1985). Though many of these are not explicitly concerned with clinical questions, it is often straightforward to see how the methods described could be applied in mental health research.

REFERENCES

Alaszewski, A. (1986). *Institutional Care and the Mentally Handicapped*. London: Croom Helm.

Allport, G. W. (1965). *Letters from Jenny*. New York: Harcourt, Brace and World.

Austin, J. L. (1962). *How to Do Things with Words*. Oxford: Clarendon Press.

Baddeley, A. D. & Wilson, B. (1986). Amnesia, autobiographical memory and confabulation. In D. C. Rubin (ed.) *Autobiographical Memory*. Cambridge University Press.

Barker, C. (1985). Interpersonal process recall in clinical training and research. In F. N. Watts (ed.) *New Developments in Clinical Psychology*. Leicester: British Psychological Society.

Bauman, Z. (1978). *Hermeneutics and Social Science*. London: Hutchinson.

Becker, H. S. (ed.) (1981). *Exploring Society Photographically*. Evanston, Ill.: Mary & Leigh Block Gallery, Northwestern University.

Bogdan, R. (1974). *Being Different: The Autobiography of Jane Fry*. New York: Wiley.

Bromley, D. B. (1977). *Personality Description in Ordinary Language*. London: John Wiley.

Bromley, D. B. (1986). *The Case Study Method in Psychology and Related Disciplines*. Chichester: John Wiley.

Campbell, D. T. & Fiske, D. W. (1959). Convergent and discriminant validation by the multitrait-multimethod matrix. *Psychological Bulletin*. **56**, 81–105.

Caskey, N., Barker, C. & Elliott, R. (1984). Dual perspectives: clients' and therapists' perceptions of therapist responses. *British Journal of Clinical Psychology*, **23**, 281–290.

Colby, K. M., Weber, S. & Hilf, F. D. (1971). Artificial paranoia. *Artificial Intelligence*, **2**, 1–25.

Davidson, P. O. & Costello, C. G. (eds) (1969). *N=1: Experimental Studies of Single Cases*. New York, Von Nostrand.

de Waele, J.-P. & Harfe, R. (1979). Autobiography as a psychological method. In G. P. Ginsburg (ed.) *Emerging Strategies in Social Psychological Research*. Chichester: John Wiley.

Dewald, P. A. (1972). *The Psychoanalytic Process: A Case Illustration*. New York: Basic Books.

Douglas, J. D. (1976). *Investigative Social Research*. Beverly Hills: Sage.

Ericsson, K. A. & Simon, H. A. (1984). *Protocol Analysis*. Cambridge: MIT Press.

Festinger, L., Riecken, H. W. & Schacter, S. (1956). *When Prophecy Fails*. New York: Harper Row.

Foulkes, D. (1978). *A Grammar of Dreams*. Hassocks: Harvester Press.

Friedrichs, J. & Ludtke, H. (1975). *Participant Observation: Theory and Practice*. Farnborough: Saxon House.

Garfinkel, H. (1967). *Studies in Ethnomethodology*. Englewood Cliffs: Prentice-Hall.

Geertz, C. (1983). *Local Knowledge*. New York: Basic Books.

Goffman, E. (1961). *Asylums*. Harmondsworth: Penguin.

Halliday, M. A. K. & Hasan, R. (1976). *Cohesion in English*. London: Longman.

Hand, D. J. (1985). *Artificial Intelligence and Psychiatry*. Cambridge University Press.

Harré, R. (1979). *Social Being: A Theory for Social Psychology*. Oxford: Blackwell.

Havens, L. (1986). *Making Contact: Uses of Language in Psychotherapy*. Cambridge, Mass.: Harvard University Press.

Horowitz, M. J. (1979). *States of Mind: Analysis & Change in Psychotherapy*. New York: Plenum Press.

Kagan, N. (1984). Interpersonal process recall: basic methods and recent research. In D. Larsen (ed.) *Teaching Psychological Skills*. Monteney: Brooks/Cole.

Katz, D. (1953). Field Studies. In L. Festinger & D. Katz (eds) *Research Methods in the Behavioural Sciences*. New York: Holt, Rinehart & Winston.

King, R. (1978). *All Things Bright and Beautiful? A Sociological Study of Infants' Classrooms*. Chichester: Wiley.

Kraut, R. E. & Lewis, S. H. (1982). Person perception and self-awareness: Knowledge of one's influences on one's own judgements. *Journal of Personality and Social Psychology*, **42**, 448–460.

Kreckel, M. (1981). *Communicative Data and Shared Knowledge in Natural Discourse*. London: Academic Press.

Labov, W. & Fanshel, D. (1977). *Therapeutic Discourse*. New York: Academic Press.

Maanen, J. Van (ed.) (1983). *Qualitative Methodology*. Beverly Hills, Cal.: Sage.

Marsh, P., Rosser, E. & Harré, R. (1978). *The Rules of Disorder*. London: Routledge & Kegan Paul.

Marton, F., Hounsell, D. & Entwistle, N. (1984). *The Experience of Learning*. Edinburgh: Scottish Academic Press.

Miles, M. B. & Huberman, A. M. (1984). *Qualitative Data Analysis: A Sourcebook of New Methods*. Beverly Hills, Cal.: Sage.

Nisbett, P. E. & Wilson, T. D. (1977). Telling more than we can know: Verbal reports on mental processes. *Psychological Review*. **84**, 231–259.

Packer, M. J. (1985). Hermeneutic inquiry in the study of human conduct. *American Psychologist*, **40**, 1081–1093.

Patton, M. Q. (1980). *Qualitative Evaluation Methods*. Beverly Hills, Cal.: Sage.

Pelto, P. C. & Pelto, G. H. (1978). *Anthropological Research: The Structure of Enquiry*. Cambridge University Press.

Pittenger, R. E., Hockett, C. F. & Danehy, J. J. (1960). *The First Five Minutes*. Ithaca, New York: Paul Martineau.

Pollock, L. A. (1983). *Forgotten Children: Parent–Child Relations from 1500 to 1900*. Cambridge University Press.

Reason, J. & Mycielska, K. (1982). *Absent-Minded: The Psychology of Mental Lapses and Everyday Errors*. London: Prentice-Hall.

Reason, P. & Rowan, J. (1981). *Human Inquiry*. Chichester, John Wiley.

Rochester, S. & Martin, J. R. (1979). *Crazy Talk: A Study of the Discourse of Schizophrenic Speakers*. London: Plenum.

Runyan, W. K. (1982). *Life Histories and Psychobiography*. Oxford University Press.

Russell, R. L. (ed.) (1987). *Language in Psychotherapy: Strategies of Discovery*. London: Plenum.

Schegloff, E. A. (1968). Sequencing in conversational openings. *American Anthropologist*, **70**, 1075–1095.

Schegloff, E. A. & Sacks, H. (1973). Opening up closings. *Semiotica*, **8**, 289–327.

Schegloff, E. A., Jefferson, G. & Sacks, H. (1977). The perference for self correction in the organisation of repair in conversation. *Language*, **53**, 361–382.

Schlenck, K-J., Huber, W. & Willmes, K. (1987). 'Prepairs' and repairs: Different monitoring functions in aphasic language production. *Brain and Language*, **30**, 226–244.

Semin, G. R. & Manstead, A. S. R. (1983). *The Accountability of Conduct*. London: Academic Press.

Silverman, D. (1985). *Qualitative Methodology & Sociology*. Guildford: Gower.

Spence, D. P. (1982). *Narrative Truth and Historical Truth: Meaning and Interpretation in Psychoanalysis*. London: Norton.

Strauss, A. L. & Glaser, G. B. (1970). *Anguish: A Case Study of a Dying Trajectory*. London: Martin, Robertson.

Toch, H. (1969). *Violent Men*, Chicago: Aldine.

Vetere, A. & Gale, A. (1987). *Ecological Studies of Family Life*. Chichester: John Wiley.

Walker, R. (1985). *Applied Qualitative Research*. Guildford: Gower.

Wootton, A. (1987). Remarks on the methodology of conversation analysis. In D. Roger & P. Bull (eds) *Conversation: An Interdisciplinary Approach*. Bristol: Multilingual Matters.

Wright, P. & Rip, P. D. (1981). Retrospective reports in the causes of decisions. *Journal of Personality and Social Psychology*, **40**, 601–614.

Yin, R. K. (1984). *Case Study Research*. Beverly Hills, Cal.: Sage.

12 Single Case Research

Stephen Morley
Department of Psychiatry, University of Leeds, Leeds LS2 9LT.

For the clinician single case research has one overwhelming advantage; the material for research is the same as their clinical work. There is no need to seek out special populations, control groups and large numbers of subjects. Research can be completed within a matter of months rather than years and there is every opportunity for the investigator to build up expertise and data rapidly and sequentially. Furthermore, some single case research can be carried out relatively cheaply without the taxing need to devote time and resources to applying for and administering research grants. But single case research should not be approached casually, there are many pitfalls and difficulties. Care must be taken over the articulation of the research question, development of measures and the implementation of the interventions.

A compelling reason for adopting single case methods is that they can be useful aids to satisfying a clinician's everyday curiosity about clients. Most clinicians are curious about their clients and ask questions about the aetiology and maintenance of problems, the effect of treatment, whether another treatment is more effective or why a treatment fails (Table 12.1).

For clinicians who approach case work as an applied scientist single case methods provide a flexible and logical way of evaluating their clinical activity. Nevertheless, there is a tension between the approach one must take as a clinician and the ideal which is expressed in the literature. Much of the published work is derived from applied behaviour analysis (ABA) which espouses single case methodology as the methodology for investigating behaviour. ABA researchers have selected to investigate potent treatments which produce rapid changes in behaviour in carefully defined

TABLE 12.1
Questions for curious clinicians

Questions about formulation:
  What contributes to the development and maintenance of a problem?
  What are the controlling factors for the target variables?

Simple outcome question:
  Has the client improved?

Simple treatment question:
  Is the improvement a result of treatment?

Complex treatment question:
  Does the treatment have a specific effect or do the non-specific components of the treatment account for the change?

Comparative treatment question:
  Is one treatment more effective than another?

Questions about a theory:
  Does the therapy work for the reasons given in the theoretical rationale?

---

problems in research settings. This represents an ideal that many practising clinicians will not be able to attain. Many of the examples cited in this chapter come from the behavioural tradition and are used because they illustrate particular points clearly. There are, however, sufficient published accounts of single case work carried out in ordinary clinical settings using treatments not derived from ABA (Barlow & Hersen, 1984; Peck, 1985) to encourage the use of single case methods in routine clinical work: especially if the clinician has access to a relatively homogeneous population which will enable the development of techniques and replication across individuals.

A PROTOTYPE CASE STUDY

Deriving a testable hypothesis is the key activity of any research enterprise. Arriving at a clinical formulation is the end product of a complex cognitive process whereby the clinician constructs a model of the patient's problem, but even simple problems can produce elaborate formulations (see Hallam, 1976) with several interrelated hypotheses. Developing a formulation is a creative enterprise involving several sources of information, as follows:

1. Prototypicality judgements (induction): case is like a previous class of problems.

2. Hunches (intuition): gut feeling that certain ideas are right.

3. Historical correlation: there is evidence of a relationship between events and the target problem.

4. Passive observation: prospective record keeping reveals a correlation between events and the target problem.

5. Accidental manipulation: the pattern of behaviour changes with a concurrent change in the person's environment.

6. Deliberate manipulation: investigator makes a deliberate attempt to manipulate events which are thought to be causally related to the target problem.

Only the tactic of deliberate manipulation is a true experiment but it will be apparent that some or all of the preceding items are necessary prior steps to deliberate manipulation. The following case illustrates this and other features of single case research.

Case Study 1: The Case of Mrs S (Turkat & Carlson, 1984).   Mrs S reported a sudden onset of a cluster of anxiety and dysphoric symptoms (sleep and mood disturbance and some avoidance activity) following the diagnosis of her daughter as a diabetic. After several interviews the therapists were unable to arrive at a satisfactory explanation of why Mrs S should be so anxious. On the basis of past experience with anxiety cases (prototypicality, hunches) they decided to treat the patient by relaxation and hierarchically determined *in vivo* anxiety management. The initial success of this treatment was followed by rapid relapse for reasons which could not immediately be discerned. The therapists reasoned that her relapse might be connected with factors that had caused the onset of the problem. During treatment the therapists observed that Mrs S continually sought reassurance that she was performing anxiety management properly (passive observation). This reassurance had been withdrawn at the termination of treatment. They reformulated the problem postulating that the main functional determinant of the Mrs S's behaviour was a hypersensitivity to independent decision making. Re-examination of Mrs S's history (historical correlation) revealed that her decision making about trivial things such as buying food was accompanied by anxiety and reassurance seeking. She reported being made anxious when reassurance was denied or when her decision making was approved of by one person but criticised by another. Finally the therapists discovered that her early upbringing showed that the patient had been characterised by a lack of independent decision making and a surfeit of criticism and anxiety surrounded her attempts at independence. Some objective evidence (passive observation) for this formulation by obtaining measures of 'Autonomy' and 'Emotional reliance on others' from a standardised personality questionnaire. As a result of the

FIG. 12.1.   The effects of formulation based treatment on the anxiety ratings of Mrs S. The graph illustrates an A-B 'design' with a short baseline (A) and a treatment phase (B).
(Reprinted with permission from: Turkat, I. D. and Carlson, C. R. (1984). Data-based versus symptomatic formulation of treatment: the case of a dependent personality. *Journal of Behaviour Therapy and Experimental Psychiatry*, **15**, 153–160. Copyright 1984, Pergamon Journals Ltd.)

formulation the therapists designed an intervention to reduce her anxiety about decision making. They constructed a hierarchy and obtained daily ratings of her anxiety on the items. These data were used as the main outcome measure. The results are shown in Fig. 12.1.

SOME BASIC ISSUES IN SINGLE CASE RESEARCH

Case study 1 illustrates three important features of single case experimentation.

1. Data Driven Experimentation

Single case experiments can be 'data driven'. The results of one phase of the experiment can provide information which will determine the course of action to be taken in the next phase allowing scientific curiosity to be indulged (Sidman, 1960). This approach has ecological validity for the practising clinician as it encourages active monitoring of clinical problems and the investigation of serendipitous findings. The emphasis of data driven, or exploratory, experimentation, should not detract from the use of single case experiments as a method for confirmatory investigation (Elashoff & Thoresen, 1978).

2. Repeated Measures and Variability

The second feature of single case research is the emphasis on repeated measurement within one subject and the investigation of variability within a person. The Achilles' heel of group-based research is the problem of generalising from group data to an individual; a functional relationship shown in group data is not necessarily reflected in an individual. A similar issue arises with respect to time. Behaviour, whether it be overt responses or thoughts and feelings, fluctuates in time, and it is assumed that in some way it is caused by preceding events. Group research assumes that the dependent variable is the result of the same preceding processes in all individuals and aggregates data to control error processes. Little attempt is made to assess or control what may be important sources of variability within individuals. That variability between subjects is not the same as variability within subjects is a truism which is nevertheless worth emphasising. Sidman (1960) and Johnston and Pennypacker (1980) argue that the most appropriate way to study behaviour is to identify and isolate the determinants of an individual's behaviour. Generalisation proceeds by replicating functional relationships across individuals, i.e. the reverse order from group research.

Variability is a two-edged sword. On one hand minimum variability within each phase of the experiment is required so that inferences about the impact of an intervention can be made by comparing sets of data points obtained under different conditions. On the other hand a certain degree of variability is required to facilitate the development of a clinical formulation. Variability is the 'window through which to observe the workings of basic controlling relationships' (Johnston & Pennypacker, 1980, p. 70). A practical resolution of this conflict is shown in Turkat and Carlson's (1984) study. Variability in Mrs S's anxiety led them to a formulation concerning her difficulties in decision making. If we examine the baseline phase of Fig. 12.1 in which daily ratings were averaged there is very little variation in anxiety. This enables us to be reasonably confident that the change in anxiety occurring in the treatment phase is not just part of the random variation displayed by the patient. In this case the simple tactic of averaging data reduces the variability. On the other hand experimental analysis of this variability might have cast light on potentially controlling variables.

Sidman (1960) pointed out that variability can be regarded as either an *intrinsic* feature of individuals, or due to *extrinsic* controlling factors. Uncritical acceptance of the intrinsic hypothesis precludes the investigation of variability. This affects measurement tactics and the type of variables which one seeks to investigate. (See Johnston & Pennypacker, 1980, pp. 207–8 for detailed discussion of these points.) The assumption that behavioural variability is extrinsically controlled leads one to search for and isolate the sources of control. This will ensure that accurate measurement is obtained and controlling influences on the behaviour determined where possible. The following common potential sources should be investigated in every case:

1. Individual; e.g. diurnal rhythms, fatigue, drugs, age effects.
2. Experimental setting; e.g. variations in the environment, setting events.
3. Measurement; e.g. poor definition of variables, untrained raters, instrumentation effects.

Unless treatments are carried out in highly contrived environments there is a high probability that the experimental setting will contribute considerable variation to the target problem. Understanding this variability can lead to productive clinical hypotheses about the determinants of behaviour. For example, Wahler (Wahler, 1980; Wahler & Graves, 1983) demonstrated that mothers could successfully implement behavioural strategies to control their childrens' oppositional behaviour but gains were often not maintained. Further analysis revealed that the mothers' own social environment determined whether they would implement the therapeutic strategies. Discovery of this source of variability in the treatment environment has led to a better understanding of the problem and development of new methods for helping families.

3. Levels of Measurement

The third feature of single case research concerns the type of measure employed. Herbst (1970) argues that individuals live in their own 'behavioural worlds'; they have unique ways of interacting with the environment. This is reflected by the fact that they have unique sets of measurement scales which are only partly related to others. For example, a standardised 10-item hierarchy in a behavioural avoidance test will not capture the critical features for all subjects. Careful scaling of the subjective distances between the items would reveal considerable differences between subjects. While much effort in measurement technology has gone into devising ways of maximising the common variance contained in scales one must question whether many issues of interest to psychologists and especially clinicians can be satisfactorily tackled using measurement techniques that throw away individual variation as error (Shapiro, 1975, 1985).

What is required are measures of criterion variables scaled for individuals. Operant psychologists routinely do this by counting frequencies of specified target events. The measurement strategy ensures that the accuracy and reliability of measurements taken on particular occasions for a single individual are assessed (Cone, 1988; Hartmann, 1984). It should not be assumed that psychometric characteristics established for a population will apply to an individual. Indeed to make that assumption is to commit a logical error: population characteristics cannot be applied to an individual. Fortunately there are procedures that can be used to develop unique measurement scales for subjective states (Philips, 1977; Shapiro, 1961). Ratio scales that measure the psychological distances between intervals on a scale can be obtained using techniques such as cross modal matching (Lodge, 1981).

Set against the need to use sensitive individual measures is the requirement that useful experiments should be generalisable to other individuals.

FIG. 12.2. The assessment–evaluation measurement funnel. The figure depicts a general strategy for selecting measures and determining when to take them. *Standard–global* measures are those that have been developed for known populations and problems. Ideally they have well-researched psychometric properties and can be used to index a person to known populations. By design these measures are often not suitable for rapidly repeated administration. They contain items selected for the population as a whole and they may not be sensitive to an individual's target problems. *Target* measures are measures developed for a particular individual and are the main outcome measures in single case research. The psychometric characteristics of target measures should be determined for each case. *Process* measures are taken more frequently than target measures and may not be taken during baseline phases or throughout treatment. They are deployed to monitor treatment sessions. They very often have a spurious validity, e.g. SUDs (subjective units of discomfort), so that the investigator is lulled into thinking that they have the properties of standard–global measures. Little attention is usually paid to their psychometric properties.

This issue is ultimately resolvable only by empirical replication. However, it is prudent to take other measures of variables which one suspects might be important determinants of generalisation across cases. Commonly these measures concern the classification of subjects into homogeneous groups representing some type of pathology or common psychological process. The measures have two characteristics:

1. They are standardised on specified populations so that several psychometric features are known, e.g. test-retest reliability, concurrent validity.
2. They measure 'global' variables such as depression which are made up of a series of items which are not perfectly correlated and which may be functionally separate in individuals.

For these reasons they may not be the most sensitive measures of individual pathology.

To meet the requirements of specificity and generality it is suggested that investigators should adopt an assessment strategy which uses the assessment funnel shown in Fig. 12.2. An excellent example of its use in an experimental clinical investigation is given by Salkovskis and Warwick (1985).

ELEMENTS OF EXPERIMENTAL DESIGN

The purpose of experimentation is to eliminate alternative explanations for a phenomenon. Common alternative explanations, or threats to the validity of experiments, are discussed by Campbell and Stanley (1966) and Cook and Campbell (1979). Kazdin (1982) discusses these issues with respect to single case experiments. The central feature of experimentation is the comparison of two or more conditions. In single case research these comparisons are made within an individual. Formal single case designs have been developed that specify sequences of baseline and treatment comparison, but within this framework investigators must make decisions about implementing and withdrawing treatments. These decisions should be governed by the data collected during the experiment, and the lengths of different phases of the experiment are not necessarily pre-planned as in conventional group research.

When Should the Intervention be Applied/Withdrawn?

In laboratory experiments it is usual to wait until the baseline behaviour has stabilised within prescribed limits. While every effort should be made to obtain stable baselines there are many clinical situations where complete control is not possible. Other criteria for introducing treatments may be used.

1. Treatments may be introduced as quickly as possible to reassure the client. This is not good experimental practice and has dubious clinical validity because there will be inadequate baseline data and no testable formulation.

2. Treatments may also be applied as soon as the therapist is convinced that an adequate formulation has been made but this may be before adequate baseline data has been collected.

3. Treatments can be introduced or withdrawn in a *reactive* manner (Glass, Willson & Gottman, 1974). In this case the therapist makes a decision to manipulate the treatment on the grounds that the target behaviour is 'out of control'. This is often a misguided decision. Extreme behaviour is rare and usually returns to a median value without intervention (Glass *et al.*, 1974). Reactive interventions are likely to be confounded with naturally occurring changes in the behaviour and they also preclude the opportunity of investigating and understanding the problem as illustrated in case study 2.

Case Study 2: A Reactive Intervention. T was a young woman with a long history of schizophrenia. Her most distressing symptoms were hallucinations in which voices told her to harm herself. She had fractured both legs and her pelvis after jumping in front of a bus. At times she appeared very distressed and her behaviour made staff anxious and protective. T was an inpatient for 5 days a week, returning to her mother's home at weekends. Invariably on her return to the ward she showed signs of distress. The staff responded to this by increasing or changing her medication. T improved during the next few days, thereby reinforcing the staffs' belief in the efficacy of the intervention and the implicit hypothesis that her behaviour was determined by neurochemical mechanisms. The data are plotted in phase A of Fig. 12.3.

Three alternative hypotheses were considered:

1. That T forgot to take her medication during the weekend. Analysis of blood serum levels and careful questionning of T and her mother invalidated this.

2. That T's distress had a 7-day periodicity for unknown reasons (intrinsic variability).

3. That the social environment at the weekend was a causal factor. Clinical records and interviews suggested that T's mother might be considered over protective and provide a high EE environment (Leff & Vaughn, 1985).

FIG. 12.3.   Fluctuations in T's psychological distress (case study 2). Distress was measured as the sum of a checklist of symptoms derived from an analysis of T's problems and rated by nursing staff 3 days a week; monday (M), wednesday (W) and friday (F). T's visits to her mother's home are shown by the arrows. Phases A, B, C, and D are described in the text.

Three tests of the hypotheses were made. Firstly no drug changes were made on her return to the ward. The data plotted in phase B show that T returned to her usual level of activity without the drug intervention. Secondly, weekend leave was deferred and T was sent home mid-week. This resulted in increased distress after her return from leave and not during the weekend (phase C); suggesting that hypothesis 2 was wrong. Finally hypothesis 3 was tested by asking T to return to her mother's home for shorter periods but more frequently (phase D). This procedure was satisfactory for T, her mother and the staff.

The final criterion for deciding when to implement treatment is based on statistical design considerations. Randomisation tests (see below) require that the interventions should be implemented and withdrawn at randomly chosen points in the experiment. This approach to single case experiments is particularly powerful when the investigator wishes to test a treatment of known efficacy and where the likely time course of the treatment is known. Under these conditions the investigator can pre-plan the experiment in some detail. Clements and Hand (1985) investigated the impact of a programme to help parents manage sleeping problems in young handicapped children. The length of the baseline was set in advance and because the investigators anticipated that treatment would not take effect for several days, decisions about the form of data analysis could be specified in advance. Also in experiments where two or more conditions are repeatedly administered it is necessary to plan the order of presentation to ensure that there is no confounding with extra-experimental events.

For How Long Should the Treatment be Applied?

Three factors must be considered:

1. Stability in the baseline.
2. The magnitude of the treatment effect.
3. The speed of the treatment effect.

Figure 12.4 illustrates some of the effects of baseline variability, and treatment strength and magnitude on the interpretability of the data. For example, if the data displays considerable variability during the baseline, (Fig. 12.4A), treatment should be extended for at least the length of the baseline. With a variable baseline and a relatively weak treatment long baseline and treatment phases are essential. In contrast to this if the

FIG. 12.4. The effects of baseline variability on the interpretation of changes in a target variable following the introduction of treatment. In (A) there is a highly variable baseline. The effect of a treatment for the period a is uninterpretable. If the treatment were extended for the period b greater confidence in its effects would be justified. In (B) there is a short treatment phase but because the baseline is stable and longer than the treatment phase it is easier to judge the impact of the treatment. (C) illustrates the effect of the magnitude of treatment. With a small effect it is necessary to obtain more measures, extending the period a to a'. (D) illustrates the role of the speed of change in interpreting the impact of treatment. Slow changes (a) will require longer periods of observation than fast-acting changes (b).

baseline is stable and the treatment is powerful (Fig. 12.4C) a short treatment phase will suffice. As a general rule baselines should always be longer than the time in which it is expected that the treatment will take effect: slow acting treatments require long baselines, fast acting treatments can be evaluated against shorter baselines.

Decisions about withdrawing or changing treatments will depend on the nature of the target behaviour, the treatment and the experimental design. Treatments can also be withdrawn for clinical reasons. A common one is when the treatment is counter-therapeutic. It is advisable to analyse why this effect has taken place. It may be apparent that the change is transient and that treatment should not be withdrawn, e.g. an increased response rate during extinction. Treatments may also be withdrawn because they appear not to be working; there may be a lag between the start of the treatment and its effect. For example some antidepressives and psychological interventions, such as relaxation for headaches, may take several weeks before their effects are felt. Investigators should guard against *reactive withdrawal* of treatments.

Specifying the Treatment

In experimental work treatments are specified in advance. While this is usually true in clinical work there will be occasions when changes in treatment are made as a function of client feedback. In all cases investigators should take great care to document exactly what treatment strategies and tactics are employed. A conceptual analysis of the differences obtaining in each of the different phases should be conducted as part of the analysis of the experiment. This should include an analysis of events occurring during baseline phases. An excellent example of this process is given by Youell and McCollough (1975).

Is the Treatment Being Applied? (Manipulation Validity)

It is necessary to obtain evidence that the treatment is actually being applied as stipulated. Where overt environmental manipulations are part of the treatment there is no apparent difficulty in ensuring that the treatment is intact. The monitoring of covert treatments (psychotherapy and cognitive therapy) is more problematic. One strategy is to use brief within-session manipulations of the treatment to determine functional relationships between the treatment and a target variable. For example, in exposure sessions for phobic anxiety, changes in subjective anxiety measured by the fear thermometer can be tracked as the intensity of the exposure is varied. This strategy of course depends on the presence of a functional relationship. If the expected changes do not occur it should not be assumed that the treatment is not in effect; it may be that there are moderating variables that mitigate its impact. With obsessional patients it is not uncommon to find that exposure to the anxiety provoking stimulus is managed by a form of covert avoidance. Careful interrogation of the patient usually reveal this and counter-measures can be taken. In general manipulation validity must be inferred from a number of sources of evidence which will vary from experiment to experiment.

BASIC EXPERIMENTAL DESIGNS

Simple Time Series; A-B Design

Measurement before and after an intervention does not enable causal inferences about an intervention to be made. Changes in the measures might reflect changes in variability, the conditions of measurement, the sensitivity of the measure, or be due to a coincidental extra-treatment event. Increasing the number of measurements taken during baseline (A) and treatment (B) phases can partly override these alternative explanations. The extent to which alternative explanations can be eliminated depends largely upon the length and stability of the baseline and the rapidity with which treatment takes effect. Long stable baselines followed by a rapid change on the introduction of the treatment are more believable than other patterns of data. If the baseline phase has remained stable despite the presence of other documented changes in the client's life then the likelihood that the change occurring with the introduction of treatment is due to anything but treatment is reduced.

Several experimental designs have been developed to overcome the problems of eliminating alternative explanations. These designs all have the same underlying logic. The logic is that if the introduction of the intervention is uniquely associated with changes in the target variable, i.e. there are no changes in the target variable at other times, then the likelihood that other explanations for the change in behaviour are true is reduced. Several basic designs are illustrated below but the reader should be aware that these represent prototypes from which countless variations can be developed in order to suit particular circumstances.

The A-B-A-B Design

The causal effect of an intervention is more believable if the effect can be replicated. The obvious way to achieve this is repeatedly to withdraw and re-introduce the intervention. If the target behaviour changes consistently in association with changes in treatment alternative explanations become less plausible.

Case Study 3: An A-B-A-B Experiment. P was a 6-year-old boy with mild asthma. He had a persistent dry cough which was especially prominent just before bedtime. An attempt was made to bring the cough under control. During the experiment all sessions were scheduled during the reading of a bedtime story and were carried out by his father. During the baseline P and his father recorded the frequency of coughing. Treatment was a time-out procedure contingent on coughing. After a cough the father turned the book over and he and P counted slowly to 10. If there was no cough during this period reading was resumed. Treatment was subsequently reversed and reinstituted. Figure 12.5 shows that the cough was suppressed by time out. At follow-up the father reported that several booster sessions had been necessary following recovery from asthma attacks.

The A-B-A-B experiment has a simple elegance about it but in clinical research there are many occasions when it cannot be used. An intervention may not be reversible, either because the person has learned new behaviour which is now under self-control, or when it is ethically inappropriate to withdraw treatment.

FIG. 12.5. The effect of time-out on the rate of coughing in P (case study 3). This graph shows the results of an A-B-A-B experiment. In this case the treatment was powerful and took effect rapidly. These factors coupled with its reversibility produced results which are easily interpreted.

Changing Criterion Design

This can be used is there is one target variable and when treatment is considered irreversible. Experimental control is demonstrated by manipulating some aspect of the treatment other than its total withdrawal. After a baseline phase several treatment phases are introduced sequentially. Each treatment phase differs with respect to the amount of change in the target behaviour expected. For example, the investigator may ask the subject to meet a specified target and only to reward behaviour which meets this criterion target. Once the behaviour has met this target and is stable a new criterion can be introduced. Experimental control is demonstrated if the changes in the target behaviour closely follow the changes in treatment conditions.

This design was originally applied to overt behaviour under the control of external reinforcement contingencies where systematic changes in parameters of reinforcement schedules could be studied (e.g. Handen, Apolito & Seltzer, 1984). Setting target criteria is a common example of the changing criterion design but any systematic change in the therapy, provided that it is variable along the same dimension, can be used to manipulate the behaviour and demonstrate experimental control. For example, it would be possible to demonstrate the effect of increasing accurate empathy on the amount of self-exploration. Certain guidelines should be considered for changing criterion designs.

1. The minimum number of changes is two although increasing this number is advisable.

2. It is important to vary the length of each treatment phase. This will ensure that the changes are not coincidental with cyclic extra-treatment events.

3. Wherever possible the magnitude of the criterion should be varied. Although for some problems large changes may be impossible, at least in the early stages of treatment, e.g. addictive behaviour.

4. It is advisable to consider whether the direction of criterion changes can be reversed. This may be possible in the later stages of the experiment and adds to the power of the design. If a full reversal cannot be considered brief probe withdrawals should be attempted. There are many published examples of the changing criterion design reviewed by Barlow and Hersen (1984). Recent examples include applications to rehabilitation medicine (Hegel, Ayllon, VanderPlate and Spiro-Hawkins, 1986).

Case Study 4: A Changing Criterion Experiment (Bernard, Dennehy & Keefauver, 1981).   Mary was concerned about her excessive drinking of coffee and tea. She reported a number of unsuccessful attempts to reduce

FIG. 12.6. The results of a Changing Criterion experiment (case study 4). This graph illustrates the step like nature of a Changing Criterion experiment. Notice the irregular spacing of the criterion changes which contributes to good experimental design. The power of the experiment would be improved by varying the magnitude of the criterion changes and by reversing the direction of the criterion changes on one or more occasions. (Reproduced from Bernard, M. E., Dennehy, S. & Keefauver, L. W. (1981). Behavioral treatment of excessive coffee and tea drinking: a case study and partial replication. *Behavior Therapy*, **12**, 543–548. Copyright 1981, the Association for the Advancement of Behavior Therapy. Reproduced with permission of the publisher and author.)

her intake. During baseline the average number of cups drunk per day was 11.54. She agreed to a response-cost programme whereby she would be fined $5.00 if she exceeded the criterion by one cup. Additional cups were fined at $2.00. The final target was 6 cups per day and the first criterion was set at 11 cups. Figure 12.6 shows the course of treatment. Each criterion was set at one cup less than the previous one. The data reveal that Mary was able to meet each criterion without incurring a penalty. The step-wise nature of the data is apparent as is the variable duration of each criterion. Follow-up data collected some three months after the end of treatment showed that Mary had successfully reduced her consumption to less than 4 cups per day.

Hayes (1981) has suggested a variant of the changing criterion design, the *periodic treatment design* where the treatment is applied only at the start of each phase. In this case changes in behaviour should be observed only at the onset of treatment. Hayes has suggested that this design could be used in outpatient work where sessions are irregularly spaced. To date there appears to be only one extant example of this design given in Hayes's original paper.

Multiple Baseline Design

This design uses control variables to demonstrate the effect of an intervention. The variables can either be other measures taken on the subject, the same target variable observed in other settings or the same measure observed in other persons in under the same conditions (Harris and Jenson, 1985; Hayes, 1985). Experimental control is demonstrated if the target variable changes with the introduction of treatment but there are no corresponding changes in the control variables. Further demonstration of experimental control is obtained by sequentially applying the treatment after a delay to the control variables. The logic of this design is that if treatment is responsible for change then change will be observed in the target variable only. If, however, the introduction of treatment corresponds with an extra-treatment event then concurrent changes will be seen in the control variables. The logic of this design is clearly inconsistent as it is supposed that treatment will produce specific changes in behaviour while non-treatment events will produce general changes. In practice results from multiple baseline designs can only be unambiguously interpreted when there is only change in target variables when treatment is introduced. When other patterns of data are observed it is impossible to know whether the results are due to a generalised treatment effect or to the coincidental effect of an extra-treatment event.

Case Studies 5 and 6. Multiple Baseline Experiments (Barmann & Murray, 1981; Barmann & Vitali, 1982). These studies by Barmann report the use of facial screening to suppress undesirable behaviour in mentally handicapped children. During treatment the subject wears a terry cloth bib which is pulled up the face for 5 seconds following the production of the target response. Barmann and Murray (1981) treated one subject in three different settings; home, the school bus and the classroom. Jimmy was a mentally handicapped boy with a record of sexually inappropriate behaviour. He rubbed his crotch and displayed his penis. Treatment was sequentially introduced into the three settings. Figure 12.7 shows that the introduction of treatment corresponded with a reduction in self-stimulation in the situation where it had been implemented but not in other situations.

In the second study Barmann and Vitali (1982) treated three mentally handicapped children who displayed trichotillomania (compulsive hair pulling). The data shown in Fig. 12.8 come from 90-minute sessions collected at home and show the frequency of hair pulling.

Although Fig. 12.8 shows that the treatments were successful in reducing the frequency of hair pulling there is one feature about the graph which is notable. Unlike the previous case (Barmann & Murray, 1981) the facial screening technique did not produce an immediate improvement in the target response. Generally the treatment took several days before an effect was observed. In all cases treatment was introduced to the other subjects before the effect on the previous subject had stabilised. Under some conditions (i.e. where different subjects are being treated in the same setting at the same time) it would be possible to argue that the effects of

FIG. 12.7. An example of a multiple baseline experiment on one subject across different experimental settings. The graph shows the delayed sequential introduction of the treatment in the three settings. In this case the treatment produced a large and rapid change in the subject's behaviour. (Reproduced from Barmann, B. C. & Murray, W. J. (1981) Suppression of inappropriate sexual behavior by facial screening. *Behavior Therapy,* **12,** 730–735. Copyright 1981, the Association for the Advancement of Behavior Therapy. Reproduced with permission of the publisher and author.)

treatment are not specific to a single subject but dependent on a general change in the way in which therapists or attendant staff interact with all subjects, Kazdin (1982) provides a further discussion of this point.

COMPARING MORE THAN ONE TREATMENT WITHIN AN INDIVIDUAL

The experimental designs discussed so far compare an intervention with a suitable baseline control. But clinicians and researchers are often more interested in questions of whether a particular component of treatment is

FIG. 12.8.   A multiple baseline experiment on three different subjects with trichotillomania. Refer to the text for commentary on the differences between this figure and Fig. 12.7. (Reproduced from Barmann, B. C. & Vitali, D. L. (1982). Facial screening to eliminate trichotillomania in developmentally disabled persons. *Behavior Therapy*, **13**, 735–742. Copyright 1982, the Association for the Advancement of Behavior Therapy. Reproduced with permission of the publisher and author.)

effective, whether one treatment is more effective than another, or with testing theoretical predictions about the impact of certain treatment variables. Single case methods can be extended to meet this challenge but a number of important issues need to be considered.

How Many Treatments Can be Compared?   In theory it is possible to investigate an infinite number of treatments but increasing the number of treatments adds demands on the time and ingenuity of the investigator. In general a maximum of 2 or 3 treatments can be compared, especially if interaction or joint effcts are to be considered (Barrios, 1984).

How Quickly Can Treatments be Alternated Within an Individual?   The rate of change between different treatments depends on several factors:

1. Treatments which take immediate effect can be alternated more rapidly.
2. This is especially true if the treatments produce stable effects with little variation.
3. The third factor concerns the speed at which treatments cease to have an effect once they are withdrawn. Treatments whose effects do not carry over when they are withdrawn are more easily investigated.

It is not necessary for the target variable to return to baseline for mulitple comparisons between interventions to be made neither is a baseline required. For example Watts (1979) and Teasdale and Fennell (1982) used an experimental design taken from standard group experimental methods. The sequence of treatments was determined by a Latin Square to ensure that each treatment followed every other treatment in a balanced order and that the appropriate number of replications were carried out. It is easy to see how this approach can be used to test general theories on single cases or to test diagnostic formulations. For example, consider an experiment that could be carried out with Mrs S (case study 1) to check the formulation. Mrs S's anxiety ratings to different types of images could be evaluated. Images would vary with respect to the degree of independent decision making and the seriousness of outcome events pending on the wrong decision. Images might include explicit acts of criticism by others. The formulation could then be tested independently of treatment outcome.

Extensions of Basic Designs

One way of comparing different treatments is to extend the basic A-B-A-B design to include more elements. A second treatment can be included in the design to form the following sequence A-B-A-C-A; this sequence should be replicated within the subject to test the reliability of the changes. In order to control for any confounding due to the order in which the treatments are presented the replication should be in the reverse order, A-C-A-B-A. It is also possible to compare the effectiveness of different treatments using a multiple baseline design by applying the treatments to the different target behaviours or settings. This tactic has not been widely reported in the literature but an example is reported by Clark, Sugrim and Bolton (1982) and some of the limitations discussed by Morley (1987).

Alternating Treatments Design

In this design a baseline is followed by a phase in which two or more treatments are presented. The order of the treatments is carefully arranged so that they are randomly associated with factors such as the time of day, therapist and any other incidental factors. This follows the standard principle of balancing the experimental treatments with non-experimental factors. After a treatment phase the therapist should be able to select the most powerful treatment and implement it.

Case Study 7: Alternating Treatments (Ollendick, Shapiro & Barrett, 1981). Ollendick and his colleagues compared two treatments for reducing stereotypic behaviour in mentally handicapped children. In each session the children were given an opportunity to engage in simple visual-motor tasks. Physical restraint comprised a verbal warning to stop the behaviour and manually holding the child's hands on the table for 30 seconds. During positive practice the verbal warning was followed by the child being guided through the visual-motor task. No-treatment sessions were also conducted. The results of this experiment for one child are shown in Fig. 12.9. The figure clearly shows that for this child positive practice was the most effective treatment and this was subsequently introduced in all the sessions.

One feature of case study 7 is that the frequency of sterotypic behaviour was increased under the no-treatment condition. This contrast effect raises an important issue about possible interactions and carry-over effects when multiple treatments are given to one person. Barlow and Hersen (1984) provide an extensive discussion of this issue and suggest that the experimenter should follow three procedural guidelines to ensure that carry-over effects are reduced to a minimum:

1. Counter-balance the order of treatments.
2. Different treatments should be interspersed by a separating time interval.
3. Rapid alternations should be avoided until the subject has learned to discriminate between the treatments.

Although these guidelines were developed from operant psychology they are relevant to the study of other treatments. Whenever carry-over effects are suspected they should be investigated. Sidman (1960) suggested that the problem can be broached by deliberate manipulation of one of the treatments. If there is a carry over effect this manipulation will be reflected in changes measured under the second treatment. Sidman (1960) called this *functional manipulation* and an example is shown in Fig. 12.10.

The principle of alternating, or more accurately randomising, different treatments is can be incorporated into other experimental designs in order to carry out further checks on threats to the validity of experiments. Figure 12.11 shows some data from an experiment by McKnight *et al.* who

FIG. 12.9. An example of an alternating treatments design used to compare the effectiveness of two treatments to reduce stereotypic behaviour in a mentally retarded boy. The upper panel shows changes in the target behaviour under different treatments. The lower panel shows concurrent changes in the performance of motor tasks during the sessions. This behaviour was not directly reinforced but was tracked to check the hypothesis that stereotypic behaviour interfered with task performance. (Reproduced from Ollendick, T. H., Shapiro, E. S. & Barrett, R. P. (1981). Reducing stereotypic behaviors: an analysis of treatment procedures utilizing an alternating treatments design. *Behavior Therapy*, **12**, 570–577. Copyright 1981, by the Association for the Advancement of Behavior Therapy. Reproduced with permission of the publisher and author.)

Facial Screening

FIG. 12.10.   An example of functional manipulation used to check on carry-over effects in an alternating treatments design. The subject was a 2½-year-old normal girl who screamed excessively. During phase 1 facial screening was implemented with two durations, 30 seconds and 1 minute. The 1 minute condition produced the greater suppression. To check whether there was an interference effect the 30 second condition was changed to 3 seconds in phase 2. The 1 minute condition produced the same amount of suppression as in phase 1, suggesting that there was no multiple treatment interference. The authors noted that this interpretation is limited by the very low levels of behaviour under the 1 minute condition (a floor effect). (Reproduced from Singh, N. N., Winton, A. S. & Dawson, M. J. (1982). Suppression of antisocial behavior by facial screening using multiple baseline and alternating treatment designs. *Behavior Therapy*, **13**, 511–520. Copyright 1982, the Association for the Advancement of Behavior Therapy. Reproduced with permission of the publisher and author.)

investigated two treatments for depression on people with different psychological profiles. People with predominantly social skill deficits responded better to a social skills package, whereas those with predominantly irrational cognitions responded better to a cognitive therapy package. This experiment exhibits the relative sophistication and economy of single case methods.

Commentary

Barlow and Hersen (1984) and Kazdin (1982) provide detailed discussions of the basic designs and their variations. A cardinal feature of single case methods is that experimental designs are flexible—within certain limits— and can be tailored to particular situations. Table 12.2 outlines some general rules which should be followed when a single-case investigation is planned.

FIG. 12.11.   This figure shows the application of an alternating treatments component to a multiple baseline design. The study investigated the effects of cognitive therapy and social skills training on depressed subjects with either predominantly social or cognitive deficits. A third group with deficits in both domains was also treated but is not shown here. In this figure the outcome measure is a measure of depressed mood. It is clear that the patients' mood improved most when they are treated for their specific deficit. This study illustrates how single case designs can be used to conduct small group experiments. The control built into the single case strategies means that fewer subjects need to be recruited than in a standard groups design. (Reproduced from McKnight, D. L., Nelson, R. O., Hayes S. C. & Jarrett, R. B. (1984). Importance of treating individually assessed response classes in the amelioration of depression. *Behavior Therapy*, **15**, 315–335. Copyright 1984, the Association for the Advancement of Behavior Therapy. Reproduced with permission of the publisher and author.)

ANALYSIS AND DISPLAY OF SINGLE CASE DATA

Visual Analysis

Single case data have traditionally been analysed by graphing and visual inspection. Statistical analysis has been kept to a minimum with reports of means and an estimate of variability. The effects of interventions are clear when experimenters select problems which produce stability (no trend and little variation) in all phases and interventions which induce a rapid and large change in the dependent variable, e.g. Fig. 12.5

In recent years there has been considerable discussion about the role of statistical tests in the analysis of single case data. However, some authors have provided reasons for regarding the advent of statistical tests with suspicion. Baer (1977; Parsonson & Baer, 1978) argues that the thrust of

TABLE 12.2

General rules for the conduct of single case experiments

Measures:

Measure frequently.

Take measures at different levels.

Make sure the measures are sensitive to your requirements (individualise them wherever possible).

Check the reliability and accuracy of measures whenever possible.

Check on instrumentation changes over time.

Look for side effects of measurement and intervention.

Record all external events which seem to be of importance, date them carefully. This will help in the interpretation of the data.

Interventions:

Investigate baseline variability—look for trends in the mean, changes in the variance, cyclical changes:

Control it if you can.

Smooth it statistically as a last resort.

Be explicit about the criteria which guide the timing of the intervention and any manipulation:

Baseline stability.

Clinical urgency/reactive intervention.

Statistical design criteria (randomisation).

Specify the intervention:

Content.

Duration.

Expected temporal impact.

Expected magnitude effects.

Make sure the intervention is enforced for long enough to have an impact.

Monitor the intervention to ensure that it is being carried out (manipulation validity).

Manipulate the intervention whenever possible to investigate causal effects (reverse, withdraw intervention).

Change one variable (aspect of the intervention) at a time.

---

single case research in the field of applied behavioural analysis is to detect effects that are strong, consistent and dependable. He argues that graphical representation of the data will ensure that only these effects are detected whereas weak effects which may be statistically significant will be ignored. In statistical terms Baer argues that visual analysis of the data will ensure that type I errors are minimised (i.e. concluding that an effect is present when it is not) but there is a corresponding increase in the likelihood of type II errors (failing to detect an effect when it is present).

Notwithstanding Baer's arguments there are many occasions when single case data are 'messy'; displaying variability in the phases, different trends across phases and no sharp discontinuity between baseline and treatment phases. Research on visual analysis (De Prospero & Cohen, 1979; Jones,

TABLE 12.3
Features of single case data that facilitate accurate visual analysis

---

Little variability within each phase.

No trend in the data: if trend does exist the direction of the trends should be opposite in each phase.

No overlap in the data between experimental phases.

Interventions with a rapid effect: interventions that occur quickly—in a period shorter than the number of baseline observations—are more easily interpretable.

Interventions that produce large-magnitude changes in the target variable are more believable.

Interventions that can be replicated within an individual; demonstration of a functional relationship between the intervention and the target variable is preferred.

Vaught & Weinrott, 1978) indicates that judges may not reliably detect changes in the data when they are statistically present. Wampold and Furlong (1981) investigated the strategies used by judges. The results suggested that the visual information used in decision making reflected the judges' training. Judges trained in visual inference attended to large changes between phases in an A-B experiment regardless of the amount of variation present. In contrast, judges trained in multivariate analysis took more account of the relative variation in the data in making their judgements. Wampold and Furlong (1981), however, point out that neither group did particularly well in classifying the graphs presented to them.

Whether the investigator decides to rely entirely on visual analysis or to include statistical methods it is imperative that as a preliminary to any analysis the data should be represented graphically. It is important to pay attention to how the data should be presented. The investigator should give consideration to the choice of axes and their scaling and ensure that the form in which the data are presented is appropriate to the type of data collected. It is also necessary to explore the data for hidden trends or changes in variability by smoothing the series and by displaying the range and variability for different points in time. There are several excellent texts which discuss these matters in detail (Chambers, Cleveland, Kleiner & Tukey, 1983; Kazdin, 1982; Johnson & Pennypacker, 1980; Parsonson & Baer, 1978). In conclusion it would seem that unless the data meet stringent requirements when they are plotted (shown in Table 12.3) and the inferences from the plot are 'obvious' then it would be best to be circumspect about the interpretation of the data.

Statistical Analysis

When faced with messy data there are a number of options open to the researcher. Experimental replication should always be attempted, because a basic tenet of scientific enterprise is the reproducibility of effects. If the investigator considers that the experiment is too flawed methodologically to warrant analysis and interpretation then replication is essential. For example each reversal point in an A-B-A-B experiment might coincide with a detectable extra-treatment event. If the experiment was methodologically sound and if there is limited opportunity to replicate and seek a stronger effect the researcher might consider evaluating the data using a statistical method. In this case it could be argued that although the effect is not outstandingly strong it might be detectable by statistical methods. Demonstration of an effect would then provide a spur to further investigations and the development of intervention and experimental technique.

Time Series Analysis. Several statistical methods of analysing single case data have been employed. The use of standard parametric tests, e.g. Student's 't' and analysis of variance, has been criticised on the grounds that the fundamental assumption of uncorrelated errors in the observations is likely to be violated in single case data. If this is the case the error term used to constuct the statistical test will be incorrect and will lead to an inflated estimate of the statistic; e.g. the 't' value will be larger than it should be. The interpretation of the result will then be misleading, with the researcher concluding that there is an effect when there is not (a type I error).

It has been proposed that time-series analysis (TSA) should be applied to single-case data (Gottman, 1981: Jones, Vaught & Weinrott, 1977) in order to deal with the problem of correlated errors. The techniques in TSA are complex and cannot be detailed in this chapter, readers are referred to Kazdin (1984) for an introductory outline and to Gottman (1981) for a comprehensive account of the various techniques of TSA. Although TSA has been widely advocated it not been used very frequently. The methods required considerable statistical prowess which may deter clinicians from learning to use them. Another barrier to their use is that relatively large sets of data (N > 50 per experimental phase) are required before any confidence in the results is justified. Some research suggests that TSA may not be necessary with single case data. Huitema (1985) re-analysed data presented by Jones *et al.* (1977) and found that correlated errors were the exception rather than the rule. In conclusion Huitema (1985) stated that 'complex time series models are neither necessary nor appropriate for serially uncorrelated data from these brief time series,' but, 'whenever a sufficient amount of time series data is available . . . time series models should be considered.'

Simpler, Non-parametric Tests for Investigating Trend. A more pragmatic approach to analysing and interpreting single case data is to use simpler statistical tools requiring less 'sophistication' which are easy to calculate and appropriate as an aid to summarising and describing the data. These statistics do not compare different experimental phases but they enable the investigator to detect and describe trend and variability within phases. Several of the statistics can be used with small sets of data (N ⩾ 6). Kendall (1976) describes a number of non-parametric tests for randomness and trend in time series data. The Records test (Foster & Stuart, 1954) is a test of trend in mean and variance. These tests are described more fully by Morley and Adams (1989).

Tryon (1982) has described the C statistic for changes in trend across different phases. This statistic makes use of the fact that the variance in a set of successive points can be calculated in two ways. The standard variance, S^2, is familiar to most readers. The second method is known as the mean successive square difference, D^2, and takes the temporal order of the observations into account. If there is no trend in the data it is expected that $2S^2 = D^2$. This relationship can therefore be used to test for trend. Tryon provides full detail of the calculations and a worked example. (Blumberg (1984) has provided a critique of this method and indicated a typographical error in Tryon's original paper. Readers should refer to this and to Tryon's (1984) reply.)

Randomisation Tests. These tests are underpinned by a different logic from parametric tests. Their conduct does not depend upon the assumption that observations are drawn from a population with a known distribution. The test estimates the probability that a more extreme set of scores than the obtained pattern of results would occur if the data were to be rearranged in all possible combinations. Randomisation tests require that the investigator should randomly select an intervention point *before* the start of the experiment. For example, Clements and Hand (1985) decided that a minimum of 5 days baseline was required with a maximum of 25 days and randomly selected to begin the intervention after 21 days. A total of 44 data points were collected in an A-B design. The statistical significance of the intervention was computed by calculating the difference in the means between successive sets of data representing all the baseline points and all the treatment point that were theoretically possible. (The first difference was between the first 5 days and the last 39 days, the second between the first 6 and last 38 days, and so on up to the first 25 and last 19 days.) Inspection of the resulting set of mean differences showed that the actual baseline treatment difference obtained was the third largest out of a total of 21, giving a probability that this result could be obtained by chance for this set of data of $p < 0.14$. With only a total of 21 possible sets of means, to attain conventional significance only one of the possible 21 sets could have produced a result $p < 0.05$. It is easy to see that if there were only 10 possible intervention points that the 'maximum' significance that could be obtained would be p < 0.10.

Randomisation tests can be applied to the median, an estimate of trend or virtually any other summary statistic which it is reasonable to calculate in the particular case. Hand (1982) provides a clear introductory discussion of randomisations tests, while Edgington (1984) provides a fuller discussion of their application to single case data with many worked examples. Pechacek (1978) and Wampold and Worsham (1986) show how the principle can be extended to the analysis of multiple baseline designs.

Other statistical tests.   There are many other tests that can applied to single case data. Kazdin (1982, 1984) provides an excellent discussion of the split middle technique and Revusky's R test for multiple baseline data. Gottman and Notarius (1978) demonstrate how Markov models may be used to examine sequential data. The interested reader is referred to these sources.

CONCLUSION

Faced with the dilemma of whether to use statistics or visual inference what should the researcher do? In the first instance it is clear that the data should be summarised and displayed to highlight the existence of trend, stability, changes in means and the inherent variability. These features should be summarised with simple descriptive statistics. Only after this has been done should a statistical test be selected; its conduct should supplement the previous two stages. The whole process has been delightfully expressed by Johnson and Pennypacker (1980, p. 330): 'Quantitative summarisation should occur concurrently with the creation of visual displays' and, 'As in amorous foreplay, the process of exploring one's data should proceed from the general to the particular, aided at every step by enhanced visualisation.'

ACKNOWLEDGEMENTS

I thank Peter Morley for his help in data collection.

REFERENCES

Baer, D. M. (1977). Perhaps it would be better not to know everything. *Journal of Applied Behavior Analysis*, **10**, 167–172.

Barlow, D. H. & Hersen, M. (1984). *Single Case Experimental Designs*, 2nd edn. New York: Pergamon Press.

Barrios, B. A. (1984). Single subject design strategies for examining joint effects: a critical examination. *Behavioural Assessment*, **6**, 103–120.

Barmann, B. C. & Murray, W. J. (1981). Suppression of inappropriate sexual behavior by facial screening. *Behavior Therapy*, **12**, 730–735.

Barmann, B. C. & Vitali, D. L. (1982). Facial screening to eliminate trichotillomania in developmentally disabled persons. *Behavior Therapy*, **13**, 735–742.

Bernard, M. E., Dennehy, S. & Keefauver, L. W. (1981). Behavioral treatment of excessive coffee and tea drinking: a case study and partial replication. *Behavior Therapy*, **12**, 543–548.

Blumberg, C. J. (1984). Comments on 'A simplified time-series analysis for evaluating treatment interventions'. *Journal of Applied Behavior Analysis*, **17**, 539–542.

Campbell, D. T. & Stanley, J. C. (1966). *Experimental and Quasi-experimental Designs for Research*. Chicago: Rand McNally.

Chambers, J. M., Cleveland, W. S., Kleiner, B. & Tukey, P. A. (1983). *Graphical Methods for Data Analysis*. Belmont, Cal.: Wadsworth.

Clark, D. A., Sugrim, I. & Bolton, D. (1982). Primary obsessional slowness: a nursing treatment programme with a 13 year old male adolescent. *Behaviour Research and Therapy*, **20**, 289–292.

Clements, J. C. & Hand, D. J. (1985). Permutation statistics in single case design. *Behavioural Psychotherapy*, **13**, 288–299.

Cone, J. D. (1988). Psychometric considerations and the multiple models of behavioural assessment. In A. S. Bellack and M. Hersen (eds.), *Behavioral Assessment* (3rd edn.). New York: Pergamon Press.

Cook, T. D. & Campbell, D. T. (1979). *Quasi-experimentation: Design and Analysis Issues for Field Settings*. Chicago: Rand McNally.

De Prospero, A. & Cohen, S. (1979). Inconsistent visual analysis of intra-subject data. *Journal of Applied Behavior Analysis*, **12**, 573–379.

Edgington, E. S. (1984). Statistics and the single case. In M. Hersen, R. M. Eisler and P. M. Miller (eds.) *Progress in Behavior Modification*, Vol. 16. New York: Academic Press.

Elashoff, J. D. and Thoresen, C. E. (1978). Choosing a statistical method for analysis of an intensive experiment. In T. R. Kratochwill (ed.) *Single Subject Research: Strategies for Evaluating Change*. New York: Academic Press.

Foster, F. G. & Stuart, A. (1954). Distribution-free tests in time series based on the breaking of records. *Journal of the Royal Statistical Society (Series B)*, **16**, 1–13.

Glass, G. V., Willson, V. L. & Gottman, J. M. (1974). *Design and Analysis of Time-series Experiments*. Boulder, Col.: Colorado Associated University Press.

Gottman, J. M. (1981). *Time–Series Analysis: A Comprehensive Introduction for Social Scientists*. Cambridge University Press.

Gottman, J. M. & Notarius, C. (1978). Sequential analysis of observational data using Markov chains. In T. R. Kratochwill (ed.) *Single Subject Research: Strategies for Evaluating Change*. New York: Academic Press.

Hallam, R. S. (1976). A complex view of simple phobias. In H. J. Eysenck (ed.). *Case Studies in Behaviour Therapy*. London: Routledge & Kegan Paul.

Hand, D. J. (1982). Statistical tests in experimental psychiatric research. *Psychological Medicine*, **12**, 415–421.

Handen, B. L., Apolito, P. M. & Seltzer, G. B. (1984). The use of differential reinforcement of low rates of behavior to decrease repetitive speech in an autistic adolescent. *Journal of Behavior Therapy and Experimental Psychiatry*, **15**, 359–364.

Harris, F. N. & Jenson, W. R. (1985). Comparisons of mulitple-baseline across persons designs and AB designs with replication: issues and confusions. *Behavioural Assessment*, **7**, 121–127.

Hartmann, D. P. (1984). Assessment strategies. In D. H. Barlow and M. Hersen (eds). *Single Case Experimental Designs*. New York: Pergamon Press.

Hayes, S. C. (1985). Single case experimental design and empirical clinical practice. *Journal of Consulting and Clinical Psychology*, **49**, 193–211.

Hayes, S. C. (1985). Natural multiple baselines across persons: A reply to Harris and Jenson. *Behavioural Assessment*, **7**, 128–132.

Hegel, M. T., Ayllon, T., VanderPlate, C. & Spiro-Hawkins, H. (1986). A behavioural procedure for increasing compliance with self-exercise regimens in severely burn-injured patients. *Behaviour Research and Therapy*, **24**, 521–528.

Herbst, P. G. (1970). *Behavioural Worlds. The Study of Single Cases*. London: Tavistock Publications.

Huitema, B. E. (1985). Autocorrelation in applied behavior analysis: a myth. *Behavioural Assessment*, **7**, 107–118.

Johnston, J. M. & Pennypacker, H. S. (1980). *Strategies and Tactics of Human Behavioral Research*. Hillsdale, New Jersey: Lawrence Erlbaum Associates.

Jones, R. R., Vaught, R. S. & Weinrott, M. (1977). Time-series analysis in operant research. *Journal of Applied Behavior Analysis*, **10**, 151–166.

Jones, R. R., Vaught, R. S. & Weinrott, M. (1978). Effects of serial dependency on the agreement between visual and statistical inference. *Journal of Applied Behavior Analysis*, **11**, 277–283.

Kazdin, A. E. (1982). *Single Case Research Designs: Methods for Clinical and Applied Settings*. New York: Oxford University Press.

Kazdin, A. E. (1984). Statistical analysis for single case experimental designs. In D. H. Barlow and M. Hersen (eds) *Single Case Experimental Designs*, 2nd edn. New York: Pergamon Press.

Kendall, M. (1976). *Time Series*. London: Charles Griffin.

Leff, J. P. & Vaughn, C. E. (1985). *Expressed Emotion in Families: Its Significance for Mental Illness*. New York: Guilford Press.

Lodge, M. (1981). *Magnitude Scaling: Qualitative Measurement of Opinions*. Beverly Hills, Cal.: Sage Publications.

McKnight, D. L., Nelson, R. O., Hayes, S. C. & Jarrett, R. B. (1984). Importance of treating individually assessed response classes in the amelioration of depression. *Behavior Therapy*, **15**, 315–335.

Morley, S. (1987). Single case methodology in behaviour therapy. In S. J. E. Lindsay and G. E. Powell (eds.) *A Handbook of Clinical Adult Psychology*. London: Gower Press.

Morley, S. & Adams, M. (1989). Some simple statistics for exploring single case time-series data. *British Journal of Clinical Psychology*, **28**, 1–18.

Ollendick, T. H., Shapiro, E. S. & Barrett, R. P. (1981). Reducing sterotypic behaviors: an analysis of treatment procedures utilizing an alternating treatments design. *Behavior Therapy*, **12**, 570–577.

Parsonson, B. S. & Baer, D. M. (1978). The analysis and presentation of graphic data. In T. R. Kratochwill (ed.) *Single Subject Research: Strategies for Evaluating Change*. New York: Academic Press.

Pechachek, T. F. (1978). A probabalistic model of intensive designs. *Journal of Applied Behavior Analysis*, **11**, 357–362.

Peck, D. F. (1985). Small N experimental designs in clinical practice. In F N. Watts (ed.), *New Developments in Clinical Psychology*. Chichester: British Psychological Society—John Wiley.

Phillips, J. P. N. (1977). Generalised personal questionnaire techniques. In P. Slater (ed.) *The Measurement of Interpersonal Space by Grid Techniques: Vol. 2. Dimensions of Intrapersonal Space*. London: John Wiley.

Salkovskis, P. M. & Warwick, H. M. C. (1985). Cognitive therapy of obsessive-compulsive disorder: treating treatment failures. *Behavioural Psychotherapy*, **13**, 243–255.

Shapiro, M. B. (1961). A method of measuring psychological changes specific to the individual psychiatric patient. *British Journal of Medical Psychology*, **34**, 151–155.

Shapiro, M. B. (1975). The single variable approach to assessing the intensity of feelings of depression. *European Journal of Behaviour Analysis and Modification*, **2**, 62–70.

Shapiro, M. B. (1985). A reassessment of clinical psychology as an applied science. *British Journal of Clinical Psychology*, **24**, 1–11.

Sidman, M. (1960). *Tactics of Scientific Research*. New York: Basic Books.

Singh, N. N., Winton, A. S. & Dawson, M. J. (1982). Suppression of antisocial behavior by facial screening using multiple baseline and alternating treatment designs. *Behavior Therapy*, **13**, 511–520.

Teasdale, J. D. & Fennell, M. J. V. (1982). Immediate effects on depression of cognitive therapy interviews. *Cognitive Therapy and Research*, **6**, 343–353.

Tryon, W. W. (1982). A simplified time-series analysis for evaluating treatment interventions. *Journal of Applied Behavior Analysis*, **15**, 423–429.

Tryon, W. W. (1984). 'A simplified time-series analysis for evaluating treatment interventions': A rejoinder to Blumberg. *Journal of Applied Behavior Analysis*, **17**, 543–544.

Turkat, I. D. & Carlson, C. R. (1984). Data-based versus symptomatic formulation of treatment: the case of a dependent personality. *Journal of Behavior Therapy and Experimental Psychiatry*, **15**, 153–160.

Wahler, R. R. (1980). The insular mother: her problems in parent–child treatment. *Journal of Applied Behavior Analysis*, **13**, 207–219.

Wahler, R. G. & Graves, M. G. (1983). Setting events in social networks: ally or enemy in child behavior therapy. *Behavior Therapy*, **14**, 19–36.

Wampold, B. E. & Furlong, M. J. (1981). The heuristics of visual inference. *Behavioural Assessment*, **3**, 79–92.

Wampold, B. E. & Worsham, N. L. (1986). Randomization tests for mulitple baseline designs. *Behavioural Assessment*, **8**, 135–143.

Watts, F. N. (1979). The habituation model of systematic desensitization. *Psychological Bulletin*, **86**, 627–637.

Youell, K. J. & McCollough, J. P. (1975). Behavioral treatment of mucous collitis. *Journal of Consulting and Clinical Psychology*, **43**, 740–745.

13 Intensive Quantitative Methods

Paul Alexander
Principal Clinical Psychologist, Medway Health Authority
Honorary Lecturer, University of Kent at Canterbury.

There is no simple definition of intensive quantitative research, but there are a number of key themes which will provide the framework of the chapter. Intensive clinical research aims to look in depth at mental health phenomena and provide meaningful and penetrating analyses, especially of processes of change and interaction. For this purpose it usually employs the rich data base provided by repeated and/or multiple measures.

There are three key features of intensive research that distinguish it from other related methodologies. Firstly, the use of *quantification techniques* identifies a commitment to empirical measurements and statistical analysis of the collected data. This distinguishes it from the qualitative methodologies discussed in Chapter 11. Yet, as Jahoda has commented in connection with one intensive technique, the Interpersonal Perception Method . . . 'quantification need not be limited to insignificant and artificially isolated aspects of psychological phenomena' (Laing, Phillipson & Lee, 1966, p. v). The intensive research tradition shows that quantification techniques are not necessarily reductionistic and impoverishing.

A further aspect of this tradition is the use of *naturalistic* research methods. In this, intensive methods stand in contrast with the experimental single-case methods considered in Chapter 12. Naturalistic research permits the study of psychological phenomena without the potentially distorting effects of experimental manipulations. Although one consequence of not applying experimentally based methods is that some naturalistic research is less able to replicate its findings easily.

Naturally occurring data are not necessarily poorly structured. Indeed this methodology has a commitment to the *planned* elicitation of naturally occurring data in order to maximise reliability and validity. For example, the Personal Questionnaire (Shapiro, 1961), which is a self-report measure of symptoms, has been developed with a thorough concern for psychometric issues (Phillips, 1977). The subject uses the method of paired-comparisons (e.g. 'Does statement A or B best express how anxious you feel?) rather than merely giving a single numerical value ('How anxious are you' rating from 0 to 10). Shapiro's method both reduces response bias and utilises the internal consistency of ratings as a measure of reliability.

The final characteristic is the use of *idiographic* rather than nomothetic data. This reflects the focus upon the intensive study of psychological processes. There are two major problems with group-based research. It is difficult to ensure the homogeneity of subjects on all relevant parameters and these methods can obscure significant individual differences by pooling scores to provide group values. Of course, techniques that have been developed for intensive research, such as the Repertory Grid, can be employed in group-based designs, but such extensions of intensive methods are outside the scope of the chapter.

One important consequence of the focus upon idiographic data is that intensive methodologies rarely, if ever, employ control subjects, and are thus unable to enjoy benefits accruing from control groups—in particular the differentiation between an active treatment and placebo or non-specific factors. This raises the difficulty that many intensive studies assume they are discovering findings unique to the research subject without verifying this assumption. The problem is that, if person-centred measures are being used in the study, the development of a standard form, which would permit controlled comparisons, would breach the central assumptions of such measures. This reflects a methodological tension which individual researchers need to think through in their own particular research contexts. Ryle & Breen (1972a), for example, attempted to integrate both perspectives in their comparison of the Repertory Grid (RG) analyses of neurotic and control subjects, by comparing measures of *structure* rather than *content*.

SELF-REPORT AND OBSERVATIONAL MEASURES

Intensive methodologies can employ measures based on either self-report or observational data. These two approaches to measurement partly reflect the different traditions and paradigms of person-centred (or phenomenological) and behavioural psychology. Both have merits and demerits which must carefully be considered in the planning stage of any research study (Nelson, 1981). Self-report measures mainly develop from an introspectionist tradition and emphasise the individual's own account of 'internal events'—their psychological state and processes. Usually these will consist of their perceptions, attitudes or feelings. An individual can also make self-reports about their own behaviour, as in self-monitoring, but such methods derive from behavioural paradigms and will be discussed below. Henceforth in this chapter, for clarity, 'self-report' will be used for phenomenologically derived methods which consider internal experience and 'self-monitoring' for behaviourally derived approaches in which subjects appraise their own overt behaviour. The focus of the perceptions elicited by self-report measures can include other people, the self, abstract roles ('good parent'), ideals ('justice') or inanimate objects and structures (day-hospital or a proposed district addiction service). Typical self-report measures range from unstructured interviews and narrative analyses through to more formalised methods where the subject is provided with a systematised structure but they determine the unique content, e.g. the RG supplies general role-categories to which the subject provides specific named persons.

Self-report measures have the advantages of the high personal validity and depth of meaning that flow from subjects expressing their thoughts and feelings in their own words. They are potentially flexible and allow for creative responses; they are essentially ways of approaching the subject material, rather than structured 'tests'. They are also the only possible means of measuring certain clinical problems—e.g. obsessional or paranoid thoughts, sexual or sleeping behaviours. Disadvantages include demonstrating a causal relationship between such covert processes and actual behaviour, and assessing whether such 'introspectionist' data have a reliability and validity lasting beyond a very short time-span. Are a person's self-reports whimsical, fleeting impressions or more lasting and consistent? Self-report methodologies must continually address such issues.

Observational measures focus from the outside upon the subject's behaviour. They are largely derived from behavioural paradigms, which have championed the need for the thorough assessment and monitoring of behavioural change. Hersen and Bellack (1976) and Craighead, Kazdin and Mahoney (1981) provide good reviews of assessment and treatment approaches with a wide range of clinical problems, although only a few of the methods presented could be considered 'intensive'. Ethological methods are also relevant, in view of their emphasis upon detailed observation and description of behaviour—usually in naturalistic situations—and the recent extension of such approaches to mental health research and developmental psychology is worth noting (Bateson & Hinde, 1976; Snowdon, 1983). A particualrly useful discusion of observational and ethological paradigms is provided by Martin and Bateson (1986).

Behavioural psychology stresses its concern with all three systems of behaviour—the motoric (behavioural), physiological and cognitive. All can be assessed with observational measures but different modes may require varied specific procedures. The majority of observational measures focus upon overt behaviour, but physiological measures (e.g. penile plethysmograph) are gaining in popularity although they are often expensive and time consuming. Furthermore, such measures are rarely appropriate for intensive methodologies. The cognitive mode is mainly assessed by self-monitoring techniques (Ciminero, Nelson & Lipinski, 1977). Typical observational measures include counts of behavioural magnitude, frequency, intensity or duration and the use of ratings or checklists completed by observers. Data can be collected on a continuous or sampling (fixed or randomised) basis. Occasionally it is possible to use indirect measures e.g. tranquilliser prescription as a measure of anxiety.

Observational measures have the advantages of clear operational definition and enhanced reliability, both within and between observers. Assessment can be made in either the clinic or natural environment, the advantage of the former being better control of variables and convenience, whereas the latter provides greater validity. However, there are a number of potential difficulties with such measures. A key requirement is that the unit of observation is meaningful (not too small or too large), but can also be identified reliably. Sometimes, reliability is purchased at the cost of excluding aspects of the broader context that make a unit of observation meaningful. Thus in a study of 'negative verbal interaction', should only single words be rated, or sentences or paragraphs; and should preceding and consequent statements be considered, to provide a context? Should non-verbal qualifiers, which may indicate that the verbal statements are not to be taken seriously, be taken into account—and if so, how? A further issue is that the relevant behaviour has to be adequately sampled to ensure that the important target events occur whilst observations take place. High-frequency behaviours will require reliable sampling procedures whereas low-frequency behaviours may require unrealistically vigilant observers.

The process of taking observational measures often has important implications for both the subject being observed and the observer (Lipinski & Nelson, 1974). Subjects' behaviour may well change significantly with the knowledge that they are being observed ('reactivity'); self-monitoring can also be affected by subjects knowing that their accuracy is being monitored (Nelson, 1981). Similarly, observers' reports can be influenced by a knowledge of the results expected, feedback from the experimenter, and reactivity—awareness that their own performance is being monitored. One final consideration with observational measures is the need to ensure adequate links between behavioural descriptions and the person's subjective experience.

Particular traditions of research have often used only one class of measurement, apparently failing to see the potential for extending the application of intensive methodologies to other data domains. For example 'studies of structure' (see next section) have largely employed self-report measures to provide structural models of an individual's psychological functioning, whereas 'response' strategies have tended only to use observational measures as a consequence of focusing solely upon overt behaviours as the responses under study. One intention of this chapter is to show that a wider range of application is possible for both these measurement procedures and to illustrate the commonality of methodological issues. A welcome research trend has been the use of a combination of self-report and observational measures, in an attempt to extract maximum benefit from each. Thus Elliott's (1984) 'event-based' phenomenological approach (discussed in detail later) uses behavioural events (observational) to act as cues for the exploration of subjective internal processes.

Intensive methodologies are applicable to a wide range of mental health issues and questions. Historically, many studies have been concerned with psychotherapy process research, but pleasingly investigations are increasingly taking place in other clinical domains. Particularly fertile areas appear to be medical psychology, neuropsychology and the special needs of children and mentally handicapped people. Increased concern with community-based services, especially for clients requiring continuing care, offers further challenging research opportunities.

Finally, it is important to consider some more general strategic issues. The more that researchers test out specific, derived hypotheses the more likely they are to provide robust conclusions and the less likely they are to lose direction. This is not to deny the value of clinical 'hunches' in research but to emphasise that these should be translated into clear questions before the research begins. Because intensive methodologies are capable of generating large amounts of data, the researcher can easily become submerged in computer printouts. Without clear research questions the ratio of conclusions to data collected can be poor. Such considerations emphasise the value of a pilot study, wherever possible. Such a pilot study should include data analysis and interpretation as well as anticipating possible difficulties in data collection and the operationalisation of relevant variables.

Researchers need to familiarise themselves with the assumptions about the data and subject pool made by the measuring procedures and to ensure these are not invalidated. This can be particularly pertinent with intensive methodologies which typically use only a small number of subjects and repeated measures and therefore fail to meet the statistical assumptions of measures developed with large samples of subjects.

TYPES OF DESIGN

This chapter will be organised around a categorisation of intensive designs into four groups, according to the kind of analysis undertaken with the empirical data. This abstract classification will hopefully direct attention to fundamental aspects of the research strategy, and will clarify the range of research questions that can be addressed by each design. In particular, it will become apparent that the most commonly used forms of intensive research are just a sample of those potentially available.

The four categories are (a) comparisons of responses, (b) sequences, (c) studies of structure, and (d) interactions and interexperience. They must be considered as dimensions which overlap at their extremeties rather than as mutually exclusive categories, and a number of examples provided will illustrate this. Thus interactive aspects can occur in both responses and sequences designs as well as in interexperience designs. A research strategy will be classified as an 'interaction' when it is assessing mutual influence rather than simply one-way effects. Methodologies in categories (a) and (b) have been used less extensively than those in (c) and (d).

Key dimensions within the categories refer to the number of people, the number of meaurement occasions and other significant parameters concerning situational and structural variables (Table 13.1). The majority of the designs in this research tradition are individual based and only one category, that of 'interaction and interexperience', focuses upon the mutual interaction of two or more people. A number of methodologies take serial measures at different points in time in order to explicate change processes but this is not an essential feature of 'intensive' research. Alternative strategies include the comparison of an individual under two different conditions which are not significantly separated in time, or

TABLE 13.1
The four categories of intensive research

Typology	Person	Number of measurement occasions	Other
Responses	1	2 or n	Situational variance
Sequences	1	n	
Structure	1	1 or n	Structural representation
Interaction & interexperience	n	1 or n	

developing structural models of the individual's conceptual world or behaviour.

1. Comparisons of Responses

This research strategy compares the responses made by a person in
different situations or conditions. Only one variable of the person's behaviour is considered (e.g. extent of stuttering) and the intention is to
investigate whether significant associations exist between conditions (e.g.
group size) and the response. Many such studies have been carried out in a
clinical context but this is not essential and similar research is possible in
educational and occupational areas. A good example of this research
strategy is Metcalfe's (1956) investigation of an asthmatic patient, which
demonstrated a significant relationship between the patient's asthma
attacks and meetings with her mother (Table 13.2). The proposed mediating mechanism was that the meetings were negatively emotionally laden
and this triggered the underlying somatic vulnerability. The association
was demonstrated by a simple frequency count of the asthmatic attacks
over an 85-day period under two conditions of the mother's presence or
absence. A 2×2 chi-square test revealed a significant correlation.

Two central methodological issues raised by this research strategy concern the definition of the situation and the definition of the person's
responses. It is vital that both can be identified in a reliable and valid
manner. The situation requires clear operational description and, wherever possible, discrete onset and offset. Usually situations are defined by
direct observation, but self-report measures are possible in principle, e.g. a
person could indicate the range of situations in which their obsessional
thoughts do or do not occur. Similar issues exist regarding the measurement of the person's responses under different conditions. Observational

TABLE 13.2

Contact with mother versus asthma attacks (from Metcalfe,
1956)

Occurrence of asthma	Days with asthma	Days without asthma
—	15	70
Within 24 hours of being with mother	9 (60%)	14 (20%)
Not in contact with mother for preceding 24 hours	6 (40%)	56 (80%)

measures (e.g. checklist of interactional frequency) have high reliability, but self-report measures may tap more relevant variables. Both options are possible and require consideration. Obviously, there will always be a time-lag between the conditions that are being compared, though in many cases this is slight as conditions may be consecutive (e.g. movement from a small to a large group in a day hospital). Sometimes a longer time-scale will be required to demonstrate a clear causal relationship, as in the study by Metcalfe, though this research strategy is not essentially concerned with changes over time.

Studies using the response–comparison methodology often investigate situation-specific behaviour, being concerned with the identification of the conditions under which the behaviour is displayed. The empirical findings are used to provide a theoretical framework to explain the origins and development of the behaviour, and in many cases to suggest future treatment initiatives. Unfortunately for our purposes, a lot of the relevant work, including studies of temper tantrums or self-injurious behaviour, has focused upon effecting change by experimental means, rather than study-ing the response/situation correlation naturalistically. Such experimental research verifies hypotheses about the causal links maintaining behaviour by observing whether significant changes occur when reinforcement con-tingencies are altered (e.g. Carr & Newsom, 1985). Methods derived from ethological research are particularly relevant, especially because of their emphasis upon the ecological context of behaviour (Bateson & Hinde, 1976). For example, Esser (1968) describes an observational study, within an ethological perspective, of the interactional behaviour and dominance patterns of schizophrenic patients on a ward.

Generalisability studies also fall into this response–comparison category of research methodologies but their aim is to demonstrate reliability across conditions rather than investigate differences between conditions (see Levy, 1974, for an exposition of the method and some clinical examples). In a study applying generalisability theory to the observation of eating behaviours, Coates and Thoresen (1978) found that reliable measures could be obtained from studying nine variables on three separate occa-sions. Essentially such studies hope to identify a non-significant difference in the person's response between situations. Many of these studies derive from a treatment context and so may not be fully considered as 'naturalis-tic', although a tradition of naturalistic observation and assessment of patients does exist in some treatments. The literature on social skills training will provide further examples (e.g. Spence & Shepherd, 1983).

2. Sequences

The focus of research methodologies in this category is the investigation of sequences and patterns of responses. This may involve the study of changes over time, but this is not an essential characteristic; a lot of research will solely be concerned with identifying existing—often intricate—response patterns. Such patterns often include regularities in the combination and punctuation of variables, even rhythms.

Clearly, a sequence or pattern can only occur if there are at least two variables under consideration (and often more). This distinguishes these methodologies from those discussed in the previous section, where only a single variable was considered. Furthermore, all methodologies in this category will require that measures of variables are taken on at least two occasions and usually many more times. Concern is upon only a single individual—the study of the covariation of a number of people is discussed below in Section (4) (page 278). Developmental studies, which would typically investigate the growth in a child's physical or conceptual skills, could also be classified within this typology, but the longitudinal nature of such studies produces severe constaints on measurement.

It is to be expected that the complexity of measurement, analysis and data interpretation will usually increase with the number of variables and occasions of measurement. A number of sophisticated statistical analyses of sequence data have been developed and these will be mentioned below. Developmental studies, which would typically investigate the growth in a child's physical or conceptual skills, could also be classified within this typology, but the intrinsic longitudinal nature of such studies would produce severe constraints on measurement. Research methodologies can employ either self-report or observational measures, but there has been a tendency for observational data to dominate. However Shapiro's (1969) Personal Questionnaire (PQ), which uses self-report data (see below), has made a significant contribution to this area.

Within this category there are two slightly different strategies, reflecting attempts to answer differing research questions. The first concerns the sequential embedding of target responses. The behaviours before and after a previously chosen target response are investigated in order to analyse their antecedents/precursors and effects. A common concern would be to identify which behaviours show increased frequency before and after the target event. Relevant examples would be the study of the precipitants and subsequent effects of aggressive or self-injurious behaviour. Research using this strategy has often employed behavioural observational measures, yet the same methods can in principle be applied to thoughts or mood (as 'covert behaviours') but only if they have discrete onset and offset. The requirement that there be identifiable and reliable onset and offset of key responses is a central methodological constraint of the sequential embedding approach. Naturally, methodologies investigating internal processes would require appropriate self-report measures. A relevant example would be Elliott's (1984) use of his client's mood changes during therapy. Such a strategy is permissible within this tradition as long as the changes in thoughts or mood occur naturally without experimental manipulation.

The second strategy investigates the covariation of two (or more) variables over time (or situation) within a single individual to assess whether they are causally related and if so, what is the pattern of the relationship. Intensive methodologies would be particularly relevant to elucidating such complex patterns. Gershon, Cromer and Klerman (1968) employed repeated observational measures of depression and hostility to see if they were positively or negatively correlated over time. Although, in some patients, they found support for the classic psychodynamic formulation of an inverse correlation between these two variables other patients revealed a coexistence of manifest hostility and depression. Another example is Chassan's (1979, pp. 231–235) study of a female patient, diagnosed as paranoid schizophrenic. She was interviewed 17 times and on each occasion rated on 20 (observational) items e.g. coherence, affective state, mental state. Analysis of the covariation of items revealed interesting findings, in particular a significant negative correlation between her 'appearance' and her 'orientation for person'. A 2 × 2 contingency table of data from this symptom-pair showed a near-perfect inverse matching— when she had a clear picture of who she was, then her appearance was slovenly. Unfortunately, Chassan fails to identify the meaning of this relationship, but this would ideally be the intention of intensive methodologies. Self-report data were employed by Garety (1985) in a PQ study of the covariation of an individual's delusional symptoms. Two patients were independently studied and interest was focused upon monitoring any fluctuation in the intensity and fixity of the self-reported delusions. Both patients completed PQ weekly and three delusional and three control beliefs (e.g. 'the sun will rise tomorrow') were rated on a 5-point scale. Some fluctuation in the strength of the paranoid beliefs was found but the control beliefs remained entirely consistent. Only one patient showed a correlation between medication-intake and weakening of delusional beliefs. One further use of self-report data could be to investigate whether a person's perceptions correlated across different people. Thus, are ratings of 'physical attractiveness' and 'goodness' significantly related? Such a research strategy comes close to issues considered in Studies of Structure below, particularly when using the Repertory Grid, but can be placed in this present category if it maintains a narrow focus and refrains from a more elaborate structural investigation.

A related research strategy would be the investigation of changes in the covariation of variables. Of especial interest would be the study of changes after a significant event, such as psychological therapy, having a baby or management training. The PQ has been used by a number of people to study changes during psychological therapy—a task to which it is well suited as it was designed specifically to facilitate repeated measures, often over brief time periods. A dominant theme has concerned the 'immediate improvement effect' in therapy, as rated by the client. Shapiro (1969) reported this effect after behavioural therapy, especially for symptoms of depression and tension. However, Hobson and Shapiro (1970) failed to replicate this when a more psychotherapeutic approach was used. Shapiro and Hobson (1972) found clear PQ 'worsenings' during psychotherapy sessions and went on to suggest that interpretative therapy may produce short-term stress for a client by challenging existing coping mechanisms, but this may provide eventual long-term benefit. This view received mixed support from a study of group psychotherapy by Shapiro, Caplan, Rohde & Watson (1975) as many group members showed variability in PQ scores, In a study comparing exploratory and prescriptive therapy Parry, Shapiro and Firth (1986) combined repeated PQ scores with the client's perceptions of helpful events in therapy and the therapist's session notes to provide a detailed analysis of the therapeutic process. Two particularly interesting findings were that most symptom change had occurred by session eight, and that different problems changed at different rates in response to different techniques—tension and irritability being influenced by a psychodynamic approach and cognitive/behavioural methods helping concentration and work problems. All the above studies have attempted to look in detail at specific variables within the therapeutic relationship and this approach can be seen as a useful adjunct to more traditional outcome data in understanding processes of change. The potential of such methods to investigate the effect of therapy on individual variables is large. For example, it may be found that variables that were tightly correlated before therapy have now become more independent, or that variables change at different rates (as indicated by Parry *et al.*) or in systematic ways. However, one important methodological issue is the need to demonstrate that the study has identified *changes* in variables and not merely a complex but pre-existing pattern.

The investigation of sequences has produced a group of related, and sophisticated, statistical analyses which essentially test whether items in the sequence are correlated or random. Good descriptions are provided by Everitt and Dunn (1983), Bakeman and Gottman (1986) and Martin and Bateson (1986). Markov analysis is used to assess whether a sequence of events (responses) is ordered or random, and is obtained by comparison of the obtained sequence with an hypothesised random one. A first-order Markov chain is one where the probability of an event C occurring depends only on the immediately preceding event B, whereas in a second-order chain the probability depends on the two preceding events AB. Markov chains can be used to study the responses of a single individual or the correlation between the responses of two people (the latter would fall into category (4)).

If times as well as the order of events have been recorded then time series analysis can be used to provide a description of temporal correlation and interaction. One particular form of time series analysis is Fourier analysis, which was used by Grant, Yager, Sweetwood and Olshen (1982) in a 3-year prospective study assessing the correlation between life-events and psychiatric symptoms. Unfortunately, they found no significant results but their study remains methodologically interesting for our purposes. These analyses of sequences are both useful and increasingly popular but they are statistically complex and their assumptions must be fully understood and adhered to in order for the validity of the results to hold. The central methodological parameters for studies of covariation involve ensuring there are sufficient variation of element items (times, people, situations, etc.) and sufficient numbers of observations.

3. Studies of Structure

Research methodologies in this category are concerned to develop structural representations—either of a person's conceptual world or of their behaviour. This approach is most commonly associated with phenomenological theories and self-report methods, but potential exists for the development of methods based on behavioural observation. However, phenomenologically derived methods probably tend to be the more complex, time consuming and popular. One of the best example of this approach is the Repertory Grid (RG) developed by Kelly (1955) and extended more recently by other workers, and a number of examples of RG usage will be provided in this section.

Generally speaking, researchers using these methods are interested in the way different constituents relate together to form an overall structure. In most cases the structure comprises hierarchically organised components and involves techniques for elucidating these hierarchical arrangements, such as factor analysis. A structural representation of the individual's problem behaviour promotes questions about aetiology, potential for change, or comparison with 'normal' behaviour. Thus Button (1985) has illustrated how the personal meanings provided by anorexic patients help in understanding the development of their condition as well as offering potential therapeutic directions; similarly Ryle and Breen (1972a) demonstrated significant differences between the RG structures of 'normal' and 'neurotic' subjects. The latter tended to see themselves as deviant, very different from their parents and ideal selves, and to make polar judgements. The 'Resistance-to-Change' RG (Fransella & Bannister, 1977) directly assesses the constraints on change in an individual's conceptual structure, by indicating the implication for the total structure of the change of any single construct. This tradition has been expanded by interactive computer programs, such as PEGASUS (Thomas & Shaw, 1977), which permit immediate feedback and 'conversation' about the effects upon a construct system of potential changes—although this, strictly speaking, cannot be considered as naturalistic research.

A second strategy is to measure changes in structure over time. Most often this will be within a treatment context in which behavioural and conceptual change is being sought, but the methodology can also be employed to investigate more naturalistic changes occurring as a consequence of a significant experience such as learning or training. If a longer time-perspective is employed then investigations that may be viewed as more developmentally framed are possible, e.g. changes in self-identity perception by adolescents during their last 2 years at school. This strategy comes extremely close to the study of covariational change discussed in the previous section when talking of the PQ, and there is potential overlap. The crucial distinction is whether the investigation focusses upon changes in an overall structure, in which case it is rightfully included in this category, or merely the study of a small number of variables. However, this distinction may in some cases be somewhat arbitrary.

In their most complete form these methods assess the person upon multiple items in each of two dimensions (e.g. situations and persons) so that a matrix of correlations can be obtained. Factor analysis (or principal component analysis) of this matrix provides a hierarchical structure demonstrating dimensions that are more centrally important than others. The RG has already been cited as a good example of this approach, and it has fostered numerous relevant studies. Good reviews are provided by Slater (1976), Fransella and Bannister (1977), Beail (1985) and Button (1985). The Q-sort (Stephenson, 1953) can also be included in this category, but would be seen as an inferior method as only two items are considered (self and ideal self) and the dimensions are supplied rather than elicited. The methodology is rarely used today, although Rogers' early research using the Q-sort to study psychotherapy process and outcome was seminal, particularly the confirmation of his hypotheses that clients' self-esteem would increase during successful therapy and that they would come to see themselves in a more 'adjusted' manner (Rogers & Dymond, 1954; Rogers, 1961).

Whereas both the RG and Q-sort are person-centred techniques, structural methodologies using observational data are also possible, although they are rarely employed. The essential requirement would be the development of a matrix of multiple ratings of behaviour in multiple situations. Various aspects of skilled behaviour would seem a good potential area. A person's social skills could be rated upon multiple aspects in multiple situations; or in a rehabilitation context components of work performance could be appraised under various conditions. Analysis of the data matrix might illustrate, for example, that some social skills cluster around an anxiety component and others around an intimacy component, whereas work performance clusters around speed and precision components.

These research strategies provide both conceptual and practical methodological issues. At the practical level it is vital that there is adequate sampling of the relevant domain comprising the matrix, otherwise the findings will be too narrowly based and not representative and generalisable (e.g. a study of a person's 'social world' will consist solely of friends and liked people, with a complete absence of disliked people or those viewed ambivalently). Thus it is necessary to ensure a sufficient number and range of elements and constructs. Consideration must be paid to the relative merits of elicited and supplied constructs, and to the statistical assumptions of the rating procedures employed, particularly in terms of the distribution of the scores and scales of measurement. This is particularly salient if factor-analytic procedures are to be employed as their statistical assumptions must not be breached. The RG literature contains a number of good discussions on these issues (Slater, 1976, 1977; Fransella & Bannister, 1977; Beail, 1985). If observational data are utilised, decisions must be made concerning the number of observers used, the criteria for ratings and the effect upon the subject of being rated (reactivity).

At the conceptual level the central issue for self-report methodologies is to demonstrate a clear link between the conceptual structure derived and the person's actual behaviour. Can the relevant behaviour be understood? Can it be predicted? Often these questions fail to be adequately answered. Observational methodologies suffer the converse difficulties. Although they can predict behavioural performance they largely fail to elucidate the role of the person's perception of the situation.

4. Interaction and Interexperience

This last research strategy focuses upon the interpersonal context by investigating the mutual interaction or interexperience of the participants. The element of mutuality differentiates it from those discussed in (1) and (2). Usually studies focus on the dyadic situation but this is not essential, and increased interest in family interaction and therapy has fostered studies of the triadic context (e.g. Scott, Ashworth & Casson, 1970). Furthermore a number of studies of group interaction have consistently been reported over the years (e.g. Smail, 1972; Winter & Trippett, 1977). Methodologies can employ either self-report or observational measures, although the former has been most commonly used; there is an increasing trend for individual studies to employ both.

Phenomenologically based methodologies, using self-report techniques, most commonly aim to explicate areas of match and mis-match in the participants' joint construction of the world, and to try to correlate this with aspects of their interaction—usually problems. Essentially this represents a translation of an intrapersonal method, designed for the study of the individual, to the interpersonal context by the comparison of two (or more) individual perspectives. Two good examples of this strategy are Ryle's extension of the RG technique, the Double Dyad Grid (see Ryle, 1985, for a good review), and the interpersonal perception approach discussed below. The elements of the Dyad Grid are relationships rather than people, as in the traditional RG; the Double Dyad Grid requires both partners in a relationship to complete a Dyad Grid independently and these are then compared. Ryle and Breen (1972b) provide an example of the method's use in marital therapy, identifying shared, but problematic, perceptions and projections of the couple.

A slightly different research focus is to investigate the extent to which one member can predict the views or psychological framework of the other. This is often used as an operational definition of empathy and is commonly employed in studies of therapist/client relationship (e.g. Rowe, 1971; Ryle & Lunghi, 1971; Shapiro & Post, 1974) or marital satisfaction (e.g. Dymond, 1954; Torpy & Measey, 1974; Allen & Thompson, 1984). Rowe (1971) and Ryle and Lunghi (1971), using the RG method, reported that therapists had appreciable insight into their clients' construct systems (correlations between therapist's prediction of client's RG and client's actual RG were 0.32 and 0.50 respectively) but, perhaps more importantly, also identified crucial and systematic misperceptions highly relevant to the therapeutic relationship. Shapiro and Post (1974) found that the major discrepancy between a psychiatrist and patient on PQ ratings was related to the severity with which the symptoms were experienced by the patient, rather than the psychiatrist misunderstanding which symptoms were present. Torpy and Measey (1974), in a study of marriages in which one member was agoraphobic, found a strong correlation between marital satisfaction and accurate prediction of the partner's views, a link commonly found in such studies.

The 'interpersonal perception' approach has typically combined the two preceding strategies by investigating both perceptual match ('agreement') and predictions of partner's views. A spiraliform model is conceptualised in which levels of perception exist, each at a higher level than its predecessor. Although logically there is no limit to the spiral, in practice no methodology considers beyond the third level and some only consider the first two. The dyad A and B, from A's point of view, will have three levels of perspective—the direct perspective (A's view of X (A-X)), the metaperspective (A's view of B's view of X (A-B-X)), and metametaperspective (A-B-A-X)). Comparison of the direct perspectives of A and B will indicate their agreement (A-X/B-X). Accurate metaperception (A-B-X/B-X) indicates A's understanding of B, whilst accurate usage of the metametaperspective (A-B-A-X/B-A-X), usually termed realisation, indicates A's ability to predict whether B understands A or not. Further intrapersonal measures reflecting perceived agreement and feeling understood are also possible, and Alperson (1975) provides a useful mathematical synthesis and description of this general approach.

The best known, and most influential example of this methodology is the Interpersonal Perception Method (IPM) developed by Laing, Phillipson and Lee (1966) within an object–relations framework. Each partner answers 60 descriptions of key relationship issues using three levels of perception, and the dyad is scored in terms of both overall perceptual accuracy and the spirals of agreement, understanding and realisation about each particular issue. In an IPM comparison of disturbed and non-disturbed marriages, Laing *et al.* found the latter to have significantly more accurate perceptions at all perceptual levels. The same study also illustrated the use of the IPM in an intensive case study of marital therapy. A related, but inferior, approach is the Interpersonal Perception Technique (IPT) of Drewerey (1969), which in one study indicated that male alcoholic patients were confused about their marital roles and dependency needs (Rae & Drewerey 1972). Scott, Ashworth & Casson (1970) extended the methodology to the triadic situation with their Family Relations Test (FRT) in their study of families with a schizophrenic child. The patient, their father and mother each made five ratings—their view of themselves, the other two, how the other two see them. The FRT illustrated that families which experienced frequent conflict and hospital admission were characterised by role-conflict, particularly in that the patient saw the parents as being as 'ill' as themselves, thereby apparently invalidating their long-term position at home.

Very few studies have employed these methods to assess change over time, yet the potential is vast. Laing *et al.* (1966) used the IPM to investigate marital therapy and Alexander (1981) used a development of this approach to study changes in the client/therapist relationship during psychotherapy, but considerable scope exists for other extensions. Furthermore, the developments started by the FRT can be extended to the four-person situation and beyond, with implications for the study of family and group interaction. The relatively few studies of changes in group perceptions over time have been within the RG tradition and have demonstrated interesting findings related to group processes worth developing (e.g. Fransella & Joyston-Bechal, 1971; Winter & Trippett, 1977).

Methodologies employing observational measures study the relationship between the behaviour of two (or more) people. The intention is to identify patterns of behaviour and thus deduce causal relationships. For example, in a married couple some behaviours may be positively correlated over time (i.e. behaviour A provokes behaviour B) and others negatively correlated (i.e. turn-taking occurs). Measurement issues concern the definition of the appropriate unit of behaviour and its operational description, together with considerations about the length of time for which subjects should be observed and the effects of being observed (reactivity).

AN EXAMPLE OF INTENSIVE RESEARCH

This final section will look in some detail at the work of Elliott, as it provides a good example of sophisticated intensive research methodology and is fertile ground for further conceptual and practical development. Elliott has been concerned with the investigation of the process of change in psychotherapy and has developed his 'discovery oriented approach' to significant change events. This rests on four key assumptions:

1. Psychotherapy process research should begin with the experiences and perceptions of client and therapist.
2. Phenomenological data should be anchored to specific behavioural events.
3. Psychotherapy research should focus upon significant change events.
4. Since significant events are both infrequent and highly complex they should be studied closely and comprehensively (Elliott, 1984, pp. 250–252).

Thus Elliott's research strategy is essentially to identify significant change moments/events in therapy and to link these with the participants' subjective experience, especially the therapist's intention and the effect ('impact') of the therapist's behaviour on the client. Although significant events can be defined by observational measures (change of posture or voice tone, crying, etc.) Elliott has taken them to be those responses reported by the client to be especially positive or negative (see below). This latter perspective is most in tune with the philosophy of the methodology, in that the participants define the key concerns.

Elliott has developed a number of interesting research methods, which are being increasingly combined to provide a comprehensive description of change processes. One intention of this research programme is to be able to suggest therapist intervention tactics that will promote beneficial changes. Interpersonal Process Recall (IPR) was originated by Kagan but developed extensively by Elliott (1984, 1986). A good introduction to the method is provided by Barker (1985). The essence of IPR is that a videotape of the therapy session is replayed to client and therapist separately in the presence of a trained 'inquirer', to whom they are encouraged to recall their moment-by-moment experience during the session by using the videotape as a cueing device. They can stop the tape whenever they wish and are encouraged to talk about their feelings and thoughts at that moment and their reaction to the other person's behaviour in the therapy session. This is the essence of the 'event-based phenomenological' approach, and may be an attractive method to many investigators because it mirrors the reality of clinical work. IPR can be used non-directively, by allowing the person to stop the tape whenever they wish to explore a personal concern, and this would be especially appropriate for clinical supervision, which is where the method originated. Alternatively IPR can be used in a more systematic manner as a research tool by sampling segments of client/therapist interaction at specific time points during therapy sessions. This is how Elliott has employed the technique, particularly in studying the intentions behind the therapist's responses and the impact felt by the client in terms of both empathy and helpfulness (Elliott, 1979).

Elliott (1984) went on to develop Comprehensive Process Analysis (CPA) as 'a procedure for describing significant change events systematically on a battery of process measures' (p. 254). This is a content analysis in which a transcript of a significant event identified by IPR is categorised on multiple quantitative and qualitative measures assessing five aspects of the therapeutic process (content, action, style, state–experience and quality). Both client and therapist behaviour is considered and ratings are made by client, therapist and observer. Finally all the measures are integrated in the form of a narrative or comparative analysis across cases. Elliott (1984) illustrates the use of this approach with four different case examples.

The Therapeutic Impact Content Analysis System (TICAS) is an extension of this method (Elliott et al., 1985). By using IPR the client identifies and describes in detail the most helpful and most hindering therapist interventions, which then receive content analysis. Elliott et al. employed 14 categories, derived from pilot data, and proposed these as a good eclectic framework for analysing change processes. They reflect many familiar theoretical constructs (e.g. 'negative therapist reaction'–countertransference; 'understanding'–empathy). In their study TICAS data were used with two different research strategies. The first compared client responses to different therapeutic approaches, and it was found that the dynamic therapy they studied evoked responses of insight and awareness, whereas with cognitive therapy reassurance and insight were most common. The second strategy correlated client response with specific therapist behaviour, by rating the latter on six modes derived from the CPA (question, advisement, reflection, interpretation, reassurance and self-disclosure). Two general findings emerged: (1) that therapist questions did not help the client feel understood; and (2) therapist self-disclosure enhanced client trust. However, these findings should be seen largely within the context of this particular study and not as being highly generalisable.

Elliott's studies appear to have produced interesting findings and offer considerable potential, both in terms of increasing our knowledge of psychotherapy processes and as a methodological model. One exciting aspect of this research method is the potential it offers for fine-grained microanalysis of different processes and sequences of client change. In particular, it offers the prospect of investigating a stage further back in the chain of interaction. Thus, can we identify the client behaviours that 'trigger' the therapist behaviours which the client perceives as being helpful or insight-promoting? Future research is likely to focus upon this issue. However, this will only be addressed more clearly once the assessment procedures become more structured and less time consuming. A final consideration concerns the reliability and validity of the methods discussed. Some attention has been paid to the reliability and validity of IPR. Barker (1985) raises issues about potential threats to validity arising from forgetting, lack of expressive skills, social desirability and fabrication but considers that overall the IPR has support. Elliot (1986) has reviewed the IPR literature and found evidence for good internal and temporal validity. However, the approach is still in its infancy and will require further sober investigation and consideration of its psychometric properties, and this is also true for the content analyses that have been developed.

SUMMARY

Intensive methodologies offer exciting opportunities to understand people in depth by the use of rigorous, yet sensitive, naturalistic research methods. Increasing research interest is being shown in the processes occurring during psychotherapy (Rice & Greenberg, 1984) and it is hoped that important gains will be made in the near future on the foundations presently established. A particularly fertile area appears to be the microanalysis and description of the chain of interaction between the responses of client and therapist. Methods that combine observational and self-report measures, in the manner of Elliott's (1984) 'event-based phenomenology', and which investigate 'significant events' may represent one of the best ways of approach at the present time. However, intensive research should not be solely concerned with the topic of psychotherapy and potential exists in many other areas. Two good candidates are rehabilitation and the investigation of organisational structure and change.

Hopefully, the four typologies detailed above have helped to clarify the central methodological issues in intensive research and that this will foster future empirical studies. There are undoubtedly alternative ways in which to conceptualise intensive research (e.g. methodologies employing observational versus self-report measures), but the typology presented appeared to be the most useful. It is important to separate issues concerning research strategy from the more tactical concerns in the precise methods used in the research study, although clearly the two levels influence each other. However, the influence should, in the main, be from the strategic down to the tactical. The typologies presented have tried to focus upon this strategic level to illustrate central constraints and to indicate some areas for future development.

REFERENCES

Alexander, P. T. (1981). *Cognitive Processes in Dyadic Therapy: Client and Therapist Negotiation about the Construction of Reality.* Unpublished PhD Thesis, University of Bristol.

Allen, A. & Thompson, T. (1984). Agreement, understanding, realisation and feeling understood as predictors of communicative satisfaction in marital dyads. *Journal of Marriage and the Family*, **46**, 915–921.

Alperson, B. L. (1975). In search of Buber's Ghosts: A calculus for interpersonal phenomenology. *Behavioral Science*, **20**, 179–190.

Bakeman, R. & Gottman, J. M. (1986). *Observing Interaction. An Introduction to Sequential Analysis.* Cambridge University Press.

Barker, C. B. (1985). Interpersonal process recall in clinical training and research. In F. N. Watts (ed.) *New Developments in Clinical Psychology.* London: Wiley.

Bateson, P. P. G. & Hinde, R. A. (eds) (1976). *Growing Points in Ethology.* London: Cambridge University Press.

Beail, N. (ed.) (1985). *Repertory Grid Technique and Personal Constructs* London: Croom Helm.

Button, E. (ed.) (1985). *Personal Construct Theory and Mental Health.* London: Croom Helm.

Carr, E. G. & Newsom, C. (1985). Demand-related tantrums. Conceptualisation and treatment. *Behaviour Modification*, **9**, 403–426.

Chassan, J. B. (1979). *Research Design in Clinical Psychology and Psychiatry*, 2nd edn. New York: Irvington.

Ciminero, A. R., Nelson, R. & Lipinski, D. P. (eds) (1977). *Handbook of Behavioral Assessment.* New York: John Wiley & Sons.

Coates, T. J. & Thoresen, C. E. (1978). Using generalizability theory in behavioral observation. *Behavior Therapy*, **9**, 605–613.

Craighead, W. E., Kazdin, A. E. & Mahoney, M. J. (1981). *Behavior Modification: Principles, Issues and Applications*, 2nd edn. Boston: Houghton Miflin.

Drewerey, J. (1969). An interpersonal perception technique. *British Journal of Medical Psychology*, **42**, 171–181.

Dymond, R. F. (1954). Interpersonal perception and marital happiness. *Canadian Journal of Psychology*, **8**, 164–171.

Elliott, R. (1979). How clients perceive helper behaviors. *Journal of Counseling Psychology*, **26**, 285–294.

Elliott, R. (1984). A discovery-oriented approach to significant change events in psychotherapy: interpersonal process recall and comprehensive process analysis. In L. N. Rice and L. S. Greenberg (eds) *Patterns of Change; Intensive Analysis of Psychotherapy Process.* London: Guildford.

Elliott, R. (1986). Interpersonal Process Recall (IPR) as a process research method. In L. Greenberg and W. Pinsof (eds) (1986). *The Psychotherapeutic Process: A Research Handbook.* New York: Guildford.

Elliott, R., James, E., Reimschuessel, C., Cislo, D., & Sack N. (1985). Significant events and the analysis of immediate therapeutic impact. *Psychotherapy*, **22**, 620–630.

Esser, A. H. (1968). Interactional hierarchy and power structure on a psychiatric ward. In S. J. Hutt and C. Hutt (eds). *Behaviour Studies in Psychiatry*. Oxford: Pergamon.

Everitt, B. S. & Dunn, G. (1983). Advanced methods of data exploration and modelling. London: Heinemann.

Fransella, F. & Bannister, D. (1977). *A Manual for Repertory Grid Technique*. London: Academic Press.

Fransella, F. & Joyston-Bechal, M. P. (1971). An investigation of conceptual process and pattern change in a psychotherapy group. *British Journal of Psychiatry*, **119**, 199–206.

Garety, P. (1985). Delusions: problems in definition and measurement. *British Journal of Medical Psychology*, **58**, 25–34.

Gershon, E. S., Cromer, M. & Klerman, G. L. (1968). Hostility and depression. *Psychiatry*, **31**, 224–235.

Grant, I., Yager, J., Sweetwood, H. L., & Olshen, R. (1982). Life events and symptoms. Fourier analysis of time series from a three-year prospective inquiry. *Archives of General Psychiatry*, **39**, 598–605.

Greenberg, L. & Pinsof, W. (eds) (1986). *The Psychotherapeutic Process: A Research Handbook*. New York: Guildford.

Hersen, M. & Bellack, A. S. (1976). *Behavioral Assessment; A Practical Handbook*. New York: Pergamon.

Hobson, R. F. & Shapiro, D. A. (1970). The personal questionnaire as a method of assessing change during psychotherapy. *British Journal of Psychiatry*, **117**, 623–626.

Kelly, G. A. (1955). *The Psychology of Personal Constructs* vols 1 and 2. New York: Norton.

Laing, R. D., Phillipson, H. & Lee, A. R. (1966). *Interpersonal Perception*. London: Tavistock.

Levy, P. (1974). Generalizability studies in clinical settings. *British Journal of Social and Clinical Psychology*, **13**, 161–172.

Lipinski, D. & Nelson, R. O. (1974). Problems in the use of naturalistic observation as a means of behavioral assessment. *Behavior Therapy*, **5**, 341–351.

Martin, P. & Bateson, P. (1986). *Measuring Behaviour: An Introductory Guide*. Cambridge University Press.

Metcalfe, M. (1956). Demonstration of a psychosomatic relationship. *British Journal of Medical Psychology*, **29**, 63–66.

Nelson, R. O. (1981). Realistic dependent measures for clinical use. *Journal of Consulting & Clinical Psychology*, **49**. 168–182.

Parry, G., Shapiro, D. A. & Firth, J. (1986). The case of the anxious executive: a study from the research clinic. *British Journal of Medical Psychology*, **59**, 221–233.

Phillips, J. P. N. (1977). Generalised personal questionnaire techniques. In P. Slater (ed.) *The Measurement of Intrapersonal Space by Grid Technique. Vol. 2. Dimensions of Intrapersonal Space*. London: Wiley.

Rae, J. & Drewerey, J. (1972). Interpersonal patterns in alcoholic marriages. *British Journal of Psychiatry*, **120**, 615–621.

Rice, L. N. & Greenberg, L. S. (eds) (1984). *Patterns of Change; Intensive Analysis of Psychotherapy Process*. London: Guildford.

Rogers, C. R. (1961). *On Becoming a Person*. London: Constable.

Rogers, C. R. & Dymond, R. F. (1954). *Psychotherapy and Personality Change*. Chicago University Press.

Rowe, D. (1971). An examination of a psychiatrist's predictions of a patient's constructs. *British Journal of Psychiatry*, **118**, 231–244.

Ryle, A. R. (1985). The dyad grid and psychotherapy research. In N. Beail (ed.) *Repertory Grid Technique and Personal Constructs*. London; Croom Helm.

Ryle, A. R. & Breen, D. (1972a). Some differences in the personal constructs of neurotic and normal subjects. *British Journal of Psychiatry*, **120**, 483–489.

Ryle, A. R. & Breen, D. (1972b). The use of the double dyad grid in the clinical setting. *British Journal of Medical Psychology*, **45**, 383–389.

Ryle, A. R. & Lunghi, M. (1971). A Therapist's predition of a patient's dyad grid. *British Journal of Psychiatry*, **118**, 555–560.

Scott, R. D., Ashworth, P. L. & Casson, P. D. (1970). Violation of parental role structure and outcome in schizophrenia. *Social Science & Medicine*, **4**, 41–64.

Shapiro, D. A. & Hobson, R. F. (1972). Change in psychotherapy: a single case study. *Psychological Medicine*, **2**, 312–317.

Shapiro, D. A., Caplan, H. L., Rohde, P. D. & Watson, J. P. (1975). Personal Questionnaire changes and their correlates in a psychotherapy group. *British Journal of Medical Psychology*, **48**, 207–215.

Shapiro, M. B. (1961). A method of measuring changes specific to the individual psychiatric patient. *British Journal of Medical Psychology*, **34**, 151–155.

Shapiro, M. B. (1969). Short-term improvements in the symptoms of affective disorder. *British Journal of Social and Clinical Psychology*, **8**, 187–188.

Shapiro, M. B. & Post, F. (1974). Comparison of self-ratings of psychiatric patients with ratings made by a psychiatrist. *British Journal of Psychiatry*, **125**, 36–41.

Slater, P. (ed.) (1976). *The Measurement of Intrapersonal Space by Grid Technique. Vol. 1. Explorations of Intrapersonal Space*. London: Wiley.

Slater, P. (ed.) (1977). *The Measurement of intrapersonal Space by Grid Technique. Vol. 2. Dimensions of Intrapersonal Space*. London: Wiley.

Smail, D. J. (1972). A grid measure of empathy in a therapeutic group. *British Journal of Medical Psychology*, **45**, 165–169.

Snowdon, C. T. (1983). Ethology, comparative psychology and animal behaviour. *Annual Review of Psychology*, **34**, 63–94.

Spence, S. & Shepherd, G. (1983). *Developments in Social Skills Training*. London: Academic Press.

Stephenson, W. (1953). *The Study of Behaviour: Q-Technique and its Methodology*. University of Chicago Press.

Thomas, L. F. & Shaw, M. L. G. (1977). *PEGASUS Manual*. Brunel University, Centre for the Study of Human Learning.

Torpy, D. & Measey, L. G. (1974). Marital interaction in agoraphobia. *Journal of Clinical Psychology*, **30**, 351–354.

Winter, D. A. & Trippett, C. J. (1977). Serial change in group psychotherapy. *British Journal of Medical Psychology*, **50**, 341–347.

14 Epidemiological and Survey Methods

David J. Cooke
Douglas Inch Centre, 2 Woodside Terrace, Glasgow G3 7UY.

Epidemiological methods are, by necessity, different from those adopted in the confines of the laboratory or in carefully controlled clinical trials. Epidemiological data are dirty; samples are rarely complete, independent variables are difficult to control, confounding factors may abound.

The principles and methods of epidemiology are wide ranging yet this chapter must be brief. Because of this constraint, this chapter will only provide a glimpse of some of the basic concepts, the basic techniques, and indeed, some of the basic problems in epidemiology.

Five facets of epidemiology will be considered. Firstly, what is epidemiology and what value and relevance does it have for the research-minded clinician? Secondly, what experimental designs can be applied in epidemiological research? Thirdly, how are suitable measures chosen or developed? Fourthly, having obtained results, how can they be analysed to the greatest effect? Fifthly, what practical problems might be encountered in carrying out epidemiological research and how might these problems be resolved?

WHAT IS EPIDEMIOLOGY?

A good place to begin is to consider the question, what is epidemiology? Leighton (1979, p. 235), perhaps the doyen of psychiatric epidemiology, described it as follows: 'Epidemiology is not only concerned with population rates of illness, but also with detecting factors which are associated with their origin, course and outcome.'

287

On the most basic level epidemiology is concerned with questions such as how many cases of senile dementia are there in the general population, or how many new cases of depression occur each year? Thus, epidemiology is about detecting and counting cases of disorder or illness.

Leighton's quote indicates that epidemiology goes beyond these simple counting activities. Epidemiologists are concerned with aetiological factors and factors that may ameliorate conditions. Thus epidemiologists will ask questions such as do life events cause depression, do social support networks protect individuals from the effects of stress, does the diet contribute to coronary heart disease and will exercise provide protection against coronary heart disease?

It is thus clear that epidemiology is a broad subject which deals not only with the distribution of illness but also with the causes of illness.

WHY IS EPIDEMIOLOGY IMPORTANT?

Why should the topic be of interest to those working in the field of mental health? There are three important reasons; the first relates to service planning, the second and third relate to our understanding of disorders.

The planning of health services is facilitated by estimating the level of need and demand. The case identification and counting functions of epidemiology can provide the necessary estimates. For example, in the Isle of Wight study neuropsychiatric disorders were studied amongst 2000 school age children (Rutter *et al.*, 1970). Over 6% of the children were found to require treatment or advice, and indeed, 2% were identified as suffering from severe psychiatric disturbance. Only 0.7% of the sample were receiving formal treatment or advice and, therefore, the health care services were providing support for only 10% of the cases of need.

Epidemiological research may not only describe the overall level of need but also it may identify those in greatest need. The work of Brown & Harris (1978a), for example, suggested that the risk of depression is highest amongst working-class women with young children. It could be argued that in times of limited resources, those resources that are available should be mobilised to assist this group.

Thus in prinicple epidemiological information should be of value to health care planners; unfortunately, in practice little of this information is used. Kreitman (1980, p. 41) described the reality with force: 'The policies advanced by the Department of Health and Social Security and the Scottish Home and Health Departments emerge as pronouncements which scorn the aid of data.'

The second reason to carry out epidemiological research relates to improving our understanding of disease and disorder. Patients studied in hospital and clinics may not make the best subjects. Shepherd, Cooper,

Brown and Kalton (1966) showed that only 5% of GP patients with 'conspicuous psychiatric morbidity' were referred for psychiatric consultation. Not only do such patients comprise a small proportion of all those who are disordered or disturbed, but also, they are non-representative. Fahy (1974a, b, 1975) in a series of studies, demonstrated that powerful selective factors operate. For example, of individuals with the same moderate degree of depression, men were much more likely to be referred to a psychiatrist than women.

Goldberg and Huxley (1980) argued that community cases have to pass through four filters before they receive psychiatric in-patient care (Fig. 14.1).

A variety of factors influence transition through each filter; few of these factors are related to symptomatology. Goldberg and Huxley (1980) indicated that referral from the primary care level to the psychiatric services is influenced by the GP's confidence in managing psychiatric problems, his attitude towards psychiatrists, the quality and availability of psychiatric services, the attitude of the patient and his family towards receiving psychiatric care as well as the presenting symptoms. Thus psychiatric patients are not representative of all those who are disordered: they are the small proportion who have elected or have been selected to become patients. Goldberg and Huxley (1980) argued that of every 250 community cases only six receive psychiatric in-patient care.

This is important because aetiological arguments based on such subjects can be misleading: Ingham and Miller (1976) argued that mythologies have developed about the causes of physical disease when only patients are studied. For example, epidemiological studies of iron deficiency and anaemia demonstrated the lack of a clear association whereas studies of patients had suggested its presence. Epidemiological studies have the advantage of having greater generality.

What other advantages accrue from the study on non-biased samples? Leighton (1979, p. 237) argued that 'Data generated from people in their natural habitat often contains much that is not found in clinics.' Epidemiologists who study people in their natural habitat may detect new types or new syndromes of disturbance. A community study of depression in Glasgow yeilded four types of depression which, while showing certain similarities to psychiatric types of depression, also showed marked differences (Cooke, 1980a).

More importantly, if we study people in their natural habitat, then it may be possible to clarify the association between disturbance and other factors and, indeed, between disturbance and potential aetiological factors. Paykel et al. (1969) demonstrated that 'undesirable' events and 'exit' events had a more powerful impact on depression than did events in general. Bebbington, Tennant and Hurry (1981) and Cooke (1981) have

FIG. 14.1.   Factors affecting the selection and detection of psychiatric cases. (After Goldberg & Huxley, 1980.)

demonstrated, in community studies, that life events are associated with neurotic depression but not associated with other forms of depression. Thus the associations between potential causes (e.g. life events) and particular disorders (i.e. neurotic depression) can be clarified using unbiased samples.

My third and final plea in favour of epidemiological studies is that it may be valuable to study people who are not ill or not disturbed. Psychologists are trained to study all forms of behaviour, not just disturbed behaviour. If we base our theories and procedures merely on those who are suffering from psychological disturbance or maladaptive behaviour, we will be less able to identify or evaluate those psychological mechanisms that may lead to the amelioration of problems. It has been argued that an expert on drowning may not be the best person to teach someone to swim. By studying people with no apparent mental illness or behavioural disturbance it may be possible to specify which aspects of their social support network, their lifestyle or their habitual cognitive processes lead them to avoid such difficulties. The above discussion has described what epidemiology is and why it should be of interest to the clinician. Some of the methods used will now be examined.

THE DESIGN OF EPIDEMIOLOGICAL STUDIES

Epidemiological studies are designed to count cases of disorder but, more importantly, they are designed to assess associations between risk factors and disorders. How can these associations be determined? Studies are often classified by the manner in which subjects are selected—for example, case–control studies versus cohorts studies—and in terms of the time period considered, for example, retrospective studies, prospective studies and cross-sectional studies. Inferences regarding the association between risk factors and disorder are tied to these two dimensions of design.

Case–Control Studies Versus Cohort Studies

In case–control studies, perhaps more correctly, case–comparison studies, the cases' exposure to risk is compared with that of the controls. In a case–control study the investigator may select cases from one of a variety of sources, from cases diagnosed in the community, from cases diagnosed in a hospital or cases referred to a particular clinic. Controls may be obtained from one or more sources including non-cases from a community sample, patients in hospital who do not have the disorder or any related disorder, or relatives or associates of the cases. Case–control studies are cheaper and less difficult to carry out than cohort studies. Unfortunately, the fundamental problem underlying case–control methodology is that it is not possible to determine what proportion of the total population is represented by either the cases or the controls. Thus the relative frequency of exposure amongst the cases and the controls is not necessarily the same as that in the population of origin.

This is not a problem in cohort studies as the relative frequency of exposure is known. Cohort studies are of two types. In the first type, subjects are grouped in terms of whether they have been exposed to the putative cause. The relative frequency of cases in those exposed, as compared with those who were not exposed, is determined. In the second type, a representative sample of a population is obtained and the subjects are divided into cases and non-cases using standardised techniques.

In both types of cohort design it is possible to determine what proportion of the total population is represented by the cases and the controls: thus it is possible to determine accurately the importance of any risk factor.

Firmer conclusions can be made about the relationship between exposure and a disorder using a cohort design as compared with a case–control design. Cohort studies are frequently used to increase the accuracy of findings obtained with case–control studies. As an example of this process, MacMahon and Pugh (1970) indicated that, in the research on smoking and lung cancer, some fifteen case–control studies were published before the first cohort study became available. Unfortunately, when the frequency of a disorder is low, very large cohorts are required if stable estimates of the rate of a disorder and its association with risk factors are to be obtained.

Retrospective, Prospective and Cross-sectional Studies

Time is the second dimension used to describe common epidemiological designs. Designs are either retrospective, prospective or cross-sectional in form.

In retrospective studies the investigator looks back from apparent effects at preceding causes. In studies of depression the investigator may look at life events or social support over the previous 12 months (e.g. Brown & Harris, 1978a; Miller & Ingham, 1979), in physical diseases, such as lung cancer, smoking habits over 20 years may be assessed (Doll & Hill, 1952).

In prospective studies the investigator identifies putative causes at one time point and follows the subjects to determine who becomes disordered and who does not. In addition, recovery can be examined. With depression this time interval may be 12 months or more (Brown, Craig & Harris, 1985; Surtees, Sashidharan & Dean, 1986). With physical disorders, such as lung cancer, the time period may be 20 years or more (Doll & Peto, 1976).

In cross-sectional studies, the investigator measures cause and effect occurring at the same point of time.

These different designs have their own particular advantages and disadvantages. These are outlined in Table 14.1

TABLE 14.1
Advantages and disadvantages of three common epidemiological designs

Type of study	Advantages	Disadvantages
Retrospective	1. Cost comparatively low 2. Results are obtained quickly 3. Efficient when considering rare diseases 4. Small samples are required	1. Estimates of risk less accurate 2. Recall may cause distortion
Prospective	1. Less bias—information is recorded before outcome is known 2. Efficient when considering rare risk factors 3. Multiple outcomes can be studied	1. Cost comparatively high—large samples observed over long periods 2. Delay between selection of subjects and the development of disorder 3. Inefficient when considering rare diseases 4. Periodic examination of subject may influence outcome
Cross-sectional	1. Low cost 2. Results are obtained quickly 3. Useful in studies of sub-clinical conditions where records are unlikely to exist	1. Estimates of risk less accurate 2. Cannot be used to establish the time sequence between putative cause and effect

The major advantages of a retrospective study are that they are relatively cheap to carry out because comparatively small numbers of subjects are interviewed on only one occasion. This has the concomitant advantage that results are obtained quickly. Retrospective studies are most efficient when used to study rare disorders because it is possible to compare all cases of the rare disorder with suitable controls. However, there are disadvantages with this type of study. Estimates of risk are less accurate. Also, when dealing with subject recall there may be significant distortion of recall through the active re-organisation of memory (Bartlett, 1932). Where medical records are used, there are problems of inaccurate or incomplete recording.

The advantages of prospective studies mirror the disadvantages of retrospective studies. Information obtained in prospective studies is less likely to be biased because it is recorded before the investigator knows about the onset of the disorder. Prospective studies are particularly efficient when examining risk factors which are unusual in the population because all cases of exposure can be studied. Thus it would be an appropriate design for studying people exposed to high levels of radiation.

Despite these distinct advantages, prospective studies have distinct disadvantages. The cost is comparatively high because it is necessary to study large numbers of subjects over long periods of time. The very nature of the design results in there being a considerable delay in results becoming available because of the delay between the selection of subjects and the development of the disorder. Prospective studies are particularly inefficient when rare diseases are being considered because large samples are required if a sufficient number of cases is to be identified. This problem can be overcome by selecting a sample in which there is likely to be a high inception rate for new disorders. The study of Brown et al. (1985) is a good example of this approach. On the basis of their previous work, they decided to select a sample of working-class women with one child at home. By doing this they ensured a high inception rate of new disorders in the period under which the study was carried out. A final difficulty with prospective studies is that periodic examination of subjects may affect the outcome of the study. This is particularly true in studies of psychological disorders where investigators may adopt, or may be manoeuvred into, a counselling role.

The final type of study is the cross-sectional study. Cross-sectional studies have the distinct advantage that they are quick and relatively inexpensive to carry out. They are particularly useful when an investigator is taking a preliminary look at a problem or when he or she is investigating sub-clinical conditions where reliable records are unlikely to exist. Unfortunately, cross-sectional studies suffer from the significant disadvantage that they cannot be used to establish the temporal relationship between a putative cause and a putative effect. Thus they cannot be used to evaluate causal mechanisms. For example, an investigator may study the serum cholesterol levels of subjects with coronary heart disease and compare these levels with those obtained in subjects without coronary heart disease. In general, there would be an elevation in those with coronary heart disease. It is only possible, however, to make the causal inference that elevated serum cholesterol level leads to coronary heart disease when it is demonstrated that there is an increased rate of coronary heart disease in those people whose serum cholesterol level was elevated on a previous occasion. Cross-sectional studies, therefore, can only provide suggestive evidence. They are of little value in epidemiological research which attempts to make aetiological statements.

SELECTING MEASUREMENT PROCEDURES

The investigator has chosen a design to suit his or her purpose and resources. The next step is to decide how to measure the constructs that may be of importance.

Epidemiological measurement techniques have proliferated and developed in the last decade. It could be argued that concern with method has eclipsed concern for substantive results.

There are two broad options in the acquisition of a measuring instrument; the investigator can use an instrument that is already developed or can develop his or her own. The selection of an instrument 'off the shelf' has many advantages. It is efficient in terms of time and in terms of development costs. Developed instruments are generally buttressed by evidence of reliability and validity; the investigator can thus be more certain of his results. Results obtained with such an instrument are easier to communicate. This may have the concomitant and not inconsiderable advantage that editors are more likely to publish the findings of the study.

Instruments have been developed to measure a wide range of characteristics from psychiatric symptoms (e.g. PSE–Wing, Nixon, Mann & Leff, 1977) and social support (e.g. Henderson *et al.*, 1980), through life events (Brown & Harris, 1978a) and hassles (Dohrenwend & Shrout, 1985), to demographic factors (Atkinson, 1971), vulnerable self-esteem (Mollon & Parry, 1984) and coping behaviour (Miller *et al.*, 1985).

Developing an instrument has obvious attractions for the 'hero innovator', but in addition it may be necessary if suitable instruments are not available to tap the domains that are of interest in a particular study. Further, many of the standardised instruments are based on evidence obtained from psychiatric cases. As noted above, the form and nature of psychiatric disorder in the general population may well differ from that in the population in which the measures were originally developed.

In choosing between developing and selecting an instrument, the investigator has to make a series of decisions which relate to time, cost, validity and suitability of particular measures. Whatever strategy is adopted, there are certain features of instruments that are desirable in any epidemiological study: there are certain questions that the investigator should ask about all instruments.

Is the Instrument Reliable?

If an instrument is unreliable it cannot measure variation across subjects or variation within subjects across time. Error will swamp true scores or true changes. The acceptable level of reliability depends on the purpose of the research. In basic explorative research it is often wasteful to choose instruments or develop instruments with reliability beyond 0.80 (Nunnally, 1967). Very little attentuation of associations will occur at this level of reliability and to increase reliability beyond this may require very lengthy procedures.

How can reliability be best achieved? In general, with qualitative social psychological information such as life event schedules or social adjustment scales, interviews fare rather better than rating scales (Cooke, 1985). This is probably true for most domains of interst in psychological epidemiology. Yager, Grant, Sweetwood and Gerst (1981, p. 347) indicated why this

might be the case: 'Interviews are likely to increase the subject's motivation and involvement, clarifying ambiguous meaning of items and result in
more accurate time framing of event answers.' It was once thought that
self-report questionnaires were more 'scientific' because experimenter
effects were less likely. However, the advantages of interviews as outlined
by Yager *et al.* (1981) outweigh this disadvantage. If the researcher is
developing an instrument, interview schedules will probably give the most
reliable and valid information.

What is Being Measured?

This question underpins the problems of construct validity: that is, which
constructs are operationalised by our instruments? (Cook & Campbell,
1979). This is important for practical research and for theoretical understanding. From a practical point of view if constructs are clearly specified
then it is easier to communicate and discuss results. From a theoretical
point of view, clear constructs can enhance our understanding of processes.
These two points can be illustrated using the construct of 'depression'.

Weckowitz (1973) indicated that the term 'depression' can denote three
distinct constructs; a normal affective state, a symptom or a diagnostic
entity. Confusion arises if the construct of 'depression' is not clearly
specified. Miller and Ingham (1979) and Brown and Harris (1978a) examined the effects of life events on 'depression'. Miller and Ingham used
'depression' to describe depressed mood; Brown and Harris used 'depression' to describe a diagnostic entity that not only included depressed mood
but also a wide range of symptoms from irritability to retardation, diurnal
variation and weight loss. These investigators are talking about different
constructs, different processes and, indeed, different experiences. If we
wish to understand the processes or experiences we must be clear about
which construct is being used.

The problem of construct validity exists whether 'off the shelf' or
tailor-made instruments are used. Cook and Campbell (1979) argued that
there are two broad strategies that can be used to enhance construct
validity, namely, careful pre-experimental specification of constructs and
careful data analysis.

In the pre-experimental phase it is necessary to define what is and what is
not characteristic of each core construct. For example, it may be necessary
to distinguish among life events, social support, symptoms and personality
factors. If these distinctions are not made then spurious relationships may
arise because two apparently distinct measures are really measuring the
same construct. A concrete example may clarify this point. Weissman and
Paykel (1974) reported a significant relationship between social adjustment
and depression in depressed women. Examination of their social adjust-

ment scale reveals that many of the items relate to primary symptoms of depression: for example, guilt, worry, resentment, distress, and disinterest in sexual contact. Their social adjustment construct appears to be an amalgam of symptoms and social adjustment variables. Therefore, use of their instrument in an unmodified form obscures rather than clarifies the link between depression and social adjustment. How can construct validity be improved? Derogatis, Klerman and Lipman (1972) and Ni Bhrolchain (1979) argued that clarity is increased when constructs are defined in restrictive terms. Thus 'depression' is best defined in terms of signs and symptoms and not in terms of correlated, but conceptually distinct, features such as demographic, pesonality and social adjustment variables.

Even if each construct domain is described in clear and restrictive terms, several constructs may be necessary to describe any domain in a satisfactory manner. In the symptom domain there may be reactive and endogenous depression, social support may be instrumental or expressive, life events may be exits or entrances. Thus even with restricted definitions all these domains may still be too heterogenous. Fortunately, careful analysis can come to the rescue in this situation.

Techniques such as factor analysis, principal component analysis, latent trait analysis can be useful. These techniques specify constructs by grouping related items or symptoms and distinguishes these from unrelated items or symptoms. Thus domains of interest can be refined: symptoms can be amalgamated into discrete syndromes, different types of social support can be described. The value of these techniques will be described in more detail in the section on data analysis.

In selecting or in developing an instrument it is essential that the investigator is clear about which constructs are being measured by each instrument.

Categorical or Dimensional Measures?

A final and fundamental decision, perhaps dilemma, faced by the investigator is whether the disorder should be measured in terms of cases of disorder or in terms of the degree of the disorder; that is, as a category or as a dimension. This is partly an epistemological decision dependent on how the disorder is viewed; however, it is a decision that has practical implications. Traditionally, in psychiatric epidemiology, respondents have been divided into cases and non-cases: cases represent people with symptoms similar to patients observed in psychiatric clinics, all other people are non-cases. This approach has both advantages and disadvantages. On the positive side, measures of 'caseness' provide a metric which clinicians can use to understand the nature of the disorder being described, health administrators can use to estimate the number of people who require services and statisticians can use to calculate measures of incidence, prevalence and risk. Thus, caseness measures have practical value.

On the negative side, caseness measures are of less value when aetiological analysis is desired. There are three specific disadvantages. Firstly, caseness measures are generally developed on the small and biased group of individuals who squeeze through the four filters that separate the community from the psychiatric ward (see above). This has two consequences. The syndromes of the psychiatric ward may not exist in the community. In addition, the instruments, while being reliable for rating severe levels of symptomatology, may be less reliable at lesser intensities. If caseness measures are developed they must be developed for use with community cases.

Secondly, caseness measures are frequently dimensions of disorder that have been split arbitrarily into 'case' and 'non-case' levels. Brown, Ni Bhrolchain and Harris (1975, p. 229) confirmed that the division may be arbitrary: 'There is evidently an arbitrary element in choosing a cut off point between a case and a borderline (case).' In aetiological analysis this is important; the decision of 'what is a case?' can radically affect the putative relationship amongst risk factors and caseness. Patterns of results may change depending on the cut-off points selected (Cooke, 1980b).

Thirdly, dichotomising information into cases can result in a substantial loss of information. Statistical power suffers. Larger samples are required to demonstrate the same effect.

To summarise, the concept of a case has been described as '. . . a chimera existing only in the mind of the investigator' (Copland, 1981, p. 11). It is a chimera with practical value in the description of the rate of a disorder; it has less value for aetiological epidemiology.

In conclusion, decisions about which instruments should be used are complex. These decisions depend on the nature of the questions being asked and the availability of suitable measures.

ANALYSIS OF INFORMATION

The fieldwork is complete, the questionnaires are coded and the information is safely stored in the local computer. How should this information be analysed? Epidemiological information can be analysed in a variety of ways, from the simple to the complex. The mode of analysis adopted depends on the quality of the information available and the purpose of the study. We will start by looking at some simple descriptive statistics and move on to statistics that provide a more comprehensive insight into the information obtained.

Rates of Disorder

The counting of cases is the fundamental feature of descriptive epidemiology. The number of cases is most often expressed as a rate. The simple rate of a disorder can be defined as:

$$\frac{\text{Number of disorders in a specific period}}{\substack{\text{Population at risk of disorder} \\ \text{in a specific period}}} \times C$$

Where C typically equals 1000 or 100,000.

This simple rate provides a clear description of the probability of a disorder within this population during a specific time period. Normally, two different types of rates are used: rates of prevalence and rates of incidence.

Prevalence can be defined as the number of cases of a disorder during a period or interval divided by the total population. If the period is short (e.g. a day or a week) then the rate is described as point prevalence. If the period is longer, typically a year, then the rate is described as period prevalence. Thus, for example, an investigator may describe the number of cases of schizophrenia which may be observed in a year or the number of cases of depression observed during one week. Prevalence is a comparatively simple measure to derive because the investigator does not have to determine when the disorder started: identifying the start of a disorder can be difficult particularly with mild psychological difficulties (Cranach, Eberlein and Holl, 1981). Prevalence is an important measure as it can be of practical value in the planning of services and the level of manpower and workload. It is of less value in aetiological studies because the investigator has no information about the relationship between potential causes and the onset of the disorder.

By way of contrast, incidence rates are of value in aetiological epidemiology. A comparison of incidence rates across groups that have been differentially exposed to risk makes it possible to identify which risk factors are important. Incidence can be defined as:

$$\frac{\substack{\text{Number of new cases of a disorder} \\ \text{in a specific period}}}{\substack{\text{Population at risk over a period of} \\ \text{time}}} \times C$$

where C typically equals 1000 or 100,000.

The numerator is usually the number of people who have had a disorder, and thus this measure indicates the probability that an individual will get the disorder during a fixed period. With frequent or episodic disorders, such as depression or the common cold, the numerator may be the number of episodes of disorder. This measure of incidence will describe the average number of episodes of depression or the common cold experienced per head of population.

The denominator in the incidence equation may have to be adjusted or corrected. Generally, the denominator is the population at risk; however, with fairly frequent disorders, such as psychological disorders, cases of disorder should be excluded from the denominator. If this correction is not made then the precision of the estimate will be diminished.

Simple rates of prevalence and incidence are easy to calculate and they accurately summarise the findings of a particular study. They suffer from the significant disadvantage that they are influenced by the nature and structure of the population studied. With disorders, such as depression, which are firmly tied to demographic features such as age, sex and socio-economic status, crude rates of incidence or prevalence can distort or mislead. For example, the rate of depression is generally twice as high amongst women as amongst men (Weissman and Klerman, 1977). If the investigator compares crude incidence rates across two populations then the rates may differ merely because the ratio of males to females differs across the two populations. It is necessary, therefore, to move from crude rates to *specific* or *adjusted* rates.

Specific incidence or prevalence rates are those derived, not for the total population, but rather for some sub-group of the population. Typically specific rates are derived for different demographic groups such as young and old, males and females, and middle class and working class. Specific rates can be used to identify those at greatest risk; thus these specific rates can be of value both for the planning of services and for promoting the understanding of a disorder.

Adjusted rates are used to provide a summary of the information derived from one population to facilitate comparison of information derived from another population. These rates are adjusted or standardised to take account of the differences in the demographic structure of different populations. There are two broad approaches to the calculation of adjusted rates, the direct method and the indirect method. Using the direct method the sex-specific rates in the two populations to be compared are adjusted to a 'standard' population of known sex ratio. In the indirect method the sex specific rates of the smallest or most unstable population is adjusted to the larger, and usually more stable, population (see Mausner & Kramer, 1985, for technical details).

Rates provide a simple and valuable description of the distribution of disorders. While rates are of interest, epidemiologists are generally more interested in the nature and strength of the relationship between risk factors and disorders. Approaches to this problem will now be considered.

Relationships Between Risk and Disorder

How can the significance or importance of a particular risk factor be estimated? Many researchers are still content to report the statistical significance of results. It is a statistical cliche, yet a cliche worth repeating, that statistical significance tells us little about the size of an association. Hays (1963, p. 204) expressed this point clearly: 'Virtually any study can be made to show significant results if one uses enough subjects, regardless of how nonsensical the context may be.' If we depend on statistical significance we do not know if the effect of the risk factor is significant yet trivial; or, indeed, significant yet nonsensical.

Psychologists and other research workers have tried to measure importance using measures such as variance explained. This is a seductive approach: unfortunately, it has pitfalls. It is enlightening to consider what variance explained actually indicates and an example from the field of cancer epidemiology may provide the clearest idea of its applicability. Epidemiological evidence indicates that smoking has a powerful effect on the incidence of lung cancer. The variance explained in the incidence of lung cancer by cigarette smoking, in one major study, is only 0.003% (Doll & Peto, 1976). Thus one of the most accepted epidemiological findings does not look convincing if the variance explained statistic is used as a measure. This apparent anomaly arises because variance-explained measures the accuracy with which it can be predicted that an individual smoker will develop lung cancer, it does not measure the overall impact of smoking. Although few non-smokers develop lung cancer, it is also the case that most smokers do not develop the disease. This point may be clearer if it is illustrated graphically (Fig. 14.2).

By careful calculation two graphs of hypothetical research findings on the association between life events and symptoms have been derived, with the same slope but with different correlations. Thus the overall magnitude of the effect is the same, though the level of variance explained is very different in the two distributions. In one distribution we can accurately predict an individual's symptom score from his life event score, in the other case this can be done with much less accuracy. The proportion of total variance explained, therefore, is not a good measure of the importance of a risk factor.

If this measure is inadequate, what other measures can be used? Epidemiologists have a plethora of measures. Murphy (1983) listed nine measures including positive predictive value, prior odds of disease, spe-

FIG. 14.2. Hypothetical results showing two distributions with identical slopes but with different amounts of variance explained.

cificity and relative risk. Other epidemiological indices include attributable risk, attributable risk per cent and population attributable risk per cent.

Two of these measures, namely relative risk and population attributable risk per cent, are of particular value in the estimation of the importance of risk factors.

Relative risks can be defined as the ratio of the rate of disorder amongst those who have been exposed to a risk factor to the rate of disorder amongst those who have not been exposed (McMahon & Pugh, 1970). It can be calculated as shown in Table 14.2.

The concept underlying relative risk may be easier to grasp if we return to the example of smoking and lung cancer already used above. The rate of cases of lung cancer among those who smoke 20 cigarettes a day has been estimated to be 32 times the rate amongst non-smokers. The relative risk is thus 32. Therefore, if an individual smokes 20 cigarettes a day, on average, the risk of lung cancer is 32 times that of a non-smoker. A high relative risk tends to increase the plausibility of a causal hypothesis.

TABLE 14.2
Calculation of relative risk

		Case	Non-case
Exposure to risk factor	Yes	a	b
	No	c	d

Cohort studies

Relative risk $= \dfrac{a(c + d)}{c(a + b)}$

Case-control studies

Relative risk $= \dfrac{ad}{bc}$

Relative risk is a valuable measure for experts; however, it is of less value for the general clinician who merely requires some notion of the power of an effect. To interpret relative risk one really needs to know what is a 'big' relative risk and this depends on the disorder being studied and the base risk of the disorder. Despite this minor drawback relative risk can be of a considerable value in the interpretation of epidemiological information.

Population attributable risk per cent, by way of contrast, does provide an immediate sense of the importance of a risk factor. Population attributable risk per cent can be defined as the maximum proportion of cases of a disorder in the population as a whole that can be directly attributed to the experience of a risk factor. This index can be calculated as shown in Table 14.3.

TABLE 14.3
Calculation of population attributable risk per cent

		Case	Non-case
Exposure to risk factor	Yes	a	b
	No	c	d

Cohort studies

$\text{PAR\%} = \dfrac{ad - bc}{(a + c)(c + d)} \cdot 100$

Case-control studies

$\text{PAR\%} = \dfrac{ad - bc}{(a + c)d} \cdot 100$

The value of this measure can be illustrated by returning to the example of smoking and lung cancer. It has been estimated that up to 86% of the deaths through lung cancer can be attributed to smoking (Doll & Peto, 1976). If all smokers stopped, then up to 86% of the cases of lung cancer would disappear. This is a measure that clinicians and health care planners can grasp instantly, this is the number of people who have a disorder because of their exposure to a particular risk.

Recent reviews of the life event and depression literature (Cooke & Hole, 1983; Cooke, 1986) have demonstrated the utility of these two indices. Relative risks were found to range from 2.6 to 6.8. Compared with the relative risks for heavy smoking and lung cancer these risks are comparatively modest; however, in the context of epidemiological studies as a whole they are significant and suggestive of a causal association. With female subjects anything between 37% and 69% of cases of depression could be attributed to the effect of stressful life events. These two measures, therefore, provide a simple yet valuable indication of the importance of risk factors. Moreover, these indices can be used to tackle two other problems of analysis in epidemiology—the problem of specificity and the problem of synergy.

Assessing Specificity

A central idea in epidemiological research is the notion of specificity. Following Susser (1973), specificity may be regarded as the extent to which one variable can be used to predict another. An example from the smoking literature may illustrate the importance of specificity (Fig. 14.3).

In the early studies on smoking and disease Doll and Hill (1952) found relationships between all forms of smoking and death due to all causes. The relative risk, however, was comparatively small (i.e. 1.3). To enhance specificity Doll and Hill refined the domain of potential causes by excluding cigar smoking and pipe smoking and examined deaths through all

Smoking	Relative risk	Disorder
Cigarettes, pipe, cigar smoking	1.3 ⟶	Death from all causes
Cigarette smoking	1.7 ⟶	Death from all causes
Cigarette smoking	32 ⟶	Death from lung cancer

FIG. 14.3. The specificity of the relationship between types of smoking and disease.

casues following cigarette smoking. The relative risk was increased to a modest 1.7. They then refined the effect side of the equation by ignoring all forms of death apart from lung cancer and they found a substantial relative risk, a risk of 32. Doll and Hill established that cigarette smoking had a specific effect on lung cancer.

Specificity does two things. Firstly, specificity increases the plausibility of a causal relationship. Secondly, specificity helps the investigator exclude irrelevancies, irrelevancies of risk and irrelevancies of disorder. This is as true of psychological data as it is of lung cancer data. In the life event field, Paykel and his colleagues found that undesirable events and events that entailed the loss of someone important had greater causal impact than events in general (Paykel *et al.*, 1969). Refining the other side of the equation, Cooke (1981) and Bebbington *et al.* (1981) showed that life events influenced neurotic or anxiety depression but not other forms of depression. Comparison of relative risks allows the investigator to evaluate the specificity of an effect.

Simple or Synergistic Effects

Relative risk and population attributable risk per cent can be used to examine the influence that more than one risk factor have on the rate of a disorder. In simple terms, two risk factors may independently produce proportional increases in the risk of a disorder or their concatenation may produce a disproportionate or synergistic increase in the risk of a disorder. For example, serum cholesterol level and smoking may independently affect the risk of coronary heart disease. Thus measures to reduce cholesterol and measures to reduce smoking would both decrease the risk of coronary heart disease in proportion to their relative risks. By way of contrast, consumption of alcohol and smoking are thought to have a synergistic effect on the risk of oesophageal cancer (Tuyns, Pequignot & Jensen, 1977). Thus the risk of oesophageal cancer for the non-smoking drinker is slightly elevated, the risk for a smoking non-drinker is slightly elevated but the risk for someone who smokes and drinks is dramatically increased.

The presence or absence of synergy is important both from the point of view of prevention and from the point of view of understanding the nature of a disorder. In the synergistic case prevention is comparatively easy because removal of one risk factor, e.g. smoking, dramatically reduces the risk of oesophageal cancer. In the non-synergistic case removal of one risk factor only reduces the risk of heart disease partially. Theoretically, the synergistic relationship implies that there is a biological interaction between smoking and alcohol which leads to oesophageal cancer. This suggests avenues that should be explored to identify the physical mechanisms underpinning the disease. In the absence of synergy it is less likely that biological interaction is present.

Synergy may be important in psychological epidemiology. In the recent British literature there has been a considerable preoccupation with the interpretation of the ways in which two risk factors may affect the risk of psychological disturbance (Tennant & Bebbington, 1978; Brown & Harris, 1978b; Everitt & Smith, 1979). Rutter (1981) has argued that this is a rather pointless controversy since any conclusion about synergy must depend on the statistical model that is assumed to underlie the relationship. By examining the appropriate relative risks it is possible to determine whether risks are additive or synergistic in nature. To illustrate this point two examples from the literature on life events will be considered (Table 14.4).

The first results are taken from a study in which the effects of life events and housing problems on the rate of depression were examined (Paykel, Emms, Fletcher & Rassaby, 1980). The relative risk for each of the four cells are tabulated. The risk when the subject has housing problems is three times more than when she does not have housing problems. The risk when she has experienced recent life events is nine times more, while the risk

TABLE 14.4

(a) Relative risks illustrating an additive interaction between two risk factors with regard to their effect on puerperal depression. Data from Paykel *et al.* (1980)

| | | Life events | |
		No	Yes
Housing problems	Yes	4.23	11.46
	No	1.00	10.31

(b) Table of relative risks illustrating a multiplicative interaction between two risk factors with regard to their effect on depression. Data from Parry and Shapiro (1985)

| | | Life events | |
		No	Yes
Lack of instrumental support	Yes	2.40	4.56
	No	1.00	1.90

when she has both life events and housing problems is just less than twelve. Given rounding error, this suggests that the effects are additive. If a synergistic effect was present, the relative risk for combined risks would be over forty. The second example comes from a study by Parry and Shapiro (1986) in which the occurrence of depression was examined in relation to life events and to the level of expressive social support (Table 14.4(b)).

In this example, the relative risk for those who lack instrumental social support is 2.4, for those who have experienced recent life events 1.9 and for those with both risk factors the relative risk is 4.64. The product of the individual risks is 4.56. It would appear, therefore, that the appropriate model in this instance is synergistic rather than additive. Thus people with poor social support are apparently at considerable risk when they experience a life event. This has important clinical and theoretical implications as it suggests that by improving an individual's social support we may reduce the impact of life events. Life events may be difficult to prevent: social support can be enhanced.

More Complex Methods of Analysis

The above forms of analysis are useful when the investigator is examining the association between one or two risk factors and a disorder. In more complex situations, where the investigator wishes to determine how a larger set of variables affects a disorder, it is necessary to use multivariate statistics. The form the analysis takes depends on the questions to be answered.

In the space available, it would be impossible to provide a detailed account of the application of these techniques, however, each of the procedures will be described briefly and examples of their application will be given.

Discriminant function analysis is a technique for refining categories of people or patients. Ni Bhrolchain, Brown and Harris (1979) applied discriminant function analysis to refine the distinction between cases of neurotic and psychotic depression. All symptoms of depression were analysed to find out which ones distinguish between cases of neurotic and psychotic depression. The best combination of discriminating symptoms was derived and cases were re-assigned to the neurotic or psychotic group on the basis of scores estimated from the discriminant function. Sharper categories were thereby achieved and individual patients were allocated to the groups with greater reliability.

Principal component analysis and factor analysis are techniques that are designed to divide variables into groups which are interrelated and distinguish them from other groups of variables (Eysenck, 1953). These are valuable techniques because they exclude irrelevancies from measures,

TABLE 14.5
The function of more complex statistical techniques

Procedure	Question to be answered
Discriminant function analysis	Which variables best discriminate 2 or more groups of people from each other? How well can these different groups be separated?
Principal component analysis and factor analysis	Which variables are correlated with each other and distinct from other variables? How may a large number of variables be expressed in terms of a smaller number of factors or constructs?
Multiple regression analysis	Which combination of independent variables predict the dependent variable (usually a continuous measure of disorder)? What are the relative contributions of the independent variables to prediction?
Log-linear analysis	Which combination of independent variables (usually dichotomous risk factors) predict the dependent variables (usually a dichotomous 'caseness' measure)?
Mathematical models	What is the pattern of effects which influence the dependent variable? What is the overall size of the multiple effect? What change would occur in the dependent variable if the level of independent variables is changed? What assumptions underpin the putative causal associations?

they generate more reliable variables (Armor, 1969) and may enhance construct validity.

Cooke (1980a) applied principal component analysis to symptom data collected in a community study. Four components or syndromes of depression emerged and were labelled 'anxiety depression', 'cognitive depression', 'vegetative depression' and 'classic endogenous depression'. This slimming down of the symptom domain allowed the demonstration of specificity in that only 'anxiety depression' was found to be associated with stressful life events (Cooke, 1981). The construct validity of the association between life events and 'anxiety depression' was thereby enhanced.

Multiple regression analysis is a technique that estimates how well a set of independent variables such as demographic factors, social support variables and measures of stress can predict the level of a dependent variable such as depression. It is a valuable technique because the relative importance of risk factors or other variables can be estimated and, also, the overall accuracy of the prediction can be estimated. Paykel *et al.* (1980)

applied this technique to predict puerperal depression. They demonstrated that five variables—namely undesirable life events, age, previous history of psychiatric disorder, post-partum blues and marital difficulties—in combination predicted 40% of the variance in puerperal depression. Each variable contributed a similar amount to the prediction. Thus the investigators could evaluate the relative importance of these variables and determine how much variability had yet to be explained.

Log-linear analysis is a technique akin to multiple regression analysis. However, it is generally used with discrete rather than continuous variables. Dichotomous risk factors are used to predict dichotomous measures of disorder.

The final set of procedures to be considered is mathematical models. Mathematical models have been used extensively in the social sciences (e.g. Wold & Jureen, 1953; Blalock, 1964; Werts & Linn, 1970). They are designed to provide over-simplified analogues of reality by describing a limited number of variables and their interrelationships.

Mathematical models have three major advantages when they are applied to the analysis of survey data. Firstly, as Dunn (1981) indicated, their application may provide a more complete understanding of results by providing a detailed explanation of the pattern of the results. Mathematical models can be used to assess the pattern of effects in complex multivariable situations. As an example of this approach Duncan-Jones (1986) was able to distinguish long-term causes of anxiety and depression such as hereditary and childhood experiences from short-term causes such as stressful life events. In addition, he was able to demonstrate the relative importance of these two types of causes. His model suggested that long-term causes were three times as important as short-term causes. This has important implications for the treatment of such disorder.

The second advantage of mathematical models is that they provide an analogue to reality and thus changes can be predicted using the model. Dunn and Skuse (1981) used a mathematical model to describe the pattern of depression found in a general practice. Using this model they were able to predict the recovery rate of patients with chronic depression and also to predict the incidence rate of new episodes of depression from past contacts at the general practice surgery.

The third, and perhaps most important, advantage of a mathematical model is that it constrains the investigator to make explicit non-ambiguous statements regarding theoretical constructs and presumed causal mechanisms. By being forced to make his model explicit the investigator may highlight unwarranted assumptions (Blalock, 1964; Dunn, 1981).

The above multivariate techniques are valuable; however, their application can be fraught with difficulties. Considerable technical expertise is required if results obtained are to be sensible. Most investigators will require expert guidance on the application of these techniques, if they are to avoid the trap of 'garbage in, garbage out'.

PRACTICAL PROBLEMS IN THE ORGANISATION OF EPIDEMIOLOGICAL RESEARCH

The final section of this chapter considers what is perhaps the most important hurdle faced by any epidemiologist, namely, organising the fieldwork. The major problems in fieldwork can be eased by the proper training of interviewers and by the careful control and monitoring of interview information as it is collected.

Training Interviewers

Training is fundamental. Most research interviewers will not have interviewed before, and if they have interviewed before, then their approach and techniques may not be those that you have chosen to use in your study.

The first task in training is to teach the details of the interview schedule and the interview procedure. Consistency in the phrasing of questioning and the application of anchor points is vital at the beginning of the project. There will be plenty of time for definitions to drift as the project proceeds! Video role play is desirable. This gives trainees confidence and it allows the investigator to ensure the appropriate application of anchor points and interview techniques. Once interviewers have learned the basics of the interview then they must be taught the pace, tone and style of questions to be used. If the approach adopted calls for semi-structured interviewing then the interviewers need to be taught such skills as reflection and prompting by the presentation of balanced alternatives.

Piloting the interview in the population of interest can reap benefits. The interviewers will develop their skills in locating the target person, they will learn how to reduce the refusal rate and they will gain confidence in using the interview procedures. Particular problems in the form of questions can be identified and resolved before the main study begins.

Quality Control

The second major hurdle faced by the investigator is that of keeping control of the information as it is received. Epidemiological studies generate large amounts of information; questionnaires are usually long and samples are usually large. Information can be degraded by non-contacts or refusals, inadequate coding and even by the falsification of data. If these problems are not minimised then the validity of the study can be threatened.

Simple steps can be taken to limit these problems. Non-contacts occur when, despite all efforts, the specified individual cannot be located and interviewed. This can be a problem because non-contacts may systematically bias a sample. For example, individuals working away from home, perhaps on the North Sea oilrigs, differ significantly from those living at home. Individuals with alcohol problems may be more difficult to contact because they are more often in public houses than others. Non-contacts, therefore, can bias results. To counter this problem it is established practice that six attempts should be made to contact the individual, at different times of the day and of the week, before they are designated as a non-contact.

Refusers can have an equally damaging effect on the validity of the study. Anxious or depressed individuals may be less likely to co-operate because of their symptoms and thus, a systematic bias enters the study. Refusals are more difficult to combat than non-contacts because people have an absolute right not to be coerced into giving personal information. Fortunately, few people are totally unwilling to co-operate with a study if: (a) they are provided with a proper explanation of its purpose; (b) they are reassured that information given will be confidential; and (c) it is demonstrated to them, by way of appropriate identification, that a bona fide organisation is carrying out the study. If the subject is showing only minor reluctance then a pleasant, reassuring and quietly persistent approach on the part of the interviewer can often pay dividends.

Once the interview schedule is returned to the research office it is important that a clerical officer checks immediately that the schedule is filled in completely. Often in the depth of an interview, the interviewer will forget to complete a section of the schedule. If they are reminded immediately they can often provide the missing information.

Traditionally, information from interviews is transferred to a computer coding sheet. This information is then typed onto computer files. During transfer of information errors inevitably creep in. It is sensible, therefore, to reduce the possibility of error by reducing the number of times information is transferred. If the interview schedule is appropriately coded, with computer columns down the righthand margin, then information can be directly transferred (Fig. 14.4). As a bonus, an extra clerical task is also avoided.

A further problem that any investigator should be aware of is the possibility that interviewers will fabricate interviews. Interviewing can be unpleasant and tedious. An interviewer may be expected to traipse the streets on cold and windy evenings and, indeed, by the time they have asked the same questions a hundred times their interest may begin to wane. The temptation to fake is always present. To prevent this the investigator should make the interviewer aware that he is conscious of the

Card no. ☐[0] ☐[1]
                    1   2

1. Referral code
                              ☐   ☐   ☐
                              3   4   5

2. Sex
        1 – male
        2 – female   ☐
                              6

3. Age
   What age were you on your last birthday?   ☐   ☐
                                               7   8

4. Household composition
   How many people live here regularly who are cared for by the same   ☐   ☐
   person as yourself?   9   10

5. Marital status
   Are you single, married or widowed?
        1 – single
        2 – married
        3 – divorced
        4 – separated   ☐
        5 – widowed   11
        6 – remarried

6. Employment category
   Were you in paid employment at the time of the offence?
        1 – yes and over 30 hrs/week
        2 – yes and under 30 hrs/week
        3 – unemployed for 3 months or less
        4 – unemployed for 6 months or less   ☐
        5 – unemployed for 1 year or less   12
        6 – unemployed for 3 years or less
        7 – unemployed for 5 years or less
        8 – unemployed for more than 5 years

FIG. 14.4. Illustration of interview schedule pre-coded for direct entry onto a computer.

problem. The procedure that is commonly used is to contact a random sample of subjects who have been interviewed to determine whether the interview actually took place.

The field of epidemiology is complex but rewarding. Many of the theoretical problems confronted by psychologists in clinical settings can only be tackled through the application of epidemiological methods. The identification of coping and adaptive mechanisms is one of several advantages of the epidemiological approach. In addition, epidemiological information can be of considerable value in the planning and development of services. The complexities of the inherent methodological problem should not deter the clinician from taking an interest in this illuminating and valuable field.

ACKNOWLEDGEMENTS

I thank Patrick Miller and David Hole for their helpful comments on an earlier draft. In addition, I would like to thank Mrs Rowena Cook for preparing the manuscript with such care.

REFERENCES

Atkinson, J. (1971). *A Handbook for Interviewers: A Manual for Social Survey Interviewing Practice and Procedures on Structured Interviewing*, 2nd edn. HMSO: Social Survey Division.

Armor, D. J. (1969). Theta reliability and factor scaling. *Sociological Methodology*, **2**, 17–50.

Bartlett, F. C. (1932). *Remembering*. Cambridge University Press.

Bebbington, P., Tennant, C & Hurry, J. (1981). Adversity and the nature of psychiatric disorder in the community. *Journal of Affective Disorders*, **3**, 345–366.

Blalock, H. M. (1964). *Causal Inferences in Non-experimental Research*. The University of North Carolina Press.

Brown, G. W., Ni Bhrolchain, M. & Harris, T. O. (1975). Social class and psychiatric disturbance among women in an urban population. *Sociology*, **9**, 225–254.

Brown, G. W. & Harris, T. O. (1978a). *Social Origins of Depression: A Study of Psychiatric Disorder in Women*. London: Tavistock.

Brown, G. W. & Harris, T. O. (1987b). Social origins of depression: A reply. *Psychological Medicine*, **8**, 577–588.

Brown, G. W., Craig, T. K. J. & Harris, T. O. (1985). Depression: distress or disease? Some epidemiological considerations. *British Journal of Psychiatry*, **147**, 612–622.

Cook, T. D. & Campbell, D. T. (1979). *Quasi-experimentation, Design and Analysis Issues for Field Settings*. Chicago: Rand McNally College Publishing Company.

Cooke, D. J. (1980a). The structure of depression found in the general population. *Psychological Medicine*, **10**, 455–463.

Cooke, D. J. (1980b). Causal modelling with contingency tables. *British Journal of Psychiatry*, **137**, 582–584.

Cooke, D. J. (1981). Life events and syndromes of depression in the general population. *Social Psychiatry*, **16**, 181–186.

Cooke, D. J. (1985). The reliability of a brief life event interview. *Journal of Psychosomatic Research*, **29**, 361–365.

Cooke, D. J. (1986). The significance of life events as a cause of psychological and physical disorder. In B. Cooper (ed.) *Psychiatric Epidemiology: Process and Prospects*. London: Croom Helm.

Cooke, D. J. & Hole, D. (1983). The aetiological importance of stressful life events. *British Journal of Psychiatry*, **143**, 397–400.

Copland, J. (1981). What is a case? A case for what? In J. K. Wing, P. E. Bebbington, and L. N. Robins, (eds) *What is a Case? The Problem of Definition in Psychiatric Community Surveys*. London: Grant McIntyre.

Cranach M. Von, Eberlein, R. & Holl, B. (1981). The concept of onset in psychiatry. In:

J. K. Wing, P. E. Bebbington and L. N. Robins (eds.) *What is a Case? The Problem of Definition in Psychiatric Community Surveys*. London: Grant McIntyre.

Derogatis, L. R., Klerman, G. R. & Lipman, R. S. (1972). Anxiety states and depressive neurosis: issues on nosological discrimination. *Journal of Nervous and Mental Disease*, **155**, 392–403.

Dohrenwend, B. P. & Shrout, P. E. (1985). 'Hassles' in the conceptualisation and measurement of life stress variables. *American Psychologist*, **20**, 780–785.

Doll, R. & Hill, A. B. (1952). A study of the aetiology of carcinoma of the lung. *British Medical Journal*, **ii**, 1271–1286.

Doll, R. & Peto, R. (1976). Mortality in relation to smoking: 20 years observations on male British doctors. *British Medical Journal*, **ii**, 1525–1536.

Duncan-Jones, P. (1986). Modelling the aetiology of neurosis: long-term and short-term factors. In B. Cooper (ed.) *Psychiatric Epidemiology: Progress and Prospects*. London: Croom Helm.

Dunn, G. (1981). The role of linear models in psychiatric epidemiology. *Psychological Medicine*, **11**, 179–184.

Dunn, G. & Skuse, D. (1981). The natural history of depression and general practice: Stochastic models. *Psychological Medicine*, **11**, 755–764.

Everitt, B. S. & Smith, A. M. R. (1979). Interactions in contingency tables: a brief discussion of alternative definitions. *Psychological Medicine*, **9**, 581–583.

Eysenck, H. J. (1953). The logical basis of factor analysis. *American Psychologist*, **8**, 105–114.

Fahy, T. J. (1974a). Pathways of specialist referral of depressed patients from general practice. *British Journal of Psychiatry*, **124**, 231–239.

Fahy, T. J. (1974b). Depression in hospital and in general practice: a direct clinical comparison. *British Journal of Psychiatry*, **124**, 240–242.

Fahy, T. J. (1975). Some problems of method in the study of depression in general practice. *Cambridge Medical Publications*, **82**, 82–89.

Goldberg, D. & Huxley, P. (1980). *Mental Illness in The Community: The Pathway to Psychiatric Care*. London: Tavistock Publications.

Hays, L. W. (1963). *Statistics*. London: Holt, Rinehart and Winston.

Henderson, S., Byrne, O. G., Duncan-Jones, P., Scott, R. & Adcock, S. (1980). Social relationships, adversity and neurosis: A study of associations in a general population sample. *British Journal of Psychiatry*. **136**, 574–583.

Ingham, J. G. & Miller, P.McC. (1976). The concept of prevalence applied to psychiatric disorders and symptoms. *Psychological Medicine*, **6**, 217–225.

Kreitman, N. (1980). Epidemiological Psychiatry: the present and the future. In M. Lader (ed.) *Priorities in Psychiatric Research*. Chichester: John Wiley & Sons.

Leighton, A. H. (1979). Research directions in psychiatric epidemiology. *Psychological Medicine*, **9**, 234–247.

MacMahon, B. & Pugh, T. F. (1970). *Epidemiology: Principles and Methods*. Boston: Little, Brown & Company.

Mausner, J. F. & Kramer, S. (1985). *Epidemiology, An Introductory Text*. Philadelphia: W. B. Saunders.

Miller, P.McC. & Ingham, J. G. (1979). Reflections on the life-event-to-illness link with some preliminary findings. In I. G. Sarason and C. D. Spielberger (eds.) *Stress and Anxiety*. Vol 6. New York: John Wiley.

Miller, P.McC., Surtees, P. G., Kreitman, N., Ingham, J. & Sashidharan, S. P. (1985). Maladaptive coping responses to stress: a study of illness inception. *Journal of Nervous and Mental Disease*, **173**, 707–716.

Mollon, P. & Parry, G. (1984). The fragile self: narcissistic disturbance and the protective function of depression. *British Journal of Medical Psychology*, **57**, 137–146.

Murphy, J. R. (1983). The relationship of relative risk and positive predictive value two by two tables. *American Journal of Epidemiology*, **117**, 86–89.

Ni Bhrolchain, M. (1979). Psychotic and neurotic depression: I. Some points of method. *British Journal of Psychiatry*, **134**, 87–93.

Ni Bhrolchain, M., Brown, G. W. & Harris, T. O. (1979). Psychotic and neurotic depression: 2. Clinical characteristics. *British Journal of Psychiatry*, **134**, 94–107.

Nunnally, J. C. (1967). *Psychometric Theory*. New York: McGraw Hill Book Company.

Parry, G. & Shapiro, D. A. (1986). Social support and life events in working class women: stress buffering or independent effects? *Archives of General Psychiatry*, **43**, 315–323.

Paykel, E. S., Myres, J. K., Dienelt, M. N., Klerman, G. L., Lindenthal, J. J. & Pepper, M. P. (1969). Life events and depression: a controlled study. *Archives of General Psychiatry*, **21**, 753–760.

Paykel, E. S., Emms, E. M., Fletcher, J. & Rassaby, E. S, (1980). Life events and social support in puerperal depression. *British Journal of Psychiatry*, **136**, 339–346.

Rutter, M. (1981). Stress, coping and development: some issues and some questions. *Journal of Child Psychology and Psychiatry*, **22**, 323–356.

Rutter, M., Tizard, J., Yule, W., Graham, P. & Whitmore, K. (1976). Research reports: Isle of Wight studies 1964–1974. *Psychological Medicine*, **6**, 313–332.

Shepherd, M., Cooper, B., Brown, A. C. & Kalton, G. W. (1966). *Psychiatric Illness in General Practice*. Oxford University Press.

Surtees, P. G., Sashidharan, S. P. & Dean, C. (1986). Affective disorder amongst women in the general population: a longitudinal study. *British Journal of Psychiatry*, **148**, 176–186.

Susser, M. (1973). *Causal Thinking in the Health Sciences*. New York: Oxford University Press.

Tennant, C. & Bebbington, P. (1978). The social causation of depression: A critique of the work of Brown and his colleagues. *Psychological Medicine*, **8**, 565–575.

Tuyns, A. J., Pequignot, G. & Jensen, O. M. (1977). *Annual Report*. Lyons: International Agency for Research on Cancer.

Weckowicz, T. (1973). A multidimensional theory of depression. In A. Boyle (ed.) *Multivariate Analysis and Psychological Theory*. London: Academic Press.

Weissman, M. M. & Klerman, G. L. (1977). Sex differences and the epidemiology of depression. *Archives of General Psychiatry*, **34**, 98–111.

Weissman, M. M. & Paykel, E. S. (1974). *The Depressed Woman: A Study of Social Relationships*. Chicago: University of Chicago Press.

Werts, C. E. & Linn, R. L. (1970). Path analysis: psychological examples. *Psychological Bulletin*, **74**, 193–212.

Wing, J. K., Nixon, J. M., Mann, S. A. & Leff. J. P. (1977). Reliability of the P. S. E. (ninth edition) used in a population study. *Psychological Medicine*, **7**, 505–516.

Wold, H. & Jureen, L. (1953). *Demand Analysis: A Study in Econometrics*. New York: Wiley.

Yager, J., Grant, I., Sweetwood, H. L. & Gerst, M. (1981). Life event reports by psychiatric patients, non-patients, and their partners. *Archives of General Psychiatry*, **38**, 343–347.

15 Research in Service Planning and Evaluation

Geoff Shepherd
Department of Psychology, Fulbourn Hospital, Cambridge.

An interest in collecting data rarely intrudes into the process of planning or evaluating services. Most professionals in the health service seem to presume to know already without any data, not only what services are required, but also how they are currently functioning. To question either often seems pointless and faintly tedious. Yet the role of the sceptic is an important one. Of course, I am not suggesting that anyone who provides services can stand completely outside their prejudices and take a truly 'objective' view of what is going on. However, they can at least try to put their prejudices alongside their data and attempt to clarify to what extent the one has permeated the other. They can also remind people of the true nature and extent of the difficulties when these blantantly contradict the plans and proposals that are being put forward. There is a natural tendency to be drawn to easy (and cheap) solutions to what are complex personal and social problems and when this happens someone has to nudge the planners and politicians with a little reality.

This is particularly important given the dramatic changes that have occurred—and that will continue to occur—in the overall pattern of psychiatric services. The need for intelligent and realistic advice has never been greater and the problems of running a dispersed, multi-agency, multi-site service have yet to be really faced. Planners and administrators have been under pressure to close hospitals, but under less pressure to develop a comprehensive and co-ordinated network of alternatives in the community. Where specific residential or community projects have been set up, a whole new set of problems with regard to research methods and evaluative techniques has arisen.

There are thus two distinct kinds of planning and evaluation exercises: the one is concerned with planning and evaluation at the level of *overall service development*, while the other is concerned with planning and evaluation at the level of *specific projects*. These will now be discussed separately. Most of the examples I will use are drawn from the field of adult mental health, particularly the care and rehabilitation of those with long-term social and psychiatric disorders, since this is the group with whom I am most familiar. However, there are some general implications for service planning and evaluation with other client groups—e.g. the elderly and the mentally handicapped—and I hope that these will also emerge.

RESEARCH AND PLANNING OVERALL SERVICE DEVELOPMENTS

This section will be concerned with the planning and evaluation of a complete service or network of facilities, such as in the rundown of a large mental hospital or the creation of a new district service. Three principal questions will be considered:

1. What is the estimated overall magnitude of the population requiring this service? *How many?*
2. What is the nature and range of facilities that are likely to be required? *What kind of service?*
3. Once in place, how will the new service be monitored and evaluated? *How do we tell if it is working?*

How Many?

The problem of accurately identifying the overall numbers of people to require a particular kind of service is a daunting one. If we are simply concerned with the existing population of a mental hospital and the task is reprovision of services on another site (or sites), it should be relatively easy to obtain an estimate of the numbers (e.g. Levene, Donaldson & Brandon, 1985). However, such simple 'head-counts' run into difficulties if the population under study is not clearly defined. Apart from specifying obvious parameters as age, length of stay, etc., more complex 'boundary problems' may arise. For example, do you include people from the existing catchment area of the hospital, or only those from the catchment area as planned in the future? Boundary problems of this kind mean that plans from other districts may need to be taken into account.

But the fundamental difficulty with cross-sectional survey data is that they tell you little about the *dynamics* in the population under study. For planning purposes it is these dynamics that are often the most important. Thus, you need to know not only how many people require services now, but also how many are likely to require services in 'x' years time. Making these predictions constitutes one of the most difficult aspects of planning and it has led to some of the most celebrated blunders. The most famous of these is probably the prediction about future bed numbers made by Tooth and Brooke (1961). These were based upon existing trends in hospital populations which had begun to fall rapidly after the 1959 Mental Health Act following the introduction of more 'open-door' policies and the widespread use of new neuropeptic drugs. Using these data Tooth and Brooke predicted that there would be no long-stay patients left in mental hospitals by the mid-1970s! These predictions were based on an extrapolation from current practice which is only valid where conditions are stable, or where the factors affecting accumulation or rundown are clearly understood (preferably both). This was obviously not the case regarding mental hospitals 20 years ago and it is still not the case today.

Recent surveys of mental hospital populations indicate that the age of the population is gradually increasing (Bewley, Bland, Mechen & Walch, 1981; Early & Nicholas, 1977; 1981). This is understandable given the correlation of age and disability, and the tendency to discharge the less disabled patients first. Most authors conclude from this that the rate of rundown in existing long-stay populations is likely to decrease assuming that there is no dramatic increase in the availability of alternative accommodation for disabled elderly people in the community. The rundown of the existing old long-stay population will then depend largely upon their mortality. This in turn will depend upon the precise characteristics of the population under consideration. Since each hospital has its own unique history and each has been influenced by a unique set of factors, the age composition of its residents and their rates of decline will vary depending upon specific local circumstances. This is reflected in the variation of mortality rates from study to study (although in nearly all cases the rates among psychiatric patients tend to be 2–3 times higher than comparable 'normal' controls). What is really required is therefore a specific modelling exercise for each population as described, for example by Moore (1985).

As indicated, this kind of projection also assumes that rates of decline through other mechanisms (e.g. discharge to alternatives in the community) will remain relatively stable and this may prove to be incorrect. For example, in the UK there has recently been a massive increase in private nursing homes for the elderly (House of Commons, 1985) which has been brought about mainly through the increased availability of funding (DHSS

TABLE 15.1
Number of hospital beds for 'new' long-stay
inpatients per 100,000 total population occupied
in seven Register areas (1981)

Area	No. of beds occupied for between 1 and 5 years
Camberwell	56
Salford	58
Cardiff	46
Nottingham	38
Southampton	37
Oxford	16
Worcester	20

Adapted from Wing (1984).

benefits) combined with local factors. If any of these parameters were to change suddenly, particularly the availability of funding, then clearly the predictions would alter. Exactly the same kind of arguments can be made with regard to the *accumulation* of 'new' long-stay inpatients (NLS) in the future. In the UK the annual incidence of NLS varies quite considerably from region to region with a median of around 3–4 per 100,000 per year (Jennings, 1982). This produces widespread differences in prevalence as illustrated in Table 15.1.

Once again, variation is explicable partly by local factors, e.g. demography (rural versus urban); existence of an active rehabilitation service; availability of alternative places in the community; and partly by national policies to shorten lengths of admission and not to rely on the mental hospitals to provide long-term care. Such factors also contribute to the heterogeneity of the population concerned. (Thus, in some places the NLS will constitute only the most severely disabled people who cannot manage outside the hospital, whereas in other places the mix may be rather different.) Variations in prevalence of this kind underline the need to understand how the total service system operates and how one kind of service element may 'substitute' for another.

In epidemiological terms, the categorisation 'new long-stay' refers to service use, not to the distribution of a specific kind of disorder. Data on service use are therefore not the same as traditional epidemiological data. Thus if one particular kind of service can be substituted for another (e.g. beds in private nursing homes for beds in hospital) then the apparent 'prevalence' of the disorder will decrease. Of course, the true prevalence has not changed, it has simply shifted from one place to another in the overall system. If service usage is confused with true prevalence in this way, then it may create the illusion that the service is being more effective when, in fact, it is not. As an example, in the United States it has been estimated that between 1969 and 1973 the resident population of nursing homes (aged 65 and over) with chronic mental disorders increased by more than 100% and over the same time similar residents in state hospitals decreased by 30–40% (Goldman, 1983). 'De-institutionalisation' can therefore become 'trans-institutionalisation'.

Of course, estimating the true prevalence of a disorder is extremely complex (see Chapter 14) but it may be useful to have some basic epidemiological facts at your fingertips. For example, cross-cultural studies of the prevalence of schizophrenia suggests that most populations contain around one in two hundred persons with the disorder (Warner, 1985). This stands in marked contrast to the 1-year period prevalence for total recognisable psychiatric disorder in the community which has been estimated at around 250/1000, of which 230 present to General Practitioners, who recognise 140, and refer on to psychiatrists just 17. The number at risk of admission per year is 6 per 1000 (Goldberg & Huxley, 1980). Of course, these kinds of figures are subject to local variation, and having some idea of the local factors may help to apply appropriate 'multipliers' to give some estimate of overall numbers.

In trying to plan services for total populations, we also come up against the fundamental problem of defining who psychiatric services are for. Are not there many people 'out there' who never come into contact with services, but who also have psychological needs? The answer is probably 'yes', but we would do well to be cautious about just how far we intend to open the 'floodgates' to them. As Goldberg and Huxley's figures remind us, for every person referred to a psychiatrist there are likely to be another 8 who continue to be cared for by their GPs (and another 5 whom the GP does not even recognise as a 'case'). Furthermore, it is generally the most severe disorders who pass the 'filters' most easily and enter the system.

Richman and Barry (1985) suggest that the concept of 'unmet need' is often a myth perpetuated by those who wish to justify the diversion of resources from existing services, rather than devoting them to the correction of existing problems in the delivery of care. They also comment upon the associated tendency to 'medicalise' problems of everyday life and the professional neglect of those with the most serious disorders in favour of better functioning individuals on the edge of what would normally be regarded as 'patienthood'. One needs to be careful, therefore, when attempting to define the magnitude of the problem to take qualitative, as well as quantative, factors into account. The apparently simple question,

'How Many?' thus turns out to be a difficult one to answer. Getting accurate figures on population sizes, and especially making accurate predictions about future needs, is not easy. But, approximate figures, particularly if they are based on local data, are certainly better than no figures at all (and also probably better than attempts to extrapolate from inappropriate national norms).

It is also important that some of the factors that are liable to influence the size of the error are clearly identified and that an attempt is made to allow for them. One must always be on guard against the tendency to employ overoptimistic assumptions and to underestimate need. Everybody wants to believe that demand for health services in the future will be less than it is today, but as yet this has never happened. In purely pragmatic terms, there may also be an advantage in erring on the side of overgenerous resource allocation since at least it allows for redeployment. You cannot redeploy resources that you have not got.

What Kind of Service?

There are essentially two approaches to defining service needs. These may be characterised respectively as *service-led* and *client-led*. Service-led planning attempts to create a comprehensive range of services based on a 'shopping list' of service elements. These are then deployed according to some set of general national norms. Service needs are thus defined according to an overall concept of what would constitute a comprehensive range of provisions. In the USA, the National Institute of Mental Health has attempted to provide such a model (Stroul, 1984, 1986), and in the UK MIND'S Manifesto 'Common Concern' (MIND, 1983) provides a similar list of facilities which health districts might wish to consider in their planning of services. Part of this list is reproduced in Table 15.2.

Various DHSS planning documents can then be used to provide guidelines as to the levels of provision required for each different kind of facility, for example:

Service element	*Norms from DHSS (1975; 1985)*
Acute beds in general hospitals	30–50/100,000
Short-stay hostels	15–24/100,000
Long-stay hostels	4–6/100,000
Day hospitals (excluding in-patients)	30/100,000
Day centres	60/100,000
Day hospitals (psychogeriatric)	30/100,000

TABLE 15.2
Services for chronic mental illness (taken from MIND, 1983)

Rehabilitation and resettlement team
Social services area teams
    either generic social work for a defined local population or specialist social work arranged
    in client groups
Occupational therapy department with ADL
Hospital rehabilitation unit or wards
Progressive hospital accommodation—
    cubicles, single rooms, group living, flats, rehabilitation homes within hospitals

Day hospitals: special arrangements for chronic mental illness

Day centres: provided by local authority

Local authority old persons' homes

Sheltered lodging scheme: landlady groups

Supervised accommodation:
    1. Jointly with housing department
    2. Housing allocation for mentally ill people

Staffed group homes

Group homes:
    1. Run by District Council
    2. Run by voluntary associations, e.g., MIND, housing associations

Halfway homes, run by, e.g., Richmond Fellowship.

Hospital hostels: the experimental schemes

Mental illness hostels
    1. Residential
    2. Assessment and crisis
    3. Rehabilitation

Special hostels: run by, e.g., St Dismas, the Cyrenians

Rehabilitation houses

Sheltered housing: warden supervised

Very sheltered housing:
    1. Warden supervised and with augmented home care services
    2. Managed jointly by social services and housing departments

Independent housing: special housing schemes and housing associations

Industrial therapy (graded work)

Sheltered work:
    1. Local authority
    2. Voluntary bodies, e.g., Psychiatric Rehabilitation Association
    3. Department of Employment
    4. Industrial rehabilitation units
    5. Industrial therapy organisations
    6. Enclave working

Social rehabilitation groups—literacy, social skills, domestic management

Joint health and social services resettlement scheme

This may sound crude and mechanistic, but it is how much planning is done and it does have some merits. At the very least, it should ensure that basic, minimum levels of provision are met. For example, if a survey of local available services is completed and this is compared with the guidelines, then certain deficiences may be highlighted. Are there sufficient (or too many) acute beds? Are there both short- and long-stay hostel places? How many? Where are they situated in relation to the populations in need? Is there a day hospital facility? Are there adequate day-care provisions for long-term support day centres? What do they provide? Is there a balance of work-orientated day care and social support? etc. This identification of gaps in service provision can be very useful and may assist in the creation of a more comprehensive system. Of course, it does not solve the problem of priorities. It may also ignore the specificity of local conditions highlighted earlier and it can place too great an emphasis on quantitative aspects of provisions at the expense of more subtle considerations about the qualitative nature of services. (The question should not be how many hostels/day centres, etc. do we need, but what *kind* of services do we require to meet individual's needs?) Despite these reservations, normative planning should not be rejected out of hand.

The alternative approach starts from the opposite end, i.e. it purports to be 'client-led'. It can be sub-divided into a '*deductive*' model in which service needs are deduced from a general set of principles or axioms and an '*inductive*' model in which services are constructed on the basis of a detailed consideration of individual clients' needs.

The 'deductive' model usually starts by defining service needs according to certain basic axioms. Thus, the principles of 'normalisation' provide an overall conceptual framework within which a range of services may be planned and evaluated (O'Brien and Tyne, 1981). The use of 'socially valued means', the attempts to reduce stigmatisation, the avoidance of age inappropriate activities, etc., provide broad parameters within which service developments may proceed. Normalisation theory has also developed systematic methods to assess individual clients and to evaluate services according to specific criteria, e.g. the 'PASS' system (Wolfensberger and Glenn, 1975). These ideas provide a conceptual framework for directing service developments and perhaps it is the need for such an overall framework in relation to the run-down of large institutions that partly accounts for their recent popularity.

Normalisation theory is not, of course, the only set of principles that can be used to provide a rationale for service developments. Other principles may be gleaned from the work of researchers like Leona Bachrach (1980) and Stein and Test (1978; 1985). Based on an analysis of the social functions served by institutions and the practical experiences of setting up a community service, they identify two central principles:

1. The service system should be adequate to ensure that the individual's unmet needs are met, i.e. the system should be sufficient to ensure that each individual gets the amount and type of each service required.

2. The service system should not meet needs the person is able to meet him/herself, i.e. a comprehensive mental health service must assume responsibility for those aspects of an individual's functioning which have, for whatever reason, broken down. On the other hand, it must preserve and support those aspects that are still intact.

These principles, together with ideas like accessibility, quality of care, comprehensiveness, continuity, and the importance of co-ordination, can then be used to provide a framework for the strategic planning of services, e.g. Cambridge Health Authority (1984). It must be recognised that such general principles can lead to problems of interpretation in particular instances. For example, what do you do if you want to build a service on the principles of normalisation and clients' expressed choice is for segregated facilities? The interpretation of such general principles in specific instances may therefore require additional expertise.

On the other hand, the *'inductive model'* begins with a detailed assessment of individual clients' needs. This often supplements statements of general principles and may be achieved in a number of ways. The most common is probably to use a standardised rating scale such as REHAB (Baker and Hall, 1983) or the CAPE (Clifton Assessment Procedure for the Elderly; Pattie and Gilleard, 1979). Some illustrative data collected using the CAPE are shown in Table 15.3.

They suggest that the numbers of patients who are likely to be able to function in relatively unsupervised accommodation is fairly small (around 25 per cent). The majority appear to need levels of supervision at least analagous to Part III homes for the elderly. Of course, these proportions will vary in different hospitals, dependent upon their own unique history of rehabilitation services. They should also not be seen as strictly *predictive* of behaviour across settings. Given all that we know concerning the specificity of behaviour, results like these are probably best regarded simply as an indication of the numbers in specific sub-groups who are currently functioning at a particular criterion level. They should certainly not be used to predict the 'potential' of individuals. That can only be done by the careful process of assessment, treatment and review, which lies at the heart of good clinical practice.

Survey data of this kind also have other limitations. Although such scales may be reliable, their content validity may still be questioned. The items they contain may have been selected carefully, but our knowledge about what contributes most critically to functioning in the community is still very imperfect and there is no guarantee that these scales necessarily tap the

TABLE 15.3
CAPE scores for 130 long-stay patients at Fulbourn Hospital (1983)

CAPE dependency levels	No.	(%)
A. No impairment: independent elderly, comparable to those living without support in the community.	11	(8)
B. Mild impairment: low dependency, likely to include those needing some support in the community, warden-supervised accommodation and the better residents in residential accommodation.	22	(17)
C. Moderate impairment: medium dependency, people functioning on this level are likely to need residential care or considerable support and help if at home.	44	(35)
D. Marked impairment: high dependency, it is within this category that there is greatest overlap between those in social services accommodation and those in hospital care.	37	(28)
E. Severe impairment: maximum dependency, this level is seen most often in psycho-geriatric wards and the ones who remain in the community homes/EMI hostels often present considerable problems to staff in terms of their demands on staff time.	16	(12)

Mean age: 63 years (range 30–85)

Mean length of admission: 21 years (range 1–54 y)

most important dimensions. For example, Kingsley, McAusland and Towell (1985) argue that the social networks of long-stay patients should be considered as just as important as their instrumental or social abilities. Similarly, clients' own wishes and ambitions need to be assessed and standardised rating scales are usually not very adequate for this purpose. An alternative approach is to ask staff to judge directly patients' suitability for various kinds of residential or day facilities. A recent example of this approach is the Bexley Hospital Patients' Needs Survey (Clifford & Szyndler, 1986). In this study all the patients who have been in Bexley Hospital for more than 1 year were rated on a number of scales covering the amount of supervision required to perform a range of basic living skills (shopping, cooking, personal hygiene, etc.). staff were then asked to make recommendations concerning the most suitable type of accommodation and day programme. Some of these data are shown in Tables 15.4 and 15.5.

TABLE 15.4
Recommended accommodation

	No.	(%)
Independent living	2	(0.7)
With family	2	(0.7)
Independent group home	1	(0.4)
Supported group home	14	(5.1)
Rehabilitation unit	23	(8.4)
Low staffed home	30	(10.9)
High staffed home (24 hour cover)	102	(37.1)
Very sheltered nursing home	87	(31.6)
Other	14	(5.1)
Total	275	(100)

From Clifford and Szyndler (1986).

TABLE 15.5
Recommended programme of day activities

	No.	(%)
Maintenance—low pressure low expectation. Some training in self-care and daily living skills.	162	(58.9)
Maintenance 'plus'—low pressure, but with greater emphasis on training and higher expectations of independence	59	(21.4)
Socialisation—strong emphasis on development and maintenance of self-care skills. Social activities/sheltered work encouraged.	37	(13.5)
Socialisation 'plus'—as above, but strong emphasis on social integration. High level sheltered work/Adult Education/Paid employment.	12	(4.4)
Follow-up only	5	(1.8)
Totals	275	(100)

From Clifford and Szyndler (1986).

Rather like the CAPE data shown earlier, these results suggest that the majority of these residents are judged to require fairly highly supervised residential accommodation (over 70% with 24 hour cover) and fairly low pressure day programmes. Clifford and Szyndler present other data to support the validity of these judgements and they also report some attempts to get the patients to express their preferences. (Only 37% expressed a clear preference, and of these 40% wished to remain in hospital.) One therefore has to weigh up the advantages of developing new questionnaires and a new format for recording staff judgements when reltively quick and easy standard instruments like the CAPE and the REHAB scales already exist which appear to serve very similar purposes. There is also the danger that staff judgements, even if reliable, will lack validity and will be contaminated through over-influence of the institutional setting, or lack of knowledge of the alternatives.

What about asking the patients directly? We noted earlier that this can be difficult. In the Bexley survey less than 40% expressed a clear preference. Similarily, in Mann and Cree's (1976) study of new long-stay only 60% expressed a definite preference. (In both cases, it is interesting that just under half expressed a preference to remain in hospital.) However, MacCarthy, Benson and Brewin (1986) report a study where a group of disabled long-term patients in the community gave very clear and consistent views as to what they saw as being problematic and difficult in their lives and what they wanted help with. Needless to say their perceptions and priorities were sometimes very different from the staff who were looking after them. Obtaining reliable information from patients, particularly some of the most disabled long-stay is difficult, but it may be possible. It is clearly worth the effort.

A final source of information to consider when assessing service needs are the patients' close family and relatives. It is only fairly recently that relatives' views have been considered important in the care and management of adult psychiatric patients. For too long they were simply blamed rather than being seen as a resource (Kuipers and Bebbington, 1985). As an example of their value in service planning Creer, Sturt and Wykes (1982) report the results of interviews with a sample of 52 relatives of long-term patients (mainly schizophrenic) living in the community, 34 said they would like some additional or modified service. These suggestions are shown in Table 15.6.

Interestingly, there is a relatively high priority attached to day care, short-term admission, additional social work help (financial assistance?) and greater involvement with hospital staff. The relatives did not seem to be requesting additional social activities, domiciliary or home-help. These results have clear service implications.

Thus we have looked at a number of methods to assess service needs and

TABLE 15.6
Additional services desired by relatives

Service desired by relative*	No. of patients	(%)
Day care, employment rehabilitation, sheltered work, etc. to suit patient's specialised needs	8	(15)
A break (includes holiday for patient to give relative a rest)	7	(13)
Social worker	7	(13)
More inclusion by hospital staff, or opportunity to speak to patient's doctor	7	(13)
Change in some aspect of patient's current night-care setting	7	(13)
Money and material help	5	(10)
Change in some aspect of patient's day-care setting	5	(10)
Domiciliary psychiatric services (e.g. community nurse)	4	(8)
Alternative residential care or sheltered accommodation for patient	4	(8)
More responsive emergency services	4	(8)
Re-housing	4	(8)
Social activities for patient	3	(6)
Home help	1	(2)

*34 relatives (65% of those interviewed) wanted some change in services currently provided and/or some additional help; the number of patients totals in excess of 34 as many desired more than one change.

From Creer *et al.* (1982).

it is clear that no one approach is sufficient on its own. Each has advantages and disadvantages and we need to be aware of their strengths and limitations. Ultimately the definition of 'need' is usually ideological, i.e. it is not based on empirical knowledge about how a particular kind of service provision will lead to a specific outcome. So, how can the 'process' of care be more closely examined?

How Well is it Working?

At a technical level the best tool for service evaluation is probably the case register. This is a data-linkage system, usually computerised, which records individual's contacts with the services. Case registers are usually restricted to psychiatric services and only operate with regard to the population of a given geographical area. (For a good introduction to the use of case registers in monitoring and evaluation, see Walsh, 1985.) A number of different types of contact may be recorded and cross-referenced (e.g. out-patient attendances, day attendances, in-patient admissions, see Wooff, Freeman & Fryers, 1983). Because case registers can monitor specific kinds of contacts they may also be used to study particular groups of patients. They may then be used as a sampling frame for more in-depth investigations e.g. Sturt, Wykes and Creer's (1982) study of 'high-contact' users in Camberwell.

Case registers are thus the most sophisticated device available for evaluating the impact of new service developments. However, they are also time consuming and expensive to set up and maintain and they provide only quantitative information about service use. They cannot tell you anything about the *quality* of service being provided or anything very meaningful about outcome. In these days of micro-computers, the trend is therefore to employ much smaller, more specific information systems (e.g. Gibbons, 1986). These 'mini' systems can provide qualitative as well as quantitative information and enable one to keep a track of individual care plans, review dates, case management responsibilities, etc., as well as monitoring contacts with the service by a specific client group (in this case schizophrenia). They are thus valuable not only as a research tool, but also for direct practical and clinical purposes.

Of course, fairly simple 'book-keeping' data may be collected without sophisticated systems providing that someone is willing to help develop a suitable data sheet and supply the motivation for its completion. For example, the development of day services in a particular district can be monitored with a simple form which each unit completes on a three-monthly, or six-monthly basis, covering:

1. Number of new clients referred.
2. Sources of referral.
3. Number accepted from each source.
4. Number currently attending.
5. Number leaving over the specified time period.
6. Changes in activities/programme offered.
7. Changes in staffing.
8. Any other developments.

Regular sharing of this kind of information between units can also help the service develop in an integrated and co-ordinated fashion.

RESEARCH AND PLANNING SPECIFIC PROJECTS

I will now turn to research regarding specific projects and consider how we can answer questions such as:

1. Is the project meeting its aims?
2. What is the quality of care being provided?
3. Does the project fit into the overall aims of the service?

Is The Project Meeting its Aims?

In order to answer this question, there must be a clear initial statement of aims. Usually, this takes the form of an 'operational policy', and this should describe such features as:

1. General aims and objectives.
2. Details of client groups to be served (including selection criteria).
3. Location.
4. Staffing.
5. Internal management arrangements.
6. Lengths of stay.
7. How aims and objectives will be achieved (details of treatment programme).
8. External management structure (who supervises?).
9. Methods of evaluation.

The purpose of an operational policy is to define, in as detailed a way as possible, the overall aims and objectives of the unit. An alternative to a formal Operational Policy is simply to try to define the nature of the service to be provided. For example, Anthony, Cohen and Farkas (1982) have attempted to 'operationalise' the necessary ingredients of a rehabilitation programme (Table 15.7). It is obviously important, if the effectiveness of the project is to be monitored, that this kind of clear operationalisation of aims is achieved.

What is The Quality of Care Being Provided?

'Quality of care' (QOC) can be defined at a number of different levels (Shepherd, 1984; Lavender, 1985). First, we need to consider the physical structure of the facility. Ever since institutions were built we have been concerned with the most suitable environment in which to offer care, though concepts of what is suitable have changed very much over time.

TABLE 15.7
The essential ingredients of a psychiatric rehabilitation programme

Ingredient	*Examples of how observed*
1. Functional assessment of client skills in relation to environmental demand	1. Client records show a listing of client skill strengths and deficits in relation to environmental demands; strengths and deficits are behaviourally defined and indicate client's present and needed level of functioning
2. Client involvement in the rehabilitation assessment and intervention	2. Record forms have places for client signoff and comments; percentage of clients who actually sign off; sample of audiotapes of client interviews indicate client understanding of *what* programme is doing and *why*
3. Systematic individual client rehabilitation plan	3. Written or taped examples of objective, behavioural, step-by-step client plans; a central 'bank' of available rehabilitation curricula; client records specify on which plans client is working
4. Direct teaching of skills to clients	4. Practitioners can identify the skills they are capable of teaching, describe the teaching process, and demonstrate their teaching techniques. Programme's daily calendar reflects blocks of time devoted to skill training
5. Environmental assessment and modification	5. Practitioners can describe characteristics of client's environment to which client is being rehabilitated and how the environment may be modified to support the client's skills level. Functional assessment should have assessed unique environmental demands
6. Follow-up of clients in their real-life environment	6. Client record indicate a monitoring plan and descriptions of monitoring results; audio-tapes of practitioner and feedback sessions; record-keeping forms provide spaces for changes in the intervention plan. Percentage if clients whose plans have changed; number of appointments for 'follow-along' services
7. A rehabilitation team approach	7. Team members can verbally describe each client's observable goals and the responsibilities of each team member in relation to those goals (may refer to client's records for this information)
8. A rehabilitation referral procedure	8. Client records indicate referral letters requesting specific outcomes by specific dates; telephone referrals demonstrate these same rehabilitation referral ingredients
9. Evaluation of observable outcomes and utilization of evaluation results	9. Agency records show the pooled outcome data for all clients; agency directors can verbally describe their setting's most significant client outcome
10. Consumer involvement in policy and planning	10. Administrators can list the number of joint meetings with consumers; consumer ratings of satisfaction with the rehabilitation programme

From Anthony *et al*. (1982).

The standards outlined by the Welsh Office in their Appendix to the Nodder Report (DHSS, 1979) and by the DHSS in 'Home Life' (Centre for Policy on Ageing, 1984) provide useful guidelines. However, one cannot equate quality of care with the adequacy of the physical environment. Like other aspects of QOC a good physical environment offers a necessary, but not sufficient, condition for a good quality of care.

The second level at which quality of care may be evaluated concerns the 'process' of care, i.e. the organisation and management practices within the unit and how these are reflected in the amount and nature of staff–client interactions.

Organisation and management practices may be analysed in a number of different ways. For example, Norma Raynes and her colleagues tried to operationalize Goffman's concept of the 'total institution' (Goffman, 1961). They developed instruments to measure organisation and management practices along four dimensions: rigidity of routine, block treatment, depersonalisation and staff-patient distance (King, Raynes & Tizard, 1971). More recently they have included staffs' perceptions of their involvement in the running of the unit as an important variable (Raynes, Pratt & Roses, 1979). Raynes' ideas have been used by Shepherd and Richardson (1979) and Gartey and Morris (1984) to study management practices in day and residential settings for the care of long-term patients. These studies showed considerable variation in the extent to which such settings are organised to meet the needs of individual clients. There also seemed to be a correlation between client-orientated management practices and levels of staff–client interaction. Where organisation and management practices were more client-orientated, staff were likely to interact with clients more frequently and in a more positive way. Both client-centred management practices *and* high levels of positive staff–client interaction seemed to be correlated with perceived staff involvement in decision-making.

An alternative way of looking at management practices is the Hospital-Hostel Practices Profile (HHPP) developed by Wykes, Sturt and Creer (1982). This assesses the restrictiveness versus permissiveness of the environment based on ideas first set out by Wing and Brown (1970) and later used by Hewett, Ryan and Wing (1975) and Ryan (1979). It surveys practices under a number of headings, e.g. restrictions on activity (bedtimes, rising times, etc.), personal possessions, meals and snacks, health and hygiene, care of rooms, and contact with services (GP, hairdresser, etc.). Wykes *et al.*, report results from a number of day and residential units, and the HHPP provides a useful way of assessing 'restrictiveness', particularly in residential settings. However, it measures many of the same dimensions tapped by the scales of King *et al.* (1971) and there is little to choose between them. Perhaps there may be slightly more comparative data available for the HHPP at present. The similarity of these measures is illustrated by Wykes' (1982) study of the hospital hostel which also figured in the study by Garety and Morris (1984). Wykes found that the hostel ward was significantly less restrictive on the HHPP than comparable hospital wards; furthermore, staff considered many more of the residents' problems as requiring intervention. This is consistent with the resident orientation identified by Garety and Morris.

The final level on which QOC may be considered concerns the outcome of care, i.e. the actual functioning of the clients themselves. A good physical environment, with client-orientated management and relatively 'permissive' practices, should facilitate high levels of positive staff-client interaction which in turn should be reflected in good outcomes with high levels of functioning. So, how may these be evaluated? Once again, client functioning has a number of different aspects and each of these needs to be considered separately. First, there is 'objective' functioning as assessed by rating scales or by other methods of direct observation. Choice of appropriate measures will depend upon a number of specific criteria such as the aims of the unit, the amount of training required, length and sophistication of the instrument, etc.

In general, it is probably best to concentrate on one or two fairly simple measures which reflect the fundamental aims and objectives of the project. For example, the simple time-budget measure used in the Wykes (1982) study showed how hostel-ward residents spent less time doing nothing compared with residents living in a traditional hospital ward. Similarly, evaluation using instruments like the REHAB 'General Behaviour' scores and Wykes and Sturt (1986) 'Social Behaviour Schedule', provide good overall indications of observer-rated functioning. Client satisfaction is another important measure, although, as we saw earlier, it may be difficult to obtain valid assessments. Relatives' satisfaction might also be considered, particularly where new services are being developed that place additional responsibilities onto the relatives. Finally, the importance of staff attitudes should not be forgotten. All new projects depend upon the enthusiasm and commitment of staff and their expressed satisfaction, whether measured directly or indirectly (through sickness, absenteeism, etc.) is crucial.

Thus, quality of care is a complex construct. It cannot be defined by a single measurement and its various aspects may have to be given different weights in different settings. The central question when assessing QOC remains an understanding of the *process* whereby features of the care provided have a direct influence on the outcomes obtained.

Does The Project Fit into The Overall Aims of The Service?

This takes us back to the interface between the overall services and the operation of a new development. Those groups who have an overall responsibility (Health Care Planning Teams, Joint Development Teams, etc.) clearly do not require large amounts of detailed information as to what is happening in every specific project, but they do require some information to ensure that new developments are staying within the strategy outlined in the original plan. One way to achieve this is for the overall planning team to set up a number of working sub-groups each with responsibility for a particular area of service development (e.g. day care, accommodation, sheltered work, crisis and emergency, etc.) If they establish regular reviews with written reports to the 'parent' planning team then they can monitor progress in each of the sub-groups.

RESEARCH DESIGNS

We have seen repeatedly how the problems of evaluation hinge around identifying relationships between particular facets of the service and the various outcomes. Unravelling such causal questions is the task of research designs. This topic is fully discussed elsewhere in this book but it may be worth making one or two comments here.

The starting point for any evaluation must be the formulation of a clear question about the relationship between two variables or sets of variables. Hopefully, the measures reviewed in this chapter give plenty of scope for the operational definition of specific dependent and independent variables. What one then has to do is explore their causal relationship. The traditional tool for investigating causal relationships in psychology has been the random controlled trial. However, for various reasons (small numbers, difficulties in matching, ethical problems, etc.) such designs may not be so useful in a service context. Here, different kinds of 'quasi-experiments' (Cook & Campbell, 1979) may be preferable. These do not employ conventional control groups, but rely instead on 'single case' studies, where control is obtained by using an extended set of baseline observations on a single subject (or unit). These kinds of single-subject, pre-post, designs can be very useful in service evaluation (e.g. in case registers, see Wing & Hailey, 1972). In small-scale studies, even simple pre-post evaluations can be useful. For example, Figs 15.1 and 15.2 show changes in the REHAB scores of two groups of old long-stay residents following transfer from a traditional ward to supported houses in the hospital grounds.

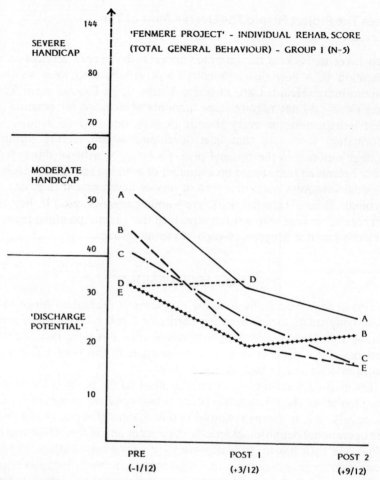

FIG. 15.1. Fenmere Project—individual rehabilitation scores for total general behaviour, group I (five subjects).

Although strictly speaking one cannot conclude that transfer 'caused' the improvements (because of the lack of adequate baseline data) the trends are nevertheless interesting. They suggest a number of more specific hypotheses. For example, why did group I apparently show a steady trend towards improvement (with one exception) while group II only began improving some time after they had been transferred? Was it because group I were better prepared? Was it due to differences in staff? Was it due to differences between the groups? (Group I were generally of a high level of functioning at the beginning.) Was it a 'floor' effect on the measure? Why did one patient in group II show such a marked deterioration in functioning? Does this suggest that there are some old long-stay residents for whom this kind of small-scale domestic setting is not suitable? The

FIG. 15.2. Fenmere Project—individual rehabilitation scores for total general behaviour, group II (four subjects).

answers to these questions need not trouble us here; the point is that such simple, uncontrolled evaluations can generate a number of useful ideas which can then be followed up in more rigorous, carefully controlled designs.

CONCLUSIONS

I have tried in this chapter to cover the basic research issues relating to service planning and evaluation, both at the level of overall service development and in connection with specific projects. Services are difficult things to do research on, they are multi-dimensional, they are complicated and they are elusive, always 'on the move'. Research methods must therefore not only be subtle and sophisticated, they must also be *dynamic* and capable of adapting to the changing characteristics of the clients and the changing perceptions of their needs. They must also be responsive to a changing social and economic climate. Empirical data can only capture a tiny fragment of this complex reality, but the challenge of trying to provide some kind of scientific basis for service development remains one of the most interesting—and potentially valuable—contributions that the social scientist can make.

REFERENCES

Anthony, W. A., Cohen, M. R. & Farkas, M. (1982). A Psychiatric Rehabilitation Treatment Program: Can I Recognize One If I See One? *Community Mental Health Journal*, **18**, 83–95.

Bachrach, L. L. (1980). Overview: Model programs for chronic mental patients. *American Journal of Psychiatry*, **137**, 1023–1031.

Baker, R. & Hall, J. N. (1983). REHAB: *Rehabilitation Evaluation Hall and Baker*. Aberdeen: Vine Publishing.

Bewley, T. H., Bland, M., Mechen, D. & Walch, E. (1981). New Chronic Patients. *British Medical Journal*, **283**, 1161–1164.

Cambridge Health Authority (1984). *Strategic Plan 1984–1994*. Cambridge Health Authority.

Centre for Policy on Ageing (1984). *Home Life: A Code of Practice for Residential Care*. London. CPA.

Clifford, P. & Szyndler, J. (1986). *Bexley Hospital Patients' Needs Survey*; available from National Unit for Psychiatric Research and Development, Lewisham Hospital, Lewisham High Street, London SE13 6LH.

Cook, T. D. & Campbell, D. T. (1979). *Quasi-experimentation—Design and Analysis Issues for Field Settings*. Chicago: Rand McNally.

Creer, C., Sturt, E. & Wykes, T. (1982). The role of relatives. In J. K. Wing (ed.) *Long-term Community Care: Experience in a London Borough, Psychological Medicine Monograph, Supplement 2*. London: Cambridge University Press.

Department of Health & Social Security (1975). *Better Services for the Mentally Ill*, Cmnd.6233, London: HMSO.

Department of Health & Social Security (1979). *Organisation and Management Problems of Mental Illness Hospitals: Report of a Working Group*. London: DHSS.

Department of Health & Social Security (1985). Government Response to the Second Report from the Social Services Committee, 1985–1985 Session, Annex I, *Mental Illness: Policies for Prevention, Treatment, Rehabilitation and Care*. Cmnd.9674, London: HMSO.

Early, D. F. & Nicholas, M. (1977). Dissolution of the Mental Hospital: Fifteen Years On. *British Journal of Psychiatry*, **130**, 117–122.

Early, D. F. & Nicholas, M. (1981). Two decades of change: Glenside Hospital population surveys 1960–80. *British Medical Journal*, **282**, 1446–1449.

Garety, P. A. & Morris, I. (1984). A new unit for long-stay psychiatric patients: organisation, attitudes and quality of care. *Psychological Medicine*, **14**, 183–192.

Gibbons, J. (1986). *Co-ordinated Aftercare for Schizophrenia: The Community Care Information Unit*. University Department of Psychiatry, Royal South Hants. Hospital, Southampton SO9 4PE.

Goffmann, E. (1961). *Asylums: Essays on the Social Situation of Mental Patients and Other Inmates*. New York: Anchor Books, Doubleday.

Goldberg, D. & Huxley, P. (1980). *Mental Illness in the Community*, London: Tavistock Publications.

Goldman, H. H. (1983). The demography of deinstitutionalisation. In L. L. Bachrach (ed.) *Deinstitutionalisation*. San Fransico: Jossey Bass.

Hewett, S., Ryan, P. & Wing, J. K. (1975). Living without the mental hospitals. *Journal of Social Policy*, **4**, 391–404.

House of Commons (1985). *Second Report from the Social Services Committee: Community Care with Special Reference to Adult Mentally Ill and Mentally Handicapped People*. London: HMSO.

Jennings, C. (1982). *Statistics from Eight Psychiatric Case Registers in Great Britain 1976–1981*. Southampton Psychiatric Case Register, Knowle Hospital, Hants PO17 5NA.

King, R., Raynes, N. & Tizard, J. (1971). *Patterns of Residential Care*. London: Routledge & Kegan Paul.

Kingsley, S., McAusland, T. & Towell, D. (1985). *Managing Psychiatric Services in Transition: Designing the Arrangements for Moving People from Large Hospitals into Local Services*. London: Kings Fund Centre.

Kuipers, L. & Bebbington, P. (1985). Relatives as a Resource in the Management of Functional Illness. *British Journal of Psychiatry*, **147**, 465–470.

Lavender, A. (1985). Quality of care and staff practices in long-stay settings. In F. N. Watts (ed.) *New Developments in Clinical Psychology*. Chichester: The British Psychological Society/Wiley.

Levene, L. S., Donaldson, L. J. & Brandon, S. (1985). How likely is it that a district health authority can close its large mental hospitals? *British Journal of Psychiatry*, **147**, 150–155.

MacCarthy, B., Benson, J. & Brewin, C. R. (1986). Task motivation and problem appraisal in long-term psychiatric patients. *Psychological Medicine*, **16**, 431–438.

Mann, S. A. & Cree, W. (1976). 'New' long-stay psychiatric patients: a national sample survey of fifteen mental hospitals in England and Wales 1972/3. *Psychological Medicine*, **6**, 603–616.

MIND (1983). *Common Concern*, London: MIND Publications.

Moore, A. J. (1985). *Long-stay Psychiatric Rehabilitation Bed Requirements in Cambridge: A Planning Model*. Unpublished MFCM Thesis, Cambridge Health Authority.

O'Brien, J. & Tyne, A. (1981). *The Principle of Normalisation: A Foundation for Effective Services*. London: Campaign for Mental Health.

Pattie, A. H. & Gilleard, C. J. (1979). *Clifton Assessment Procedures for the Elderly (CAPE)*. Windsor: NFER-Nelson.

Raynes, N., Pratt, M. & Roses, S. (1979). *Organisational Structure and The Care of the Mentally Handicapped*. London: Croom Helm.

Richman, A. & Barry, A. (1985). More and More is Less and Less: The Myth of Massive Psychiatric Need. *British Journal of Psychiatry*, **146**, 164–168.

Ryan, P. (1979). Residential care for the mentally disabled. In J. K. Wing & R. Ilsen (eds.) *Community Care for the Mentally Disabled*. London: Oxford University Press.

Shepherd, G. (1984). Quality of Care. In *'Institutional Care and Rehabilitation*. Chapter 4. London: Longmans.

Shepherd, G. & Richardson, A. (1979). Organisation and Interaction in Psychiatric Day Centres. *Psychological Medicine*, **9**, 573–579.

Stein, L. I. & Test, M. A. (1978). An alternative to mental hospital treatment. In L. I. Stein and M. A. Test (eds.) *Alternatives to Mental Hospital Treatment*. New York: Plenum Press.

Stein, L. I. & Test, M. A. (1985). (eds.) *The Training in Community Living Model: A Decade of Experience*. San Francisco: Jossey-Bass Inc.

Stroul, B. A. (1984). *Toward Community Support Systems for the Mentally Disabled: The NIMH Community Support Program*, available from the Center for Rehabilitation Research and Training in Mental Health, Boston University, Boston. Mass.

Stroul, B. A. (1986). *Models of Community Support Services: Approaches to Helping Persons with Long-term Mental Illness*, available from the Center for Rehabilitation Research and Training in Mental Health, Boston University, Boston, Mass.

Sturt, E., Wykes, T. & Creer, C. (1982). Demographic, social and clinical characteristics of the sample. In J. K. Wing (ed.) *Long-term Community Care: Experience in a London Borough, Psychological Medicine Monograph Supplement, 2*, Cambridge University Press.

Tooth, G. C. & Brooke, E. (1961). Trends in the Mental Hospital Population and their effect on Future Planning, *Lancet*, **i**, 710–713.

Walsh, D. (1985). Case Registers for monitoring treatment outcome in chronic functional psychoses. In T. Helgason (ed.) *The Long-term Treatment of Functional Psychoses*. London: Cambridge University Press.

Warner, R. (1985). *Recovery from Schizophrenia*. Lonon: Routledge & Kegan Paul.

Wing, J. K. & Brown, G. W. (1970). *Institutional and Schizophrenia: A Comparative Study of Three Mental Hospitals, 1960–1968*. London: Cambridge University Press.

Wing, J. K. & Hailey, A. (eds) (1972). *Evaluation, a Community Psychiatric Service: The Camberwell Register, 1964–1971*. London: Oxford University Press.

Wolfensberger, W. & Glenn, L. (1975). *Program Analysis of Service Systems*, 3rd edn. Toronto: National Institute of Mental Retardation.

Wooff, K., Freeman, H. L. & Fryers, T. (1983). Psychiatric service use in Salford: A comparison of point-prevalence ratios 1968 and 1978. *British Journal of Psychiatry*, **142**, 588–597.

Wykes, T. (1982). A hostel-ward for 'new' long-stay patients: an evaluative study of 'a ward in a house'. In J. K. Wing (ed.). *Long-term Community Care: Experience in a London Borough, Psychological Medicine Monograph Supplement, 2*. Cambridge University Press.

Wykes, T. & Sturt, E. (1986). The measurement of social behaviour in psychiatric patients: An assessment of the reliability and validity of the SBS schedule. *British Journal of Psychiatry*, **148**, 1–11.

Wykes, T., Sturt, E. & Creer, C. (1982). Practices of day and residential units in relation to the social behaviour of attenders. In J. K. Wing (ed.) *Long-term Community Care: Experience in a London Borough, Psychological Medicine Monograph Supplement, 2*. Cambridge University Press.

Author Index

Subject Index